# UNNATURAL SELECTION

# INTERNATIONAL STUDIES IN GLOBAL CHANGE

Edited by **Tom R. Burns**, Uppsala University, Sweden
**Thomas Dietz**, George Mason University, Fairfax, Virginia, USA

This book series is devoted to investigations of human ecology, technology and management and their interrelations. It will include theoretical and methodological contributions to the analysis of social systems and their transformation, technology, risk, enviromental problems, energy and natural resources, population growth, public health, and global economic and societal developments.

# UNNATURAL SELECTION

## Technology, Politics, and Plant Evolution

**Cary Fowler**

**GORDON AND BREACH**

Switzerland  Australia  Belgium  France  Germany  Great Britain  India
Japan  Malaysia  Netherlands  Russia  Singapore  USA

Gordon and Breach Science Publishers S.A.
Y-Parc
Chemin de la Sallaz
1400 Yverdon, Switzerland

**Library of Congress Cataloging-in-Publication Data**

Fowler, Cary.
    Unnatural selection: technology, politics, and plant evolution /
Cary Fowler.
      p. cm.—(International studies in global change, ISSN
1055-7180: v. 6)
    Includes bibliographical references (p.    ) and index.
    ISBN 2-88124-640-0 (hard).—ISBN 2-88124-639-7 (pbk.)
    1. Plant varieties—United States—Patents.   2. Seed industry and
trade—Law and legislation—United States.   3. Crops—United States—
Germplasm resources.   4. Germplasm resources, Plant—United States.
5. Plant varieties—Patents.   6. Crops—Germplasm resources.
7. Germplasm resources, Plant.   I. Title.   II. Series:
International studies in global change; v. 6.
SB123.5.F68   1994
333.95'317—dc20                            94-17304
                                                    CIP

*To My Parents*

"What we can hand over after our time of work is not just what we have managed to add to the heritage; it is the whole heritage with the little we have managed to add."

*Dag Hammarskjöld*

# Contents

# Introduction to the Series

This series brings together under one banner works by scholars of many disciplines. All of these researchers have distinguished themselves in their specialties. But here they have ventured beyond the frontiers of traditional disciplines and have developed new, innovative approaches to the study of social systems and social change.

Why? What has prompted this foray into uncharted territory? What is the reason for broadening theoretical perspectives and developing new methodologies? The impetus comes from the world we seek to understand. Scholars have traditionally made "boundary" assumptions that limited their scope of inquiry to the concerns of a discipline. Such limitations facilitate concentration, though they have always been artificial. The interpenetration of social, economic and environmental phenomena, and the precipitous pace of change in the late twentieth century make it clear that such convenient intellectual boundaries are not only unrealistic, they are untenable.

How complex waves of change sweep through the contemporary world, altering the natural environment, technology, the economy and social systems; the interaction of these forces, their impact on nations, communities, families and individuals; and the response to them by individuals and collectivities — this is the focus of the research to be presented in this series. The scholars writing in the series are themselves engaged in social change — the restructuring of our way of thinking about the world.

Dr. Fowler's Unnatural Selection is an important interdisciplinary study that shows how human action shapes both social and biological evolution. And at the same time Fowler demonstrates how the genetic constitution of plant species has influenced the law and agriculture even as the character of these species is being transformed to meet economic ends. As humans intervene in the biological world with ever greater precision and subtlety, the issues Fowler raises are becoming a critical part of national and international policy. Dr. Fowler can provide rare insight into legal, economic and biological transformations because he is not only a fine historical sociologist but also has been an active participant in the policy debates he discusses. We are very proud to include this volume in our series. It demonstrates the power of the engaged interdisciplinary scholar in revealing the dynamic interplay between the biological and the social.

*Tom R. Burns*
*Thomas Dietz*

# Preface

Some ten to twelve thousand years ago, human beings began to make the transition from hunting and gathering to the practice of agriculture. In the process, several hundred plants were domesticated, a paltry number compared to the many thousands of plant species used by gatherers. But among the plants experiencing domestication, diversity flourished as the plants traveled with people and encountered and adapted to new climates, soils, insects and diseases, and human cultures. By the time Charles Darwin set sail as a young man on the *Beagle*, thousands upon thousands of genetically distinct types of wheat existed . . . and rice . . . and corn . . . and many other major crops. Each type might be as genetically distinct from the others as a dachshund from a golden retriever! Little wonder that Darwin titled the first chapter of *The Origin of Species* "Variation under Domestication."[1]

The genetic diversity[2] "created" during twelve thousand years of agricultural history has become, arguably, the world's most valuable raw material. Genetic diversity is required for agricultural crops to continue to adapt to changes in the climate and to stronger pests and more virulent diseases. It is used by farmers, plant breeders, and biotechnologists alike. Without the diverse characteristics embodied in the genes of crop varieties which trace their ancestry back thousands of years, today's plant breeder would be incapable of adapting modern crops to new conditions. Genetic diversity is also the sustenance of the new biotechnology industry which uses it as a raw material in fashioning new crops and new products of all kinds. In the Third World, diversity is important at the farm level, enabling selection of crop varieties adapted to areas not suitable for industrial agriculture.

Genetic diversity is the foundation of evolution. And evolution is necessary for the continuation of all living things, including the crops which sustain us. The health of this resource is thus of immense ecological, social, political, and economic importance to human beings. As Jack Harlan, celebrated geneticist and crop historian at the University of Illinois, has put it, "These resources stand between us and catastrophic starvation on a scale we cannot imagine. In a very real sense, the future of the human race rides on these materials."[3] It is a tenuous perch. Genetic diversity is, according to many experts, being lost at an alarming rate as the many traditional crop varieties with their myriad characteristics are replaced by stands of the same uniform varieties.[4] Substantial amounts of diversity supposedly safeguarded in "gene banks" have also been destroyed. With the loss of this material we lose options for the future and become more and more dependent on artificial means — fertilizers, insecticides, fungicides, herbicides, favorable weather, and just plain luck — to secure food production.

Countries are not equally endowed with biological diversity or with the full range of economically important plant species. For various reasons including the effects of the Ice Age and the location of early human settlements and patterns of human migrations, most species and genetic diversity in nature and in agriculture have been found in developing countries. This "botanical inequality" has historically provided a backdrop for contests over access to and control over biological diversity which have been such an important part of our history. (Could we recount the history of the colonial era without reference to the lust for plants?[5]) People's ability to use resources including technology to obtain, develop, and exploit botanical materials has been a factor of major importance historically. It is no less so today, perhaps, than it was during earlier times.

There are no clear-cut answers to questions of who deserves credit for or ownership over the earth's biological treasures. Most answers reveal biases; most solutions appear self-serving. Can we really say that the modern plant breeder who turns out a disease-resistant tomato, wheat, or rice variety has done something more grand or worthy of reward than the farming community that first identified and conserved the disease-resistant characteristic in its fields? And what of our ancestors who domesticated these plants and in so doing created a food crop which could not just be picked in the wild, but grown over vast expanses? Should biological diversity be treated as a common heritage like the air we breathe, free for the taking? Or should it be privatized, patented, and owned? If credit and ownership are to be assigned, how can it be done? On what basis, under what rules? Who shall make the rules? How is the value of the resources to be determined? Such questions are not trivial.

Struggles over ownership of property are often at the crux of tensions in social relations and subsequent upheaval and social change. The struggle for the control of plants helped forge the world's first "geopolitics" many centuries ago. It is still the source of considerable turmoil and controversy today. If, as some say, we are now entering the "age of biotechnology" in which manipulation of living organisms will propel industry and development, then the fate of nations is tied more closely than ever to biological diversity and its control. Apart from the obvious and virtually incalculable political and economic implications, questions of ownership and control over biological resources will also influence how effectively the resources are conserved. Those who cannot ensure through ownership or other forms of control that they will reap benefits from the resources cannot be expected to go to the expense of conserving them for the use and aggrandizement of others. Thus, the very existence of the resource which feeds humanity is tied to patterns and arrangements of ownership and control and how these affect the way in which the benefits of diversity are shared, or not.

It is essential, therefore, to understand the dynamics of mechanisms of control — how these mechanisms come into existence, what forces undermine them, what influences encourage new forms of control. Issues such as these lie close to the heart of the contentious debates under way in a number of national and international fora regarding how genetic diversity will be conserved, who will own and control it, and how the benefits of the use of this resource will be apportioned. *How these questions are addressed will shape the world we live in and that of our children and theirs in the most profound ways.*

This book looks at the social construction of control over this most valuable of resources. As background, I shall discuss plant collecting and development in Europe and the United States from roughly the seventeenth to the twentieth centuries. This will set the stage for an examination of modern, legal forms of ownership of biological diversity — a topic of considerable controversy as this book is written. Patent and patent-like laws and their creation in the United States are examined in some depth. These laws are not the simple by-product of scientific or technological advance. Often as not, they are more closely related to changes in the seed and nursery industries and the marketplace. The initiative for their passage comes from companies trying in large part to secure and broaden their position in the marketplace in a context in which physical control is no longer effective.

The title *Unnatural Selection* has obvious biological allusions. But it is also meant to convey a message: that the choices human societies make about how to treat genetic resources are just that, choices. There is nothing "natural" — that is preordained, inevitable, or required — about those choices. If nothing else, I aim to show that laws concerning biological materials have "feet of clay." They do not descend from above and are not part of some "natural order" obligingly implemented by society. Property rights and other mechanisms of control of resources derive from and structure human relationships. They allocate resources. They are

creations not givens of human society. This leaves us with awesome
responsibilities. As struggles continue over the precious resources that
sustain our life, it will be increasingly important to try to understand the
dynamics of the choices being made and to become more knowledgeable
actors in the shaping of those choices. This book represents a first step in
that direction. Other steps should follow.

The subject matter here covers material which could easily be addressed by a number of disciplines: history, sociology, political science,
economics, geography, law, and even biology, botany, and genetics. Most
obviously, it could have been written as a linear history of the development of mechanisms of control or intellectual property rights (IPR) for
biological material. After all, it deals with events which span several
centuries. But no strenuous effort has been made to link each fact with
another temporally as history is so often written. Nor has any effort been
made to include "all the facts." The complexity of modern society defies
total description or overview. Instead, I have tried to explore the turning
points and the process in the development of mechanisms of control.
Thus, a reader expecting a complete history will not be fully satisfied.

Neither is this book primarily an exercise in the field of social theory. It
is informed by theory and, to a certain extent, I believe it develops and
applies that theory. (The theoretical foundations of the book are discussed
in Appendix IV, whereas theoretical conclusions are noted in the discussions at the end of each chapter.) The book's focus, however, is not on
theory development.

There are a number of alternative ways of viewing the history and the
topics covered in this book. Different authors would certainly notice and
stress different things as a natural result of their world views and theoretical assumptions. One might choose a technological deterministic or
structural deterministic approach. One might see in the development of
the law the simple unfolding of legal logic. One could look for conspira-
cies. Another might argue that it is a history of the ruling class or
capitalism working its will with almost inevitable success. Or still another
could assume that property rights come into existence due to the requirements or needs of "the system." The empirical material and my understanding of it encourage me largely to reject these alternative approaches
as too simplistic and too mechanistic, or as just plain wrong. While it was
not my purpose to "disprove" these alternative approaches, I suspect and
hope the reader will conclude that the book does so implicitly.

I have attempted to make this book accessible to the lay person without
sacrificing the detail which I think gives depth and richness to the story. In
the table of contents, the reader will find reference to abbreviations and an

appendix on definitions of technical terms used here. I draw the attention of those wishing to pursue research in this area to Appendix II on sources of information and methodology. In order to help other researchers, I have supplied rather extensive notes.

Part I, encompassing chapters 1 and 2, provides an introduction and background to the body of the study. These chapters look at early efforts to collect and use plant material. In the United States, the government was involved in plant collecting and development efforts prior to this century. But the nature and purpose of its efforts were quite different from British efforts through Kew Gardens, for example. The U.S. government made no effort to limit or control the dissemination of the plants it collected. In fact, the aim was to spread seeds widely and encourage the expansion and adaptation of American agriculture. The plant types collected and subsequently further developed by American farmers provided the genetic foundations for commercialized agriculture in the United States. Chapter 2 looks specifically at rationalization and commercialization in American agriculture. Farmers cease saving seeds, begin producing for the commercial market, and begin a shift toward dependency on purchased seed supplies and nursery stock.

The main body of this study, Part II, concerns the construction of intellectual property rights in the United States. Chapters 3 to 5 deal with the passage and later expansion (through Congress and the courts) of patent and patent-like laws to cover plants. It would be difficult to make sense of the laws passed in 1930, 1970, or 1980 without referring back to the history and developments discussed initially. Chapters 3 to 5, rather than supplying a full history, are focused on certain strategic questions. Attempts to fashion mechanisms for economic control of plants are related to commercial and technological factors explored in the earlier chapters in addition to other factors.

Part III deals with more contemporary events. Chapter 6 sees the contest over intellectual property rights taken to international arenas where the conflicts and controversies it examines are still very much ongoing and unsettled. Much of chapter 6 was written in 1990 and early 1991. It is intended to offer the reader a quick glimpse of how issues developed as they encountered very new and different arenas and actors. In this chapter, I have not attempted to develop the context or story in as detailed a fashion as in earlier chapters. More detailed information and analyses concerning these topics are available elsewhere. Instead, I have sought only to inform the curious reader as to the general direction of events that continue to unfold as this book is published. Chapter 6, therefore, should not be considered a definitive treatment of the current situation, but as only a hint of part of another book I hope to be able to write in the future.

Even in such a brief overview of the chapters, one can detect some common elements. But how can we begin to make sense of this very long, complicated history which spills over into our morning newspapers with stories of persistent controversy over the ownership and control of biodiversity? That was the task which confronted me when I began this project.

My involvement in the subject was certainly encouraged by my up-bringing. My father is a lawyer and judge; my mother a dietician; my sister received her university degree in animal sciences. All now live on a small farm outside Memphis, Tennessee. As I grew up, my maternal grandmother still managed a larger, commercial family farm. Both sides of my family were involved in electoral politics, government, and edu-cation. Thus, a study dealing with food, agriculture, law, and politics must seem in character. An unexpected benefit was the way in which my research into the commercialization of American agriculture, for instance, built a context within which I could place and begin to under-stand the details of my own family's history.

Other than a continuing fascination with tropical fish breeding and genetics which gripped me as a youngster, I had no real interest in "genetic resources" until I happened upon the writings of Jack Harlan while doing research for the book *Food First: Beyond the Myth of Scarcity,* in 1975. Long involvement in the civil rights and peace move-ments in the American South may help explain why I rather quickly concluded that the genetic resources "problem" was not just a scientific one, but a political one as well. Since my encounter with Harlan, much of my career has been spent working on genetic resource issues, including controversies over intellectual property rights. My employers were the Rural Advancement Foundation International (then through the National Sharecroppers Fund/Rural Advancement Fund), the Norwegian Centre for International Agricultural Development, and finally the United Na-tions Food and Agriculture Organization. I have also been associated, in a voluntary capacity as the chairman of the board, with the American Livestock Breeds Conservancy, a group working to conserve rare breeds of domesticated livestock. And I have served as a member of the U.S. Department of Agriculture's National Plant Genetic Resources Board, appointed by the secretary of agriculture.

It has been my great good fortune to have had the guidance of Professor Tom Burns of the Institute of Sociology at Uppsala University in Sweden from the beginning of this project until its completion. Students and colleagues of Tom know what a difference his involvement in a project makes. I can honestly say that without his help and encouragement this book would either never have been finished, or it would have been completed long before it was ready. Tom has helped me achieve one of my biggest dreams. My debt to him as a teacher and a friend is very, very great.

Much of this book was written while I was employed as associate professor and senior research scientist by the Norwegian Centre for International Agricultural Development (NORAGRIC) at the Agricultural University of Norway. Without the generous financial and personal support provided me by this wonderful institute and its staff, I would never have had the time or energy to write such a book. In particular, thanks are due to Stein Bie and Trygve Berg.

While at NORAGRIC, I was able to accept a visiting appointment with the agronomy department of the University of California at Davis. Much of my time in Davis was spent doing research for this book. I am indebted to NORAGRIC, the agronomy department of UCD and to Professor Cal Qualset for this opportunity.

The completion of this book means that I must find new excuses to visit the Dag Hammarskjöld Foundation in Uppsala. During frequent trips to Uppsala, the foundation provided me with a place to stay and an office with a view of the castle and the university library. Moreover, I benefited from many long discussions — more than a few lasting all night — with foundation staff. Some of the most productive times and pleasant experiences of my life have been spent at the offices at Övre Slottsgatan 2. For material support and for help in keeping me focused on what is important, thank you Sven Hamrell, Olle Nordberg, Gerd Ryman-Ericson, Ing-Charlotte Elfström, and Kerstin Kvist.

From 1978 until early 1990, I was in the employ of the Rural Advancement Foundation International (RAFI) and its former parent bodies, the National Sharecroppers Fund and the Rural Advancement Fund. Little, if any, of the "participant-observation" described herein was done with the notion that it would end up in such a book. Research and action were done as part of a team with my close friends, Pat Mooney and Hope Shand. What times we had! My thanks are also due to Kathryn Waller for her steadfast support and faith.

A number of people reviewed all or portions of the manuscript and graciously shared their thoughts and research with me over the years. In particular I wish to thank my friends and colleagues Trygve Berg at NORAGRIC and Don Duvick, recently retired from Pioneer Hi-Bred. For her early influence and inspiring work, Erna Bennett (retired from FAO) has my thanks. I have learned a great deal from these fine people. Tom Dietz, Stephen Turner, Merrick Tabor, Bo Lewin, and Rolf Nygren each reviewed drafts of the manuscript and provided me with thoughtful comments and criticisms. Each helped improve the final product in ways they will probably recognize. One of Stephen Turner's contributions will be easy for him to spot. It's on the cover — "Unnatural Selection." My thanks are due to Henry Shands, Åsmund Bjørnstad, Stephen Brush, the Keystone Center staff, and the many others who trusted and cared enough to help me in many different ways. Thanks must also be given to those who allowed me to interview them, including Raymond Baker, Wayne Denney, Barry Greengrass, Richard Kleindienst, Harold Loden, Clay Logan, Richard Lyng, John Pino, Dale Porter, Frank B. Robb, Robert Romig, John Sutherland, Ed Weimortz, and Melaku Worede. Their participation in this project provided me with information and insights I would never have gotten otherwise.

Sally Antrobus of Seabrook, Texas, edited the final manuscript copy. Several years ago I had the pleasure of working with her on *Shattering: Food, Politics, and the Loss of Genetic Diversity*. Once again, her eye for detail and considerable editing skills have helped improve the end product significantly.

Finally, for their encouragement over a number of years, I want to thank my parents, Betty C. and Morgan C. Fowler, and my sister, Jo F. Hargraves. Writing this book made me repeatedly aware and appreciative of the many ways in which they have influenced me. There is much of my family in these pages. I also wish to thank my friend, Natalie Hubbard, for giving more support than I ever deserved. During the final two years, there were times when it must have seemed that I was married to this project. Mette Wik put up with and encouraged it, provided frustratingly good critiques, solved innumerable computer problems, and gave me the final push. I shall always be grateful to her. All of these people sacrificed in some way simply because they knew what this project meant to me. I continue to marvel at this. Each has my gratitude and my love.

## NOTES

1. For convenience, I use this abbreviated title of Darwin's work. Numerous editions exist, the later ones containing Darwin's responses to contemporary criticisms of his work.
2. Definitions of technical terms, such as "genetic diversity," are in Appendix III.
3. Harlan, Jack. "Genetics of Disaster." *Journal of Environmental Quality* 1(3) (1972): 212.
4. See Appendix I for a discussion of this problem.
5. Note the interesting story behind the real mutiny on the *Bounty*. A group of West Indian planters had petitioned King George III of England to help them obtain breadfruit from Polynesia to feed their slaves. Captain Bligh was dispatched on the *Bounty* for Tahiti. He

obtained over a thousand seedlings which were kept in pots on board. Bligh took the care of his botanical passengers seriously, infuriating his crew by giving the plants fresh water which was in short supply. Scarcely three weeks after leaving for the West Indies, Fletcher Christian and others revolted and set Bligh adrift in a small rowboat. Bligh survived the ordeal and later completed his mission of introducing breadfruit to the West Indies in 1793. The first tree, planted by Bligh himself, was still standing in 1966 when Queen Elizabeth II visited the Botanical Gardens in St. Vincent for the ceremonial planting of a scion from Bligh's original tree. Fowler, Cary, and Pat Mooney. *Shattering: Food, Politics, and the Loss of Genetic Diversity.* Tucson: U of Arizona P, 1990. 40–41.

# Abbreviations

| | |
|---|---|
| AAN | American Association of Nurserymen |
| AASCO | Association of American Seed Control Officials |
| ABA | American Breeders Association (chapter 3) |
| ABA | American Bar Association (chapter 4) |
| ASD | actor-system dynamics |
| ASTA | American Seed Trade Association |
| BOB | Bureau of the Budget |
| CEO | chief executive officer |
| CGIAR | Consultative Group on International Agricultural Research |
| CIMMYT | International Center for the Improvement of Maize and Wheat |
| CMS | cytoplasmic male sterility |
| COAG | Committee on Agriculture (FAO) |
| CPGR | Commission on Plant Genetic Resources (FAO) |
| DNA | deoxyribonucleic acid |
| FAO | Food and Agriculture Organization (of the UN) |
| GAO | General Accounting Office |
| GATT | General Agreement on Tariffs and Trade |
| GE | General Electric |
| GRAIN | Genetic Resources Action International |
| IARC | International Agricultural Research Center |
| IBPGR | International Board for Plant Genetic Resources |
| ICDA | International Coalition for Development Action |
| IPR | intellectual property rights |
| IRRI | International Rice Research Institute |
| MIT | Massachusetts Institute of Technology |
| NAS | National Academy of Sciences |
| NGO | nongovernment organization |

# Abbreviations

| | |
|---|---|
| NORAGRIC | Norwegian Centre for International Agricultural Development |
| NSF | National Sharecroppers Fund |
| OECD | Organization for Economic Coordination and Development |
| OMB | Office of Management and Budget |
| OTA | Office of Technology Assessment |
| PBR | plant breeders' rights |
| PGR | plant genetic resources |
| PPA | Plant Patent Act (1930) |
| PVP | plant variety protection |
| PVPA | Plant Variety Protection Act (1970) |
| PVR | plant variety rights |
| RAF | Rural Advancement Fund |
| RAFI | Rural Advancement Fund International |
| UN | United Nations |
| UNCTAD | United Nations Conference on Trade and Development |
| UPOV | Union for the Protection of New Varieties of Plants |
| US | United States |
| USDA | United States Department of Agriculture |
| WIPO | World Intellectual Property Organization |

# PART I: BACKGROUND

**Distribution, Development and Early Forms
of Control of Biological Materials
and
the Commercialization of U.S. Agriculture**

# CHAPTER 1

# Seed Collection and Use: Early Examples from Europe and the United States

Plant species of economic importance have never been equally distributed around the globe. European explorers "discovered" many important species at a time when it was becoming possible to utilize the discoveries economically. Later the United States government became active in collecting seeds for use by American farmers. This chapter provides an overview of the beginnings of rationalization of plant development and commercialization on an international scale by examining certain situations in both Europe and the United States.

In Europe, institutions were established to try to make use of plant material, bring rationality to its development, and gain some degree of control over it. Systems were necessary if profits were to be made. The level of technology available influenced the means available to secure control. In fact, some technological developments (such as the Wardian case, a terrarium for transporting delicate plants shipboard) enhanced the ability of colonial powers to move plants about and control their production while at the same time enabling others to break down these primitive monopolies. Specific cases illustrating these points are discussed throughout the chapter.

Closer attention is paid, however, to the work of Britain's Royal Botanic Gardens at Kew, the largest and most important garden of the period, and to its work with two plants: cinchona and rubber. Abbreviated case studies or sketches of these crops help illustrate how the botanic gardens participated in developing an increasingly rationalized system of plant collection, study, development, distribution, and commercialization. With Kew we also see the social construction of a global system for acquiring, making use of, and controlling plant materials.

In the United States, a different pattern of seed collection, use, and control emerged in response to different problems and opportunities. Seeds were collected by the government and widely distributed in an effort to expand agriculture into new lands and make it more generally productive. Those involved were no empire builders such as at Kew. Control over seeds was held by farmers, who played an active role in developing this genetic material.

3

The role of "law," discussed in depth in later chapters, is relatively unimportant during the early period covered here. In some cases this was due to the difficulty of enforcement, which is tied to inadequacies of existing institutions and the ability of the biological material to reproduce itself. In other cases we see different goals in regard to how actors wanted the botanical material distributed and used.

As a result of the Ice Age, the northern hemisphere was left botanically impoverished relative to the south. Hunting and gathering flourished and agriculture originated in the warmer lands to the south in what we today call the Third World. It is here that agriculture's long history (which is a history of human-plant interactions) had time to produce the genetic diversity that is the very foundation of modern agriculture.[1]

Acquisition of plant genetic resources for use by colonial and nascent corporate powers is one of the enduring relationships between a number of "developed" and "developing" countries. As sailors of would-be colonial powers hoisted the canvas, they began not only the often-recounted search for glittering minerals and shorter trading routes, but the search for economically important plants as well. They were not the first plant explorers. Recorded history gives that honor to the Sumerians who sent collectors into Asia Minor around 2500 B.C. in search of vines, figs and roses.[2] Egypt's Queen Hatshepsut dispatched a collecting expedition to East Africa for incense trees in 1482 B.C.[3] The walls of a temple at Thebes graphically depict this journey.

The return of Columbus from his voyage of discovery to the New World marked the beginnings of what A. W. Crosby called the "Colombian Exchange," the mass transfer of native crops between the Americas and the outside world.[4] Columbus had discovered not just the New World, but maize. Spanish and Portuguese mariners helped spread maize eastward as far as China, where it was first mentioned by a Chinese writer in 1555.[5]

Other crops followed maize across the Atlantic: potatoes, squash, tomatoes, peanuts, common beans, sunflowers. Many of these crops found ecological, cultural and economic niches in their new homes, adding to human diets and agricultural productivity. Maize and potatoes were particularly important in this regard as they became staple crops contributing in part to dramatic population increases in Europe.[6] The diffusion of these crops was rather rapid owing in part to the ease with which they reproduced and could be cultivated. "Control," through plantation production, restriction of access to reproductive materials, or patent ownership was clearly not feasible for such crops at this time due both to the above mentioned biological characteristics and the state of the legal, administrative and economic structures of the period. Furthermore, the market for food staples was not as well developed as it is today. The costs of production, broadly defined, could not be justified by the returns. Money was to be made mostly in rarer, high-value items.

The importance of the discovery of new plants in the New World was not their discovery, per se, but the fact that the plants could be *used.* Advances in navigation and shipbuilding provided the means — part of the context in which European states could exploit the botanical wealth they were finding. According to Cipolla:

> Exchanging oarsmen for sails and warriors for guns meant essentially the exchange of human energy for inanimate power. By turning whole-heartedly to the gun-carrying sailing ship the Atlantic peoples broke down a bottleneck inherent in the use of human energy and harnessed, to their advantage, far larger quantities of power. It was then that European sails appeared aggressively on the most distant seas.[7]

> The gun-carrying oceangoing sailing ship developed by Atlantic Europe in the course of the fifteenth, sixteenth, and seventeenth centuries was the instrument which made possible the European saga. Whenever and wherever the ships of Atlantic Europe appeared, there was no power that could offer any resistance.[8]

The importance of these technological advancements was not so much that they facilitated the discovery of plant diversity, nor even in its spread, strictly speaking. Crops had already been "discovered" by their users. They had been spreading outward from their "centers of origin" for thousands of years and in any case, simple sailing craft could have accomplished simple transfers. The importance lay in the facilitation of exploitation of these new botanical resources, and in the creation of social conditions (including the imposition of slavery) which would make this exploitation profitable. This was particularly true for crops with limited geographic distribution which lent themselves to concentrated plantation production — especially in the tropics — for which naval strength was critical to establishing and maintaining control over production and distribution.

Various spices, sugar, bananas, coffee, tea, rubber, indigo, and other industrial and medicinal crops began to make their move to new production sites under the control of newly emerging colonial powers and their state-backed trading companies. The assembly of a network of botanic gardens was to prove crucial to the movement and development of crops in this botanical chess game.

Gardens designed to keep exotic plants for aesthetic and religious reasons have a long history. The gardens built by Nebuchadnezzar for his wife about 570 B.C., the famous Hanging Gardens of Babylon, are an early and particularly well known example. The Aztecs built gardens in and around their capital, which the Spaniards found to be the most beautiful they had ever seen.[9] Monastic gardens in Europe kept diverse plants as miniature recreations of the Garden of Eden. Other than various and impressive efforts to collect and describe medicinal plants, there was no organizational rationale linked to an economic purpose. These were primarily pleasure gardens.

## EUROPEAN BOTANIC GARDENS SEIZE THE INITIATIVE

The earliest botanic gardens associated with economic plants were those founded to study medicinal plants. Botanic gardens in Florence, Leiden, Leipzig, Montpellier, Pisa and Heidelberg — all founded in the sixteenth century — were connected with medical faculties at universities. In the following century, a number of gardens facilitated and promoted the study of taxonomy. The most famous of these efforts was undertaken in the 1700s by Carl Linné, who held an appointment as professor of medicine at the university in Uppsala. Some of the more notable gardens are listed in table 1, with their founding dates indicating considerable involvement in plant development beginning in the seventeenth century.

As the world beyond Europe began to be explored in earnest, new plants arrived in huge numbers. Naturalists such as Charles Darwin were routinely included on voyages financed by the Crown, scientific societies, wealthy individuals, trading companies, or botanic gardens.

By the end of the eighteenth century it is estimated that sixteen hundred botanic gardens existed in Europe alone. Plant materials were being evaluated for any and all possible uses — food, medicinal, industrial. As Brockway notes, "Botanic gardens consciously served the state as well as science, and the shared mercantilist and nationalist spirit of the times."[10] The British founder of the Calcutta Botanic Gardens, for example, stated that the gardens were established "not for the purpose of collecting rare plants as things of curiosity or furnishing articles for the gratification of luxury, but for establishing a stock for disseminating such articles as may prove beneficial to the inhabitants as well as the natives of Great Britain, and which ultimately may tend to the extension of the national commerce and riches."[11]

Arguably, the world's premier botanic garden of the nineteenth-century colonial period was the Royal Botanic Gardens at Kew on the outskirts of London. Britain was the leading industrial and colonial power of the age and Kew played a valuable coordinating and facilitating role in identifying, collecting, developing and disseminating important economic plants. Kew Gardens, as it is commonly known, was established as a state institute in 1841, though its roots trace back to 1759 when Princess Augusta, the mother of George III, established a private garden on the site.

From 1841 onward, Kew was much more than a pleasure garden. Glasshouses, also called "orangeries" because citrus trees were often grown in them, had become status symbols among wealthy noblemen in Britain in the late seventeenth century.[12] Now they provided a means for successfully growing and propagating tropical plants. The "accidental invention" and subsequent development by a London physician and amateur botanist of the Wardian case (1829), actually a terrarium, facilitated shipment of delicate tropical plants to the glasshouses at Kew. With this the stage was set for a massive transfer of botanical material the likes of which the world had never before seen. Plants (significantly those that cannot feasibly be transported or propagated as seed) could now be transferred from their native land to a glasshouse where they could be studied, developed, and multiplied. William Hooker, Kew's director in 1841 was able to import six times as many plants in 15 years as had been imported in the previous century. Whereas in 1819, according to Brockway, only one plant in a thousand had survived the voyage from China to England, in 1851, thousands of tea plants in Wardian cases made the journey from Shanghai to Calcutta to start the Darjeeling tea industry.[13]

Fewer than a hundred plants were introduced to the British Isles in the sixteenth century, but close to a thousand arrived in the seventeenth, and almost nine thousand exotic plants were brought in during the eighteenth century.[14] Developments such as those cited above opened the floodgates. At Kew the influx of plants was so great as to be described as "embarrassing" by one early curator, William Bean. Writing in 1908, Bean observed that "at the beginning of the nineteenth century the floral treasures of great areas of the globe were still not only ungathered but unknown. All Africa, saving its northern and southern extremes, almost the whole of Asia, the two Americas, with the exception of the eastern seaboard of the north — all these remained practically virgin fields, open to the plant collector." But by the end of the nineteenth century, Bean lamented that "the fact is the world has been pretty well ransacked by this time . . ."[15] The colonial botanical garden — with Kew at the forefront — was the coordinator of collecting efforts and recipient of the plants.

Kew quickly expanded in size and capabilities. A number of glasshouses with elaborate heating systems were constructed to accommodate new arrivals, the literal fruit of expeditions to the Americas, Africa, and Asia. A Museum of Economic Botany opened. It was said that visitors saw so many vegetable products of the empire there that they "wondered at which to stare."[16] Such collections provided "the material for the botanical survey of the Empire . . . the museums contained every kind of vegetable product capable of utilisation . . . " according to Kew's third director.[17] Kew was, arguably, the world's headquarters of botanical science. Indicative of its position perhaps, a photograph of its director was on Charles Darwin's fireplace mantel and it was to this man that Darwin first turned to read and comment on his early writings on natural selection which would become *Origin of Species*.[18]

In 1859, Kew upgraded its training program with formal lectures. While Kew was becoming increasingly popular as a place to visit and take in the sights, it was reserved until 1:00 P.M. each day for scientific study. Kew training usually lasted for a period of two years and prepared the student for a career in applied botany. Of these students, Kew historian Ronald King says:

> Many of them went overseas to serve in Empire countries and it was on them that the economic development of the Empire was built, since much of that development depended upon the exploitation of the indigenous plant populations, and the distribution of these around the world to test their suitability and economic value in other countries . . . [19]

Bean's history indicates the role of the Kew Gardens as seen from within:

> In the industrial development of British colonies and possessions, the Kew man has always been among the earliest workers. As soon as the *pax Britannia* has been established, and often before, he appears. He founds botanic stations where useful plants are grown for distribution, and he gives demonstrations of the best methods of cultivating them. He fostered the tea industry in India and Ceylon; he also started the cultivation of cinchona there; he helped largely in the regeneration of the West Indian Islands, and at the present time Africa is dotted over with stations he is managing, each one a nucleus of what will probably develop into the most important industries of the continent. Often he suffers the fate common to pioneers: he sows that others may reap. Many a Kew man has laid down his life in the conscientious performance of his duty, as genuine sacrifice to the cause of empire and humanity as any soldier or missionary has ever made.[20]

As the *Kew Bulletin* noted on the centenary of the gardens: "One of the functions of Kew has been to send plants of economic and horticultural value to all parts of the Dominions and Colonies where conditions might be suitable for their cultivation."[21,22]

Kew stood at the center of a network of Parliament-funded gardens in the United Kingdom. A government-appointed committee which reported to Parliament in 1841 at the beginning of Kew's modern period chartered Kew to be this center. From Kew the government expected "to obtain authentic and official information on points connected with the founding of new colonies: it would afford the plants these required."[23]

Funds for overseas gardens were drawn from the Ministry of Colonial Affairs or the India Office, for example.[24] Kew was not formally in charge of the overseas gardens, but it served as a "clearing house for the exchange of information, planning, research, and the actual exchange of plant material."[25] By custom, Kew appointed the director of the satellite gardens, the principal staffs of which were British, many having been trained at Kew. By 1889, Kew was linked to an impressive network of gardens in the British empire, including: Bangalore, Barbados, Bombay, British Guiana, Calcutta, Cambridge, Dominica, Dublin, Edinburgh, Fiji, Glasgow, Gold Coast, Grenada, Hong Kong, Jamaica, Lagos, Madras, Malta, Mauritius, Natal, New South Wales, New Zealand, Niger Territories, Northern India (Saharunpur, Lucknow, Cawnpore), Oxford, Queensland, St. Lucia, South Australia, Straits Settlements (Singapore, Penang, Malacca), Tasmania, Trinidad, and Victoria.[26]

Table 1. Selected Colonial Botanical Gardens [27]

| Botanical Garden | Country | Founding Date | Associated Crops* |
|---|---|---|---|
| Leiden | Holland | 1587 | vanilla, cinchona |
| Oxford | Britain | 1621 | |
| Jardin des Plantes, Paris | France | 1626 | |
| "Linnaeus" Garden, Uppsala | Sweden | 1655 | |
| Edinburgh | Britain | 1670 | |
| Amsterdam | Holland | 1682 | coffee |
| Pamplemousses, Mauritius | France | 1735 | nutmeg, pepper, cinnamon, sugarcane |
| El Jardin Botanico del Soto de Migas Calientas | Spain | 1755 | |

Table 1 (*Continue on next page*)

**Table 1** (*Continue*)

| Botanical Garden | Country | Founding Date | Associated Crops* |
|---|---|---|---|
| Kew, London | Britain | 1759 | cinchona, rubber, coffee, cocoa, tea ornamentals, breadfruit |
| St. Vincent | Britain | 1766 | breadfruit, nutmeg |
| Bath Botanical Garden, Jamaica | Britain | 1779 | banana |
| Calcutta | Britain | 1779 | cinchona |
| Manila | Britain | 1779/1787 | |
| Jardim de Aclimatacion, Orotava, Canary Is. | Spain | 1788 | |
| Penang | Britain | 1796 | nutmeg, clove |
| Jardim Botanico, Rio | Portugal | 1808/1811 | tea |
| Peradeniya, Sri Lanka | Britain | 1812 | cinchona, vanilla, rubber |
| Bogor, Indonesia | Holland | 1817 | African oil Palm, tea, rubber, cinchona |
| Havana | Spain | 1817 | |
| Trinidad | Britain | 1819 | |
| Washington, U.S.A. | U.S.A. | 1842** | |
| Singapore | Britain | 1859 | rubber |
| Georgetown, Guyana | Britain | 1879 | |
| Jardin Botanique de Victoria, Cameroon | Germany | 1892 | |
| Amani Botani Garden (Tanzania) | Germany | late 1800s | |
| Entebbe, Uganda | Britain | 1898 | |

* This column indicates major crops associated with the botanical garden. In most cases, the crop listed passed through or was propagated at the garden before being commercialized.
** The date given is arbitrary — when glasshouses connected with the seed introduction activity of the U.S. government were operating in Washington. A plant-testing garden was established in 1669 in a South Carolina settlement. A public experimental garden was established in 1733 in Savannah, Georgia. And a land grant was made to an individual to establish a tropical plant introduction garden in Florida in 1838. But none of these efforts, including the glasshouses, became institutions engaged in the type of organizing activities we might associate with a Kew Gardens, for example (though the Florida garden did attempt to develop economic plants). Congress did not grant funds for establishing the U.S. National Arboretum until 1927.[28]

Kew's network made the employment of staff collectors unnecessary after the 1860s.[29] Plant material was forwarded to Kew by this network. And the network provided an unprecedented opportunity for the testing and development of plants "on location." For commercial interests, botanical expertise in propagation was available from the nearest colonial garden or from Kew through the mail. In a speech to Parliament in 1898, the Colonial Secretary noted that

> there are several of our important Colonies which owe whatever prosperity they possess to the knowledge and experience of, and the assistance given by, the authorities at Kew Gardens. Thousands of letters pass every year between the authorities at Kew and they are able to place at the service of those Colonies not only the best advice and experience, but seeds and samples of economic plants capable of cultivation in the Colonies.[30]

Though Kew was involved in the transfer and commercialization of many crops, a brief sketch will be provided of only two. The examples of cinchona and rubber demonstrate clearly the relationship between colonial powers and "satellite" countries during the colonial period; the characteristics of mechanisms of control over biological materials; and the beginnings of rationalization as it affects the treatment of exotic botanical materials. In each of these areas the botanic garden is an important actor.

## CINCHONA

The use of quinine derived from the bark of the cinchona tree of the Andes as a treatment for malaria had been known for hundreds of years by indigenous peoples.[31] When the British Secretary of State for India in coordination with Kew Gardens authorized a collecting expedition to South America in the late 1850s, quinine's efficacy was well established in western medicine.[32] In fact, a reasonable amount was known about its culture. William D. Hooker had written his doctoral dissertation "On Cinchona" twenty years earlier — two years before his father took over the directorship of Kew.[33]

Kew staff helped plan the collecting expedition to four separate areas in South America, and Kew-trained personnel accompanied the missions. Previous attempts at obtaining cinchona had not met with success. Local governments were "jealous" according to British reports, and exportation of the tree or its seeds had become illegal. At this time the Andean republics were exporting two million pounds of bark annually and the British were paying 53,000 pounds sterling a year to purchase quinine just for India.[34] As the only known treatment for this extremely widespread disease, reliable supplies of quinine were becoming more and more important to the British government. Without quinine, British administration and commerce in many of the colonies would be very difficult and costly.[35]

Using a number of questionable and even illegal tactics, British collectors succeeded in returning to England with seeds and Wardian cases full of cinchona in 1860. The Treasury financed a special glasshouse for the raising of cinchona and within five years a million trees had been distributed.[36]

In cooperation with Kew, experimental plantations were established in Mauritius, Fiji, St. Helena, Tanganyika (now Tanzania), the Cameroons, Burma, Trinidad, Tobago and Jamaica. However, efforts were concentrated in India and Ceylon (now Sri Lanka). Hybridizing work was done at the botanic gardens in both countries. And at the Calcutta Botanic Garden, a method was devised to increase the amount of harvestable bark.[37]

Botanic gardens throughout the empire distributed millions of cinchona seedlings to private growers. By 1887, Ceylon alone was producing 13 million pounds of bark. Andean exports which had risen to nearly 20 million pounds in the early 1880s collapsed by seventy-five percent within a period of three years.[38]

Within thirty years of cinchona's transfer, production had been radically transformed and rationalized. The monopoly which Andean republics had enjoyed over the indigenous tree was broken by well coordinated and planned collecting expeditions which utilized the latest technology to transport trees safely back to Kew Gardens. At Kew the plants were studied and propagated. Seedlings were sent to Kew's network of affiliated botanic gardens where further work was done on hybridizing and on extraction methods in the precise locations of future production. The results of this work, both in the form of new cinchona varieties and knowledge of cultivation and processing techniques was then provided to private interests for commercialization. Through this process, the British colonial administration (through the Secretary of State for India) working with the scientific establishment (at Kew) succeeded in establishing plantation production of a crop which was extremely important to political and commercial activities in the British colonies. Cinchona supplies were increased while prices were lowered as gathering of cinchona in labor-scarce Latin America was replaced by commercial production of higher-yielding varieties on plantations in labor-abundant Asia.

## RUBBER

The story of rubber follows a pattern similar to that of cinchona. The colonial India Office financed transportation costs and collectors' fees for the rubber collecting effort in Brazil, the native habitat of rubber. At the time, the commercial importance of rubber was known in Brazil.[39] But plantation production of rubber was precluded in Brazil due mainly to disease problems associated with monoculture. Rubber was tapped from wild trees dispersed in the forest. Large regions of Brazil were tightly tied to the rubber economy. Fortunes were made as demonstrated by the existence of the famous but unlikely opera house in the Amazon forest town of Manaus.

The story of the smuggling of rubber out of Brazil has been told frequently enough. The British collector, Charles Wickham, was obviously well aware of the desire of local authorities to prevent its removal. Howard and Ralph Wolf quote Wickham as saying:

> It was perfectly certain in my mind that if the authorities guessed the purpose of what I had on board we should be detained under plea of instruction from the Central Government at Rio, if not interdicted altogether. I had heard of the difficulties encountered in the Clements Markham introduction of the Cinchonas in getting them out of the Montana of Peru. Any such delay would have rendered my precious freight quite valueless and useless. But again fortune favoured. I had a 'friend at court' . . . [40]

Wickham's ship, laden with Wardian cases full of rubber trees (which by fortuitous accident were disease-free), steamed back to England where they arrived at Kew in June, 1876. Seedlings were distributed to botanic gardens in the colonies. Brockway notes that "as with cinchona, Kew supplied the trained botanists for the colonial stations and orchestrated their research effort."[41] Again, the colonial gardens served as experiment stations and demonstration plots. At the Botanic Gardens in Singapore, the Kew-trained director, Henry Ridley, developed tapping methods which yielded a great increase in latex from the trees allowing commercial quantities to be extracted without damaging the trees. Private planters could obtain both planting materials and instruction such as this at the gardens. Bulletins were also published to further the flow of information.

Through such efforts, rubber production was successfully transferred from Brazil to Asia. Brazil lost its market suddenly and almost totally (declining from a hundred percent to five percent), precipitating economic collapse and famine in the northeast. From this point until World War

II, 75% of world rubber production was in the hands of British nationals—
69% on its own territory.[42]

Many crops in addition to cinchona and rubber were transferred. And
efforts to control and commercialize other crops took different forms. The
Dutch cut down three-quarters of the clove and nutmeg stands in the
Moluccas and concentrated production on three heavily guarded islands.
The French offered the guillotine to anyone caught stealing live indigo
plants off of Antigua. Coffee production was transferred to Latin America
and cocoa was moved from its native habitat in Latin America to Africa.
Bananas left Southeast Asia for the Caribbean, soon to give their name to
a new phenomenon, the "banana republic." China lost much of its tea
trade. Mexico lost sisal. And West Africa lost palm oil to Southeast Asia.

Crops were moved from their homelands to new production sites often
lacking the old pests and diseases which had coevolved with the crop.
Efforts were centered on high-value crops which had to be produced
outside Europe and exported back. Crops were moved from areas of low
population (Latin America) to areas offering cheap labor (Asia).[43] The
intentional movement of crops provided a measure of control and, just as
significantly, calculability, to their production.

By the late 1800s the task of placing production of exotic plants on a
scientific and commercial basis was a more pressing and realistic concern.
Rather than build armies and navies to defend island-based monopolies,
England, for example, built a scientific base upon which new crops could
be more rationally and effectively exploited.

## GOVERNMENT SEED DISTRIBUTION AND FARMER SEED SAVING IN THE UNITED STATES

For rather obvious reasons, the United States was a latecomer to the
botanical chess game of the colonial era. But this is not to say that the
country did not participate. It became a production site for a number of
crops introduced from elsewhere. And political leaders were keenly
interested in acquiring new plants. As Thomas Jefferson is often quoted as
saying, "The greatest service which can be rendered to any country is to
add a useful plant to its culture."

Jefferson and other political leaders of the new United States were
enthusiastic introducers of exotic plant material into the country. At a
time when smuggling was punishable by death,[44] Jefferson smuggled
upland rice sewn into the linings of his coat out of Italy in an attempt to
introduce it to and encourage its cultivation in South Carolina. (But
farmers there begged him to keep his rice to himself, believing their rice

to be superior to his.[45] ) George Washington imported large quantities of seed yearly from Britain and Europe and carried on a steady correspondence with Jefferson about seed crops.[46] Benjamin Franklin is credited with making several successful introductions. Meanwhile, various planters and businessmen undertook similar efforts to import seeds or to locate exotic material through the expanding American consulate system. However, with the major exception of maize, a crop native to North and Central America, most of the original seed stocks were either brought into the country by immigrant farm families or collected from abroad and imported into the United States by the government itself. (Only a few crops of commercial importance are actually native to the United States: sunflowers, cranberries, Jerusalem artichokes, hops, some nuts and berries. All other crops have been introduced.[47])

At the beginning of the nineteenth century, there was no significant seed business and seeds were undeveloped as a commodity. Obviously, farmers were saving a portion of each year's crop to use the following year as seed, a practice dating to the earliest days of agriculture. Nevertheless, farmers had a constant need — economic and biological — for infusions of plant material. Farmers used new material to adapt old crops to new regions, maintain productivity in old areas of cultivation, and test the possibility of growing new crops throughout the country.[48]

By 1800, westward expansion was in full swing.[49] When the first shots had been fired in the Civil War, the borders of the United States had greatly expanded, encompassing the additions of the Gadsden Purchase, the areas of Utah, Nevada, Arizona, California, parts of western Colorado and New Mexico, and Texas. In fewer than sixty years total land area more than tripled from 868,000 square miles to nearly 2,945,000 square miles.[50] The government and farmers alike were interested in settling this land, some of it amongst the richest and most fertile in the world. The population center of the country moved westward with each settler family, as did its center of agricultural production.

Significantly, in the early part of the nineteenth century the American government became involved in obtaining crop diversity and facilitating its testing and adaptation in order to aid in the commercial success and expansion of agriculture. In 1819 the Treasury Department officially requested American consulates to send seeds home:

> The introduction of useful plants, not before cultivated, or such as are of superior quality to those which have been previously introduced, is an object of great importance to every civilized state, but more particularly to one recently organized, in which the progress of improvements of every kind has not to contend with ancient and deep rooted prejudices. The

introduction of such inventions, the results of the labor and science of other nations, is still more important, especially to the U. States, *whose institutions secure to the importer no exclusive advantage from their introduction.* [italics added] Your attention is respectfully solicited to these important subjects.[51]

Another request for seeds and plants was made by President John Quincy Adams in 1827. This request included instructions on how to pack and ship plants.[52]

In 1836, Henry Ellsworth became Commissioner of Patents under the Department of Treasury. Ellsworth was a member of a prominent Connecticut family. His father was a framer of the Constitution and Chief Justice of the Supreme Court under Washington. Ellsworth himself was a large landowner and a backer of efforts to settle the West. He had been a Commissioner of Indian Affairs for a region southwest of Arkansas. His travels had convinced him that the West had great agricultural potential and accordingly he had accumulated great tracts of land from Iowa to Michigan, including 65,000 acres in Benton County, Indiana, alone.[53] Settlement of the West, Ellsworth realized, depended on the successful promotion of scientific agriculture to provide a living for the settlers and a basis for industry and commerce.[54] In fact, he had already made contact with and, through agricultural societies, associated himself with those advocating use of improved livestock breeds and the importation and improvement of seeds.

In his new job at the Patent Office, Ellsworth saw it as being as much his business to promote agriculture as manufacturing, even though the patent laws did not apply to living material (note the italicized section of the Treasury Department circular, above). By 1839, Ellsworth had secured funds for collecting and distributing seeds and for the collection of agricultural statistics — activities which would later lead to the establishment of a Department of Agriculture. He committed space in the new Patent Office building for the "reception and exhibition" of seeds and informed the chairman of the Committee on Patents that the Commissioner of Patents, Ellsworth himself, would make a requisition from the patent fund in order to "find a remuneration from expenses already becoming onerous to himself personally."[55]

The U.S. Navy also entered the seed business during this period. Commodore Matthew Perry's famous gunboats (with a Patent Office biologist onboard) not only opened Japan to American trade, but returned with vegetable seeds, barley, rice, beans, cotton, fruits and roses.[56] By 1842, a government glasshouse was operating in Washington to house the influx of botanical immigrants.[57]

The American seed trade had begun with the over-the-counter selling of seeds by urban merchants in Providence,[58] New York and Boston, though David Landreth of Philadelphia usually gets the credit for establishing the first seed company in 1784, because he set aside land exclusively for seed production. Soon thereafter the Shakers, a religious sect, began growing vegetable and flower seeds for sale, which they sold in small paper envelopes — a marketing first.[59] The trade remained small and while citizens were certainly beginning to experiment with and breed (or select) new varieties,[60] it is unlikely that any seed company actually had full time breeders on its payroll. The chief source of new material was not the seed industry, but the Patent Office, which had picked up the Shaker technique and by the time of Ellsworth's departure in 1849 was sending out 60,000 seed packages a year.

In the spring of 1862, as German botanist Julius Sachs was demonstrating that starch is produced by photosynthesis and as the United States was engulfed in a bloody war, a Department of Agriculture was created at President Lincoln's request. The purpose of the Department was to promote the science of agriculture and, according to the act establishing it, "to collect . . . new and valuable seeds and plants; to test, by cultivation, the value of such of them as may require such tests; to propagate such as may be worthy of propagation, and to distribute them among agriculturalists."[61] By 1878, the department was spending a third of its budget on germplasm collection and distribution[62] and trials of exotic plants were under way all over the country.

Government distribution of seed packages had grown to be very popular, the number of packages mailed out having increased from 306,304 in 1862 to a high of 20,368,724 in 1897. As each package contained a number of packets of seeds, the actual number of samples distributed was much higher. Distribution of plants and cuttings (not reflected in table 2 below) reached a high of 156,862 in 1880.

The packets did not contain enough seeds to supply commercial farming. They were instead of a size to facilitate experimentation. That,

**Table 2.** Seed Distribution by U.S. Government[63]

| Period | Seed Packages | Yearly Average |
|--------|---------------|----------------|
| 1862–1869 | 6,597,979 | 824,747 |
| 1870–1879 | 12,894,336 | 1,289,434 |
| 1880–1889 | 34,951,232 | 3,495,123 |
| 1890–1897 | 81,561,998 | 10,195,250 |

indeed, was the original purpose of the program. Additionally, Congress (as evidenced in a 1870 resolution requesting a report from the Commissioner of Agriculture) was interested in how this program might help replace foreign imports.[64] Lacking the basis for a commercial seed industry and lacking a public sector infrastructure for breeding and disseminating seeds in quantities sufficient to satisfy demand, the Patent Office and later the Department of Agriculture chose to encourage the farmer to be a selector, breeder, and multiplier of seed. In the *Report of the Commissioner of Patents for the Year 1854*, Commissioner Mason makes this point clear. By distributing small rather than large packages of seeds:

> the opportunity of experimenting can be placed within the reach of several hundred times as many persons than would be if distributed by the bushel. A small amount will, in most instances, test the adaptation of the grain to any particular soil and climate as effectually as would be done in a larger quantity.[65]

Mason, as had previous commissioners, urged farmer experimentation, selection and the crossbreeding (then termed "hybridizing") of different varieties:

> A judicious system of hybridizing might still further increase the improvement, and would be well worthy of an experiment . . . It is therefore earnestly suggested to every one who has the requisite taste and ability that he should undertake a course of experiments of the kind above contemplated, or any other which his own judgement may dictate, with a view not only of testing choice varieties of such seeds as he may procure, but also of improving the qualities of those very varieties. If the seeds distributed through this office can fall in small parcels into the hands of persons, in all sections of the country, who will pursue the course herein suggested, it may reasonably be expected that the most substantial benefits will result from such a course.[66]

In addition to the seeds sent in by consulates, private individuals, and the military, the federal government sponsored numerous plant collecting expeditions. Prior to the Civil War, a plant explorer was dispatched to collect sugarcane from "the most elevated regions of Caracas," and returned with a thousand boxes of cane cuttings, plantain, banana, and other plants.[67] During the war, one expedition went to China to collect sorghum, and a second went to Europe.[68] By the end of the century collectors had returned with seeds from Russia, Turkestan, Western China, Siberia, the Nordic countries, Japan, and many countries of Europe, Africa, and South America.[69]

Other introductions of considerable but unestimated value, which farmers made use of, included: Turkestan and Siberian alfalfas, Trebi barley,

Sudan grass, Acala and Egyptian cotton, date palms, Smyrna figs, oriental mangoes, Mexican avocados, pistache nuts and Chinese persimmons.[70]

Out of both necessity and eagerness, farmers used the seed provided them by the government (the most diversity ever assembled and distributed by a government directly to farmers) to create and adapt varieties to their own needs and ecological conditions.[71] A stream of immigrants in the latter half of the nineteenth century added to this diversity — U.S. population doubled between 1860 and 1890, a third of this attributable to foreign immigration.[72] Coming from all parts of Europe, immigrants brought in seeds of many diverse types in waves allowing for the integration of the new genetic material.

The number of varieties documented as being in use during this period rose "with almost incredible rapidity," according to A. J. Pieters who was in charge of USDA's pure seed investigations in 1899.[74] A number of apple varieties which are standards even today (for example, McIntosh and Delicious) were selected by farmers before the turn of the century. Colorfully named and still popular tomato varieties such as Mortgage Lifter also came from this period. Other farmer-bred and selected varie-

**Table 3.** Introduction of Valuable Crops/Varieties by the Patent Office and the USDA, Selected Examples[73]

| Crop or Variety | Cost of Collection | Value of Introduction* |
|---|---|---|
| Sorghum | $2,000 | $40,000,000 |
| Kafir corn | $5,000 | $15,000,000 |
| Durum wheat | <$30,000 | $40,000,000 |
| Japanese short-kerneled rice | <$20,000 | $3,000,000 increase in annual value |
| Swedish Select oats | $5,000 | $1,000,000 increase in annual value in Wisconsin |
| Excelsior White Schoenen oats | $1,000 | $15,000,000 increase in annual value |
| Chevalier barley | $1,000 | "many millions of dollars" |
| Fultz wheat | "small cost" | "millions of dollars" |
| Washington Navel orange | "insignificant" | $10,000,000 in California alone |

* Unless otherwise stated, "value of introduction" refers to total value of annual production in the U.S., circa 1912.

ties were destined to become the backbone of and raw material for the emergence of public and eventually private plant breeding programs.

Farmers in the nineteenth century were more aware of or at least had more access to useful breeding information than some might now suspect. As early as 1716, the famous Puritan, Cotton Mather, had noted that color crossing in corn was especially prominent on the side toward which the wind normally blew. Mather's experiments, which were published, apparently showed him the effect of pollen from one type falling on the silks of another.[75] Less than a hundred years later, the Philadelphia Agricultural Society published a practical account of corn crossing. Four years later, in 1812, John Lorain wrote of crossing gourdseed corns and flinty corns to produce a new variety yielding one-third more. Significantly, Lorain recognized that characteristics did not just "blend" in the breeding process. Offspring might exhibit a larger proportion of favorable traits, for example.[76]

Farm newspapers and journals carried news of such experiments. Articles exhorting farmers to choose seed carefully from the best plants were not at all uncommon. The USDA distributed free-of-charge "farmers' bulletins" offering encouragement and advice.

Through selection, farmers could be plant breeders and could exercise influence over the development of their crops. Even unconscious random selection of grain crops could result in steady improvements, as the most prolific types would be favored due to their greater numbers.[77] Many farmers, however, were engaging much more deliberately in selection and breeding activities. At the first Iowa State Fair in 1855, a speaker told the assembled farmers:

> formerly you paid but little attention to the quality of the seed you sowed or planted. If it was corn — grains of corn were sufficient — if wheat, grains of wheat were sufficient. If potatoes — the semblance of that popular vegetable was sufficient. Now, with what care the intelligent farmer selects his seed corn — desirous of obtaining that variety which is most productive in its nutritive qualities, and produces the largest results from a given quantity of ground.[78]

Parker and Decanio assert that "most early recorded experimentation" was in the Northeast. But the proliferation of small and moderate-sized farms (two million between 40 and 300 acres by 1860) meant that "many small experiments were occurring simultaneously and their results communicated among rural neighborhoods."[79]

Two keen observers, Henry A. Wallace (at various times U.S. Vice-President, Secretary of Agriculture, farm newspaper editor and founder of the first hybrid corn seed company) and his co-author William Brown (later to become CEO of the world's largest seed company) writing in 1956 about the nation's most valuable crop, stated: "We have seen how observant farmers during the first half of the Nineteenth Century recognized and put to use the benefits of crossing differing varieties of corn."[80] While many crossings were understandably undirected or even accidental (the result of the farmer mixing varieties in the field and awaiting the result of natural cross-pollination), "others were planned," Wallace and Brown stressed.

By the turn of the century, the United States had imported an immense amount of genetic material from all over the world. American diplomats and military personnel had answered the call of their government to send seeds home. Wave after wave of ethnic immigrants packed seed in their baggage as they set out for a new life in America. And government sponsored collecting trips had returned from distant lands with thousands of samples of both familiar and exotic species. Armed with ample amounts of diverse germplasm and blessed with many different growing conditions, America's farmers undertook countless "experiments" and, through mass selection, developed literally tens of thousands of varieties. During the nineteenth century American farmers had developed and grown some 7,000 varieties of apples.[81] An 1859 survey of Ohio wheats revealed 135 varieties which were or had recently been cultivated on a "significant scale" in the state.[82] By 1925, when *The Small Fruits of New York* was published, Hedrick was able to describe 1,362 varieties of strawberries, virtually all originating in the United States since 1800.[83] Over 450 varieties of radish and 350 varieties of onions had been developed or used.

Experimentation with plant breeding and adaptation of crops to new environments would have been encouraged by a number of factors including the availability of information about techniques (mentioned above) and the seeds themselves. Late in the century the USDA began publishing inventories of government seeds available for experimentation. These inventories contained as much information on each variety than is kept on many accessions in USDA seed collections today, and often more. From these lists serious farmers could choose which types they might be interested in testing.[84]

There were few viable alternatives to farmer seed-saving. New lands to settle and the absence of *good* commercial sources of seed were powerful incentives for on-farm seed breeding and saving. By the mid-1800s, itinerant seed and nursery stock salesmen plagued the countryside.[85] Salesmen made wild claims knowing that they would be long gone when unsuspecting farmers discovered the truth. Earl Hayter documented some of the claims: grapes so mild that wine made from them is not intoxicating; strawberries that grow on trees and are the size of oranges; corn with kernels the size of chestnuts (one wonders how the salesman explained the size of his seed); and Egyptian wheat discovered in a tomb and owing its great yields to "the long rest it had."[86] In fact, the salesmen rarely had anything of great merit to sell. Formal, scientific plant breeding programs were nonexistent. Many salesmen could only sell their products through deception, a practice which brought widespread mistrust of the struggling seed and nursery business. Popular culture glorifying the self-provisioning farmer simply made a virtue out of necessity and reinforced farmer control over seeds. The lack of harvesting machinery (during much of the century) also meant that farmers were forced to harvest by hand, a task which gave them ample opportunity to study their crops, choose seeds from superior plants, and notice unusual and useful recombinants and mutations.

After independence there were few attempts to control production by means of monopolizing access to breeding material reminiscent of the era discussed earlier in the chapter. Presumably, the young country could not marshal the forces necessary to accomplish this, nor did it have the kind of presence or power abroad that could give it exclusive control over valuable botanical material. The U.S. focus was on internal development of agriculture. This was done in part by appropriating seed from others and encouraging the adaptation of these seeds to American conditions. Without the complication of having to appease a commercial seed industry, both political and private interests were served by the wide distribution of diverse types of seeds. Expansion, not limitation of production, was the goal.

The picture we have painted thus far is one of farmers in control of their seeds; of farmers as plant breeders, selectors, and savers. This is not the full picture, however. To shed light on how farmers lost this control, how seeds became a commodity, and how farmers became dependent on purchased seeds, we must examine the history and some of the changes that took place in nineteenth- and early twentieth-century American agriculture in more depth than we have thus far. Chapter 2 examines, among other things, the effects of commercialization on the relationship between farmers and seeds.

## DISCUSSION

The discovery of new and potentially useful and valuable plants in the New World came at a time when European powers were beginning to have the capability of exploiting these discoveries. During the nineteenth century, colonial powers — England in particular —created scientific institutions and networks centered around botanic gardens. In this history we see the beginnings of a process of rationalization in relation to economically valuable botanical materials, involving in Weberian terms "the explicit definition of goals and the increasingly precise calculation of the most effective means to achieve them . . . "[87]

Agents creatively and intentionally constructed a system spanning the globe and involving elements of orderly classification, collection and evaluation of plants, production, marketing, and defense. In this system, botanical gardens served as staging areas for plant collecting and for introduction of plants into new regions. They helped acclimatize the new crops and develop cultural techniques and knowledge about the plants. In due course the plants left the gardens for further testing and study in associated tropical gardens or for secure production sites.

Different levels of power among actors allowed some to take advantage of the world's botanical wealth — to collect it, gain knowledge about it, transport it to their production areas, and market it. Others could not do this at all or could do it only in limited ways. The technologies and the systems created by the European powers were used in ways which profoundly altered the character of plant production systems.

This process of rationalization is most clearly evident in the examples of cinchona and rubber. These two wild (nondomesticated) trees were removed from their natural habitat against the wishes of their native "owners" and transported to Kew. At Kew they were studied and then shipped to affiliated botanic gardens in the colonies. Breeding work was undertaken. Growing techniques and methods of extraction were improved. Plant materials and methods were used to establish government and private plantations with the result that supplies of two items of extreme importance to a colonial and industrial society were greatly increased. Through this process two products previously gathered from the wild in South America came to be produced in a commercial setting with full scientific and political support. Again, notions of control and ownership were profoundly altered.

The benefits from exotic plant material were derived not just from their control, but from their development, use, and commercialization. This points to the fact that inventions (or in this case, discoveries — plants) alone are not enough if a system or a capability to facilitate use is not in place. It also brings into question the importance and meaningfulness of control in circumstances where actors do not have the capability of exploiting that which is "controlled." Physical control was attempted and was temporarily important with a few crops. However, it was ultimately the rationalization process, the development and exercise of the capability to use the material, not exclusive possession, that gave England its most meaningful form of "control."

Complete physical control was problematic and fleeting because it essentially had to be over the entire species of a crop. At this time, formal plant breeding was virtually unknown, as were stable, uniform or pure "varieties." Much diversity existed of course, but the ability to manipulate it, to combine genes to create new, customized varieties was limited prior to the rediscovery of Mendel's laws of heredity in 1900. Maintaining absolute monopoly implied the restriction of propagation not of one variety of indigo or sugarcane, but essentially of all types. To the extent that control was achieved by certain powers, it was won on a crop by crop basis. It had to be reinvented, re-established with each crop and each production site. Actors exercised power but had only tenuous control over these biological materials.

Smuggling was common and was facilitated by the fact that smugglers had only to carry out seeds or propagating material of species rather than varieties. While genetic diversity is concentrated in what are now called "Centers of Diversity," these centers cover a great deal of territory. "Centers" is not really a very useful concept, unless one is comfortable thinking of the Andes region or a band of land 1500 kilometers wide across the breadth of Africa as a center. It was difficult to keep competitors/smugglers away from such large areas. Even the plantations were not impregnable. Since the finished product in some cases was identical to the means of production (the seed), potential monopolies of some crops could be broken through normal commerce. Finally, once broken, a plant monopoly was broken for good. Attempts at plant control had a built-in, limited life expectancy. When they fell, they fell not just because another actor snitched some seeds, but because other actors were successful in creating the infrastructure to exploit those seeds commercially. While the plantations of this era still exist in some cases, their botanical control and monopoly over breeding material has long since disappeared. It was not until the advent of modern plant breeding that further concerted attempts at control over plants and their breeding material would be made, this time through the patent systems of "developed" countries.

Futile attempts were made to establish legal protection of biological property. As early as 1556, Spain's Council of the Indies (convened in Madrid) passed legislation making it illegal for foreigners to explore for plants in Spain's New World possessions.[88] A number of countries reserved ownership rights over new plant discoveries to the king. But few other countries felt even slightly constrained by such laws, and officially sanctioned smuggling was the rule rather than the exception when confronted with unenforceable laws.

With the examples of cinchona and rubber the goal of the British Colonial Office was not simply to gain control from South Americans, but to establish reliable commercial production and make that production more readily available for their purposes. (Cinchona alone had a great impact on the ability of Europeans to do business and work in malaria-infested areas.) Removal of the plants from their native habitat and the breaking of the local monopoly was a logical step in the process.

The impact of plant introductions and movements in this period was substantial. New plants changed human diets and significantly bolstered the emerging chemical and dyestuffs industry in Europe. The impact on the economies and peoples of the tropics was no less profound, though less positive. But equally important perhaps was the emergence of rational planning and systems for the acquisition, study, development, dispersal, and commercialization of exotic (non-European) crops on an international basis.

As already noted, the United States was a latecomer to the botanical chess game.[89] Immigrants brought a large amount of genetic diversity with them. But government officials also organized massive importations of genetic materials. They created systems for handling this material, including information systems to pass on what was known about a particular collection to the farmers. These officials were faced with problems such as adapting crops to the extremely varied American landscape and thereby encouraging the spread of American agriculture and people westward. Initially this was not done through establishment of a network of botanical gardens. Instead, the job of experimentation and adaptation in different environments was handed over to the farmers themselves. Tight, proprietary control over seed types would not have accomplished the government's goal. Distribution and usage were much more important than centralized control.

Farmers were largely self-sufficient in seeds and other supplies. The wide distribution of seeds helped place control of seeds and their development in the hands of farmers, who developed varieties appropriate to the many different ecosystems found in the United States. These varieties formed the biological foundation for the rise of U.S. commercial agriculture, which will be discussed more fully in the following chapter.

In summary, from the 1600s onward, European powers began to find spices and other valuable plants in far-flung lands. Ownership and control were derived from physical possession. Government and early companies traded with the gatherers and growers of these crops. These practices were steadily replaced by much more rational forms. Countries with significant naval capabilities, such as England, planned and organized expeditions to search out the best and most productive species of the crops in which they were interested. At Kew a state-funded scientific institution was built, where practical research was undertaken to facilitate the successful transfer of the crops. Species were crossed, tests made to see which were most productive. Methods of extraction and processing were improved. Institutions such as Kew coordinated much of the activity surrounding these new plants, keeping written records and publishing their research findings. Close ties were kept with commercial producers. In the United States, actors also constructed systems to collect and distribute seeds, albeit more "democratically." There was also evidence of rational planning and development, but for different ends. The contrast between the two patterns indicates the importance of viewing these events in their own distinct economic and political contexts.

What we can see in its infancy in the 1800s is the creation of a strikingly new, efficient, organized, "scientific" and rational way of working with biological materials. The haphazard nature of plant collection and commerce characteristic of precolonial and early colonial days was gone or fast disappearing. When Mendel's laws of heredity were not-so-accidentally rediscovered by three separate researchers in 1900, they entered a very different and more receptive world than he might have imagined as he tended his peas behind the monastery wall short decades earlier.

## NOTES

1. While this is true for grains and most fruits, vegetables and tuber crops, it should be noted that when agriculturalists penetrated the forests of central and northern Europe, the forest clearings were invaded by "colonizing" grasses and clovers. Over time these became the forages upon which is based much of the ruminant livestock production in the temperate world.
2. Woolley, C. L., *The Sumerians*. Oxford: Clarendon Press. 1930: p. 79. See also Klose, Norman, *America's Crop Heritage: The History of Foreign Plant Introduction by the Federal Government*. 1950: p. 3.
3. Farney, Dennis, "Meet the Men Who Risked Their Lives to Find New Plants." *Smithsonian*, June 1980, p. 134.
4. Crosby, Alfred W., Jr., *The Colombian Exchange: Biological and Cultural Consequences of 1492*. Westport, Conn.: Greenwood Press. 1972.
5. Ho, Ping-ti, "The Introduction of American Food Plants into China." *American Anthropologist*, 57: p. 194.
6. Crosby, op. cit., p. 166.
7. Cipolla, Carlo, M., *Guns and Sails in the Early Phase of European Expansion*. London: Collins. 1965, p. 81.
8. Cipolla, Carlo, M., *Before the Industrial Revolution: European Society and Economy, 1000-1700*. New York: Norton. 1976: p. 209.

9. Smith, Nigel J. H., "Botanic Gardens and Germplasm Conservation," Harold L. Lyon Arboretum Lecture Number Fourteen. Honolulu: University of Hawaii Press. February 6, 1985. p. 9.

10. Brockway, Lucile, *Science and Colonial Expansion: The Role of the British Royal Botanic Gardens.* New York: Academic Press. 1979: p. 74–5.

11. Kyd, Lt. Col. Robert, quoted in Brockway, op cit., p. 75.

12. Hepper, F. N., *Royal Botanic Gardens, Kew: Gardens for Science and Pleasure.* London: Her Majesty's Stationery Office. 1982: p. 59

13. Brockway, Lucile, op. cit., p. 86–87

14. Lemmon, Kenneth, *Golden Age of Plant Hunters.* Cranbury: A. S. Barnes and Co. 1968: p. 15.

15. Bean, William J., *The Royal Botanic Gardens, Kew: Historical and Descriptive.* London: Cassell & Co. 1908: p. 22.

16. King, Ronald, *Royal Kew.* London: Constable & Co. 1985: p. 202.

17. Thiselton-Dyer, W. T., "Introduction," in Bean, op. cit., p. xviii.

18. Bean, op. cit., p. 56.

19. King, op. cit., p. 204.

20. Bean, op. cit., p. 68.

21. Royal Botanic Gardens, "Centenary of the Royal Botanic Gardens," *Kew Bulletin of Miscellaneous Information.* 1941. p. 208.

22. Interestingly, histories of Kew by staff members almost invariably seem to stress the close link between Kew and the Colonial Office and the clear and conscious concern of Kew directors in the nineteenth century with serving colonial interests and giving practical assistance to colonial commercial/agricultural efforts. See, for example, W. J. Bean (cited above) and W. B. Turrill, *The Royal Botanic Gardens Kew: Past and Present.* London: Herbert Jenkins. 1959.

23. Thiselton-Dyer, op. cit., p. xvii.

24. Brockway, op. cit., p. 76.

25. Ibid.

26. Royal Botanic Gardens, "List of the Staffs of the Royal Gardens," *Kew Bulletin of Miscellaneous Information.* No. 29. 1889. p. 122ff.

27. A variety of sources were used for this table, chiefly "Botanic Gardens and Germplasm Conservation" by Nigel Smith (see note 9, this chapter).

28. Smith, Marvanna S., *Chronological Landmarks in American Agriculture.* U.S. Department of Agriculture. Washington: Government Printing Office. 1979: p. 2, 3, 12, 51.

29. Bean, op. cit., p. 48.

30. Chamberlain, Joseph, quoted in Bean, op. cit., p. 60.

31. King, op. cit., p. 205.

32. Brockway, op. cit., p. 104.

33. Ibid., p. 111.

34. Ibid., p. 112–113.

35. Ibid., p. 126.

36. King, op. cit., p. 205.

37. Brockway, op. cit., p. 118–121.

38. Ibid., p. 112, 122.

39. In 1839, Charles Goodyear developed a technique for processing rubber. This process greatly enhanced the significance and potential for rubber in the industrializing societies of Europe and North America.

40. Wolf, Howard, and Ralph Wolf, *Rubber, A Story of Glory and Greed.* New York: Covici Friede. 1936: p. 159.

41. Brockway, op. cit., p. 143.

42. Ibid., p. 165.

43. Ibid., p. 14.

44. de Souza Silva, Jose, "Science and the Changing Nature of the Struggle Over Plant Genetic Resources: From Plant Hunters to Plant Crafters." Ph.D. dissertation, University of Kentucky, 1989: p. 141.

45. Jefferson, Thomas, *Thomas Jefferson: Garden Book*, edited by Edwin Morris Betts. Philadelphia: The American Philosophical Society. 1944: p. 124, 131.
46. Beck, Frank Victor, *The Field Seed Industry in the United States: An Analysis of the Production Consumption and Prices of Leguminous and Grass Seeds*. Madison: University of Wisconsin Press. 1944: p. 5.
47. Gary Nabhan in numerous articles and books has correctly pointed out that native American Indians used and domesticated an impressive number of crops which, though of potential importance now, are not widely used. Many of these crops were "lost" as the people and cultures which nurtured them were disrupted and destroyed. Were it not for this tragedy, North America's "contribution" to the list of the world's major crops might be much larger.
48. Most of this adaptation was through selection in conjunction with unconscious crossing. Little conscious crossing can be assumed with self-pollinated field and horticultural crops.
49. Cochrane, Willard W., *The Development of American Agriculture: A Historical Analysis*. Minneapolis: University of Minnesota Press. 1979: p. 8.
50. U.S. Department of Commerce, Bureau of the Census. *Historical Statistics of the United States: Colonial Times to 1970*, Part 2. Washington: U.S. Government Printing Office. 1975: p. 38–9.
51. Crawford, Wm. H., "Treasury Circular," reprinted in Rasmussen, Wayne D., *Agriculture in the United States: A Documentary History*. Vol. 1. New York: Random House. 1975: p. 458–459.
52. Ryerson, Knowles A. "History and Significance of the Foreign Plant Introduction Work of the United States Department of Agriculture." *Agricultural History*. Vol. 7, No. 2. april, 1933: p. 113.
53. True, Alfred Charles, *A History of Agricultural Experimentation and Research in the United States, 1607–1925*. Miscellaneous Publication No. 251, U.S. Department of Agriculture. Washington: Government Printing Office. 1937: p. 23–4.
54. Alfred True relates that Ellsworth died leaving two wills. In the resulting court battles over his estate the question of his sanity was raised. One reason for doubting it was Ellsworth's public prediction that steam power would be used some day to operate machinery and pull plows on the Prairies — see, True, p. 24. (Steam tractors were commercially manufactured in the U.S. from 1915 to 1925.)
55. Ellsworth, Henry L., letter to chairman of Committee on Patents (from the U.S. Patent Office, Annual Report, 1839, pp. 57-59) in Rasmussen, Wayne D., *Agriculture in the United States: A Documentary History*. Vol. 1. New York: Random House. 1975: p. 500.
56. Klose, Norman, *America's Crop Heritage: The History of Foreign Plant Introduction by the Federal Government*. Ames, Iowa: Iowa State College Press. 1950: p. 33. Perry succeeded in negotiating the first U.S.-Japan treaty in 1854.
57. Kloppenburg, Jack Ralph Jr., *First the Seed: The Political Economy of Plant Biotechnology, 1492–2000*. Cambridge: Cambridge University Press. 1988: p. 55.
58. Pieters, A. J. "Seed Selling, Seed Growing and Seed Testing," in *Yearbook of Agriculture, 1899*. U.S. Department of Agriculture. Washington: Government Printing Office. 1900: p. 550. The first record of seeds for sale found by Pieters was that of Nathaniel Bird, a book dealer, who advertised seeds newly arrived from London in the Newport, R.I. *Mercury* of 1763.
59. Manks, Dorothy S., "How the American Nursery Trade Began," in *Plants & Gardens: Origins of American Horticulture*. Brooklyn: Brooklyn Botanic Garden. Vol. 23, no. 3. Autumn 1967: p. 5–6.
60. Hedrick, U. P., *A History of Horticulture in America to 1860*. Portland, Oregon: Timber Press. 1988 (original copyright, 1950, Oxford University Press): p. 432ff.
61. Rasmussen, op. cit., p. 615.
62. Klose, op. cit., p. 62.
63. Ibid., p. 57, 98.
64. Ibid., p. 60.

65. Mason, Charles. *Report of the Commissioner of Patents for the Year 1854*. 33d Congress, 2d Session, House of Representatives, Ex. Doc. No. 59. Washington: U.S. Government. 1855: p. vii.

66. Ibid., p. viii–ix.

67. Brown, Louis Joseph. "The United States Patent Office and the Promotion of Southern Agriculture, 1850–1860." M.A. thesis, Florida State University. June, 1957: p. 35.

68. Ryerson, Knowles A. op.cit., 1933: p. 118.

69. Ryerson, Knowles A. "The History of Plant Exploration and Introduction in the United States Department of Agriculture." In *Proceedings of the International Symposium on Plant Introduction*, Escuela Agricola Panamerican, Tegucigalpa, Honduras. Nov. 30– Dec, 2, 1966: p. 16.

70. Pinkett, Harold T., "Records of the First Century of Interest of the United States Government in Plant Industries," *Agricultural History*, Vol. 29, no. 1. January, 1955: p. 41.

71. Nelson Klose in *America's Crop Heritage*, chapter 6, documents the development of new varieties from selections of introduced materials. Speaking of wheat, Klose states: "Agriculturalists of the nineteenth century were keenly interested in improving the familiar varieties of wheat. Even before 1860 they were making selections from admixtures, mutants, and the natural hybrids found in their fields." p. 67.

72. Schmidt, Louis Bernard, "Some Significant Aspects of the Agrarian Revolution in the United States," *Iowa Journal of History and Politics*. Vol. XVIII. 1920: p. 376.

73. Data and quotes taken from: Galloway, B.T. *Distribution of Seeds and Plants by the Department of Agriculture*. USDA Bureau of Plant Industry Circular No. 100. Washington: Government Printing Office. 1912: p. 21.

74. Pieters, op. cit., p. 567.

75. Wallace, Henry A., and William L. Brown, *Corn and Its Early Fathers*. East Lansing: Michigan State University Press. 1956: p. 46–47.

76. Ibid., p. 54ff.

77. Alsberg, Carl, "The Objectives of Wheat Breeding." *Wheat Studies*. Vol. 4, No. 7. 1928: p. 271.

78. Quoted in Danhof, Clarence H., *Change in Agriculture: The Northern United States, 1820–1870*. Cambridge, Mass.: Harvard University Press. 1969: p. 156.

79. Parker, William N., and Stephen J. Decanio, "Two Hidden Sources of Productivity Growth in American Agriculture, 1860–1930." *Agricultural History*. Vol. 56, no. 4. October, 1982: p. 649.

80. Wallace and Brown, op. cit., p. 69.

81. Ragan, W. H. *Nomenclature of the Apple: A Catalogue of the Known Varieties Referred to in American Publications from 1804 to 1904*. Bureau of Plant Industry, Bulletin No. 56. Washington: U.S. Government Printing Office. 1926

82. Danhof, op. cit., p. 157.

83. Hendick, U. P., *The Small Fruits of New York*. Albany. 1925.

84. Cook, O. F. Inventory No. 1, *Foreign Seeds and Plants Imported by the Section of Seed and Plant Introduction, Numbers 1–1000*. Washington: U.S. Department of Agriculture, Division of Botany. undated (1898). Inventory 7, published in 1900, contains a typical description (p. 15), quoted here in its entirety to demonstrate the type of information frequently available to farmers and researchers:
"2796. *Panicum Miliaceum* Broom-corn millet. From Russia. Received March, 1899, through Mr. M. A. Carleton. *Red Voronezh*. From the government of Vopronezh. Mean annual rainfall, 20 to 21 inches; for the growing season (May to September, inclusive), 10 to 11 inches. Mean annual temperature, 41.1 degrees. Soil, sandy black loam, rather rich in humus. Sown in Voronezh during the last week of May, but probably should be sown a little earlier in this country — soon after May 15. Period of growth about 115 days. It is best drilled in at the rate of 12 to 15 pounds per acre. Yields anywhere from 18 to 50 bushels per acre, depending upon treatment and the season. A red-seeded millet, but having the compacted form of panicle. Grown chiefly for the seed, which, besides

being good stock feed, is extensively used in Russia for human food in the form of grits or gruel and with soups. Well adapted for trial in almost all the prairie States, but especially the drier, colder districts. Amount obtained, 3 bushels. Reprinted from Inventory No. 4. See Carleton, Bull. 23, Div. Bot.: 29.

85. The Shakers had a small itinerant business as this time, which was not immune to bad publicity. In 1819 they discontinued their practice of buying seeds "of the world" to mix with their own saying that this practice threatened to bring "dishonor upon the gospel." See: *The Shaker Garden Seed Industry* by Margaret Frisbee Somer, Old Chatham, New York: The Shaker Museum. (M.A. thesis, University of Maine — Orono, 1966) 1972: p. 12. However, the Shakers were still being criticized years later. See Walter Elder's 1854 book, *The Cottage Garden of America*, Philadelphia: Moss & Brother. p. 169

86. Hayter, Earl W., "Horticultural Humbuggery Among the Western Farmers, 1850–1890." *Indiana Magazine of History*. Vol. XLIII, no. 3. September, 1947. And, "Seed Humbuggery Among the Western Farmers." *Ohio Archaeological and Historical Quarterly*, Vol. LVIII, 1949: p. 52–68.

87. Beetham, David, *Max Weber and the Theory of Modern Politics*. Cambridge: Polity Press. 1985: p. 68.

88. Haughton, Claire Shaver, *Green Immigrants*. New York: Harcourt Brace Jovanovich. 1979: p. 76–77.

89. It has not been the purpose of this chapter to delve into the obvious differences in the patterns of plant collection and development between the United States and some European countries. Instead I have tried to provide a background and setting for upcoming struggles over the control of plants in the United States. But obviously the pattern was different, more democratic. Perhaps it was because the United States did not have the military or economic might to do what England had done. Perhaps it was because the most easily exploited, controlled, and valuable plants had already been "taken," or there were few American territories suitable for production of high-value, monopolized crops. In any case, I find no evidence that the British model was ever seriously discussed or considered. It is more likely that the actors involved existed in a different context and had different priorities, as discussed here.

# CHAPTER 2

# From Seed Saving to Seed Buying: The Rise of Commercial Agriculture and Scientific Plant Breeding in the U.S., to 1930

We begin this chapter at the turn of the nineteenth century in the United States, with farmers firmly in control of seeds and other planting materials. Like generations before them, these farmers selected and saved their seed from year to year. Farmers might acquire some seeds from neighbors through barter, but for the most part farmers supplied their own seed by saving a portion of each year's harvest just as they had done since Neolithic times. In so doing farmers maintained individualized control over seeds. There was no sizable commercial market for seeds at the beginning of the century and seeds were undeveloped as a commodity form. The level of scientific development provides no particular impetus of its own to the emergence of a scientific or professional elite — there was no such thing as a professional plant breeder during much of the period.

As seen in chapter 1, the government helped facilitate the expansion and development of agriculture by distributing huge quantities of free seed to farmers. This was seed of many species and many varieties collected around the world — precisely the type of diversity farmers could use to fashion new crop varieties adapted to the numerous environments and emerging markets. The availability of "breeding" materials and farmers' success in using them would appear to strengthen their *de facto* control over their own seed.

This chapter does not proceed chronologically from the last. I return to the beginning of the nineteenth century to examine developments in agriculture and the broader economy and society which will come to have a profound impact on the self-provisioning farmer and the relationship between farmers and planting materials. This is a story of the commercialization and rationalization of agriculture, of the "extension of the market economy" and the beginnings of "bureaucratization," in Weber's words.[1] Here we find actors endeavoring to bring more calculability, order, professionalism, fixed rules — in short, rationality — to their sphere of work. These are conscious problem-solving efforts. Not surprisingly, these actions create tensions and encourage opposition.[2]

To the extent that previous writers have touched on this specific topic at all, the replacement of the farmers' traditional varieties has been viewed as coming at the hand of the superior scientifically bred seeds introduced in the early 1900s.[3] Farmers simply "traded in" their old seeds to get better varieties in an act which simply and politely ended thousands of years of farmer seed saving. But the process was much more complicated than this. The United States did not experience a "Green Revolution" like that in the Third World, where the introduction of new seeds was seemingly the single biggest factor in the replacement of farmer varieties. When new scientifically bred seeds were introduced in the United States, they entered an agricultural system which was to a great extent already rationalized, developed and market-oriented — indeed, the seeds were produced by this system. The new seeds still replaced the old seeds in the literal sense. But old relationships between farmer and seed were already well on the way to being transformed before the advent of the modern varieties. The decline of farmer seed-saving, the emerging commodification of seed, and the erosion of farmer control over seed began occurring prior to there being any convincing scientific advantage for commercial, scientifically bred seed. Farmer seed-saving was undermined primarily by the commercialization of agriculture and secondarily by the reduction in the amount and the change in the quality of breeding materials made available to farmers from the government, the development of hybrids and other scientifically bred varieties, and the lobby against farmer seed-saving by the industry.

I look at the increasing rationalization of agriculture as the context (1) in which the farmers ceased to save seed, and (2) out of which the seed industry came to life, gained economic strength, and began to act politically (a topic further explored in following chapters). When scientific advances came in the early 1900s, they could be used in ways dramatically different than they could have been a hundred years earlier.

My goal here is not to offer a complete, definitive history of the commercialization of agriculture. It is to describe the process in order to explain sufficiently how and why farmers began to have a different relationship to the seeds they used and how a commercial seed industry might have started to gain a foothold in this period. I shall deal with the expansion of agriculture during the nineteenth century and its increasingly commercial focus facilitated by the development of transportation, postal, and marketing systems, among others. The rise of the seed industry shall therefore be placed within the context of the commercialization of agriculture and this in turn will enable us to make more sense of the steady erosion of farmer control over seeds through the decline in farmer seed selection and saving.

A number of scientific discoveries and rediscoveries were made in the early part of the twentieth century. These were used and developed by both public and private sectors, particularly in relation to hybrid corn. In the process, plant breeding became a science to be practiced by professionals. It clearly also became more directed and goal-oriented, and less haphazard. It was an activity which could be *planned* and *controlled*. These events gave practical power to certain actors and further undermined the farmer-as-plant breeder and the farmer-as-seed saver. In this chapter we can begin to see — particularly in the case of hybrid corn — the beginnings of a redefining of the nature of and the ownership and control over planting materials. This sets the stage for the following chapter which deals with attempts to pass a law giving patent rights to "inventors" of certain new plant varieties.

## THE COMMERCIALIZATION OF AMERICAN AGRICULTURE

At the beginning of the nineteenth century, the main regions of the United States were each agriculturally self-sufficient.[4] At the household level, farm families were also largely self-sufficient. They endeavored to produce what was needed, but were not averse to selling any surplus.[5] Only a quarter of farm production in rural northern communities — the most developed region — was sold as late as 1820. Even per capita production of home-produced textiles kept rising until 1825. In Henretta's words, this was the "heyday of domestic manufacture."[6] Merrill goes further and speaks of a "household mode of production."[7] The breakdown of this self-sufficiency, according to Henretta, awaited the growth of nonagricultural populations and the creation of markets.

Rapid growth of cities and of markets was indeed under way. "The growth of manufacturing and related urbanization in the New England and Middle Atlantic states substantially increased the demand for western staples," according to Douglas North. Rapid development of western states "reflected primarily this expansion in demand for food stuffs."[8]

Transportation posed problems for farmers. An overnight trip —12 to 15 miles — was as far away as a farmer could be from a market and still maintain regular contacts. Milk could only be hauled four or five miles on a daily basis.[9] Nevertheless, farmers living near population centers in the Northeast found increasing opportunities to engage in commerce. Not only were there opportunities, but there were also pressures in the form of rising land values and prices in rural areas near cities.[10] For the first time, farmers in significant numbers began to specialize and seek the marketplace for much of their production. Repeal of the Corn Laws in England in 1846 added a bigger export market to the growing domestic market and further "stimulated specialization in wheat farming."[11] American agriculture was in a period of great growth and transition. A subsistence agriculture was being commercialized and farmers were specializing more and more.

In the cities, booksellers and hardware and general merchandisers began selling imported or farmer-bought seed to an urban clientele in the eighteenth century. Sometime prior to 1825, seedsmen in Connecticut, New Jersey, New Hampshire and Pennsylvania started seed farms for the sole purpose of raising seed to sell.[12] As noted, the religious group called the Shakers also produced seed for sale. These developments are more important now to seed industry history than they were at the time to the relationship between farmer and seed. In the first quarter of the century, probably no more than six or eight seed merchandisers were raising their own seed for sale. Farmers were largely untouched by this development and were still self-sufficient in seeds. (Early exceptions to this statement might have occurred with seed of some vegetables for commercial farmers near cities, but there is no firm evidence which would prove farmer reliance on purchased seed.) Understandably, urban gardeners were more dependent on purchased seed.

We know that commercialized agriculture gained its first foothold in the Northeast. In many other areas farmers had to wait for the development of markets and marketing infrastructure and especially for better transportation to be created. Westward expansion and the building of railroads played a large part in this.

As noted earlier, the U.S. incorporated a large area — over two million square miles of territory in the first half of the century. Westward expansion was underway and with it the railroads. From a modest beginning of 40 miles of track in 1830, American railroads were laying thousands of miles of track on average each year from 1848 through 1917 (with the exception of the Civil War years).[13]

In the early stages of railroad development, the U.S. government gave large grants of land to new railroad companies. The companies, in turn, promoted settlement and development by selling directly (or indirectly through land companies and speculators) to farmers. In 1856 the Illinois Central Railroad had 700 miles of line, but few paying customers. It had received two and one-half million acres of land from the government and was busily selling it to raise capital. The directors of the railroad saw it as in their interests to promote agriculture — commercial agriculture, which would produce commodities for shipment to cities, and would require supplies and equipment for shipment to rural areas. The railroad actively supported the Illinois State Agricultural Society and its fair. To encourage mechanization it offered a $3000 prize for the invention of a successful steam-driven plow. Additional cash prizes were offered for the invention of corn cutters, stackers and a ditching machine.[14]

The Illinois Central (IC) line soon ran from Chicago to New Orleans. In 1850, Chicago was a town of only 30,000 people, but it stood at the center of western agriculture and was strategically situated as a processing and onward-shipping site; New Orleans was the gateway to foreign exports. The first railroad to operate in Chicago (the Galena and Chicago Union) was founded in 1848 by the city's first mayor, a business partner and financier of Cyrus McCormick. McCormick, who invented the mechanical reaper in 1831, began building his manufacturing operation in Chicago the year the railroad arrived.[15] He established a steam-operated plant and pioneered in modern sales and organizational methods including the institution of a spare-parts department.[16] The Chicago Board of Trade was also founded in 1848 to accommodate futures trading in grain.

The IC's fortunes were linked with the development of commercial agriculture and with the position of Chicago (and to a lesser extent, New Orleans) in that trade. Between 1857 and 1900, IC shipments of grains and grain products rose from 126,270 tons to 3,217,202 tons. During the same period the IC increased its hauling of fruits and vegetables from 6,000 tons to 372,031 tons, a clear reflection of the steady growth in commercial agriculture.[17] The IC began shipping strawberries in refrigerated cars from southern Illinois to Chicago in 1867. Its 25-car "Thunderbolt" was described as the "first all-strawberry train in the nation" in 1892. Eight years later, the IC had 1,101 fruit cars and 730 refrigerator cars. A total of 60,000 refrigerated railway cars were operating in North America by 1901 and it is estimated that such cars handled 95 percent of California's deciduous fresh fruit production (the first successful shipment from California had been made in 1869). Furthermore, 600 establishments with a combined 50,000,000 cubic feet of refrigerated space were now storing fruits and produce for the market.[18]

While typical of the region's railroads, the IC still only managed to be the fourth or fifth biggest railroad in terms of grain shipments to Chicago during the period.[19] Indicative of the growth of the period, Illinois population almost quadrupled between 1850 and 1880. Iowa population rose more than eightfold.[20] Along the Atchison, Topeka and Santa Fe Railway route, farms increased from 6,000 to 21,500 between 1870 and 1880.[21]

Other railroads followed suit, promoting agriculture — and their own expansion — even more enthusiastically. The Burlington and Rock Island railroads began "agricultural colleges on wheels" in 1904. These educational trains soon became quite common. In 1905 there were trains in 21 states and by 1911 there were 62 educational trains operating.[22] The Burlington line had a "Seed and Soil Special" in Missouri in 1905. The train would pull into small communities and offer lectures and demonstrations extolling modern, standardized, commercial agriculture. At every stop:

> speakers emphasized the necessity of using seed corn having grains of equal size and shape in order that the (mechanical) planter might drop them evenly and thereby produce a proper distribution of grain on the ground; they also urged farmers to select carefully the ears to be used for seed, taking care to examine the quality of the stalk as well as the ear itself, and to test the germinating power of the seed before planting.[23]

Crowds were said to be "immense."

The Frisco, Burlington, and Wabash railroads sold seed corn and cowpeas when their "Seed and Soil Specials" called on farming communities. Others distributed alfalfa to encourage cattle raising. The Frisco and Burlington, as well as many other trains, also promoted improved breeds of livestock. The Frisco train carried "Missouri Chief Josephine," the world record milk-producing cow. It was claimed that she could draw bigger crowds than the president.[24] The Burlington railroad even offered to swap a pure breed bull or boar for a non-pure breed in a number of towns in Colorado one year.[25]

Formal lectures were reinforced with entertainment. The railroads offered free food, music, and contests, and often reduced shipping rates for farmers producing for the urban market. Some towns held mock trials convicting farmers of owning "scrub" bulls. In Nebraska, farmers prepared the following pedigree for such a bull:

> This official document is intended to serve in a dual capacity, first as a bill of sale and a conveyance in fee simple, and also a pedigree to one red, white-faced semi full-blooded Hereford scrub bull, with an age of about three summers and as many winters but with a size and dimensions of a ten months' old dogie, whose mother died of starvation while he was yet an infant and whose unfaithful inbred father unceremoniously ran away with a nice young three-year old heifer.
>
> We warrant this bull to be an inbred calf.
> His style and form will make you laugh.
> He will take no prize at a livestock show,

But will eat and drink, and maybe grow.
He was born by chance in a suspicious way;
His mother died, his dad ran away.
He's lousy as hell and somewhat thin,
But a damn good bull for the shape he's in.[26]

The trains thus functioned as an extension service, distributing improved stock and crop varieties, and helping to create a popular culture supporting "scientific" agriculture. They declined in importance only when government services — the extension service, agricultural experiment stations, and agricultural colleges — began to be effective (and in the face of financial crises for many railroads).

The government postal system made use of new railroad lines to improve and expand its service. It was using 2,300 miles of line — 82 percent of the total — in 1840.[27] Twenty-four years later, the Post Office had increased its use almost tenfold in terms of mileage.[28] Now tens of millions of letters were being carried yearly.

The postal service not only delivered the government's "free seed," it also "brought the seedsman to every door."[29] Commercial firms of the day now began selling their seeds by catalog through the mail. The rise of the mail order seed business provided the setting for an early attack on the USDA's free seed program in 1859. It was voiced by the Commissioner of Patents (who because of the past importance of the program had become a political appointee). He said the government had no business distributing seeds because farmers could "obtain everything . . . from the seed-stores."[30] Congress emphatically rejected this idea, initiating a sixty-year battle on the part of seed firms to eliminate government competition.

After the Civil War, color illustrations began appearing in seed catalogs. Business boomed. The mail-order business was still directed toward an urban market, but increasingly it reached into rural areas to supply farmers with vegetable and flower seed. Even Sears, one of the country's pioneering mail-order houses, established a seed division. Such sales leaped. Whereas in the 1870s a firm receiving a hundred letters a day during the season would have been considered large, by the end of the 1890s some firms were receiving 6,000 letters a day.[31]

The seed companies themselves were becoming more specialized and more focused on the business of producing and selling seed. The Civil War encouraged domestic vegetable seed production (by cutting off European imports) and laid to rest the apparently widespread notion that most vegetable seeds produced in America were inherently inferior to imported seeds. Shortly after the war some 2000 acres were devoted to the commercial production of vegetable seeds. Over the course of the next 11 years, 5000 acres were added. However, the 1890 Census shows 96,500 acres devoted to commercial seed production with 596 firms involved. The acreage figures are conservative because they exclude company contracts with farmers for producing seed. One firm had 13,000 acres under contract for vegetable seed in 1892.[32]

The institutional structure for a more scientifically based commercial agriculture was also being created. Congress had helped establish a number of agricultural colleges through land grants in the 1860s and broadened the system with grants for experiment stations in the late 1880s, and a strengthening of federal in-house research. Graduate enrollments in agricultural sciences, which had stood at less than two dozen in the entire country at the turn of the twentieth century, shot up to nearly 400 just 15 years later.[33] The 1914 Smith-Lever Act put federally sponsored extension activities on a firm footing as a way of disseminating scientific research to the farmers. The act allowed for both public and private support of extension activities. The American Farm Bureau Federation (the first chapter of which was started by the Chamber of Commerce) was founded originally as a way of supporting these extension activities which some business people thought would bring farmers increasingly into the marketplace. A Sears & Roebuck Company executive (Sears had a large mail-order business with significant rural interests) offered $1000 to each of the first 100 counties that employed extension agents. Railroad and banking figures also enthusiastically supported the service. Harry Cleaver documents the influential role of Dr. Seaman Knapp in the development of the extension service and in so doing connects that service solidly with business interests. Knapp was a former president of Iowa State Agricultural College and served on the Rockefeller Foundation's General Education Board. He helped shape both the extension service's approach and its financing, orchestrating funding from industry including the railroads and farm input and machinery companies like International Harvester, in which the Rockefeller family had a financial stake.[34] (It is notable that a number of professional societies were founded in the late 1800s which supported education, professionalism, and scientific agriculture. Proposals such as the Hatch Act establishing experiment stations received the support of such groups.[35])

Agricultural fairs also helped nudge farmers toward commercial agriculture. Supported by the Patent Office, agricultural societies were formed across the country.[36] After the Civil War the number of agricultural fairs exploded. In 1868 there were 1,367 agricultural societies sponsoring fairs. By 1913 the number had doubled.[37] According to Wayne Neely, a sociologist who studied the fairs, they were intended to promote "modernization."[38] Competitive displays were an essential element of the fair and were intended to interpret standards to the farmer — they helped educate the farmer as to the ideal in a given crop. "Here," according to Neely,

> the farmer is aided immensely by the direct visual demonstration of the standards which the market more or less compels him to meet. New measuring sticks are set up from time to time in response to changing factors; the fair is often the quickest and most effective avenue by which the farmer may be reached.[39]

In the Midwest, fairs gave premiums for new crops. "The experimentation thus fostered by the fairs made of them essentially a sort of popular testing ground for the trial of many kinds of products, in the hope of determining those most suitable for adoption in their respective communities," said Neely.[40]

Like education trains, agricultural fairs helped educate farmers and build a popular culture around commercialized agriculture. Farmers did not make the transition to commercial-oriented agriculture purely because of the push or pull of economic factors. Social factors were involved as well. At the fairs, for example, farmers coming home with blue ribbons for their corn and cattle gained bragging rights and social prestige. The certificate my great great grandmother won for having the best butter at the first Madison County (Tennessee) Fair in 1871 still hangs in the dining room of my parents' home, for example. Such nonmonetary rewards in competitive small farm society induced "locality-wide rather than merely single farm advances in plant and animal breeding."[41]

Farmers were under social pressures to "better themselves," but of course there were socially acceptable ways of doing this and sanctions for transgressors. In the early part of the nineteenth century, a farmer was expected first to supply his family with the necessities of life. In practice this meant producing them on the farm with as little dependence on the commercial world as possible. Needed goods and services were often bartered for rather than purchased. These "rules" came into conflict with the farmer-as-entrepreneur, with the farmer as one who specializes, maximizes profit, serves the marketplace. However, self-improvement was defined as including the accumulation of land, which promoted commercial agriculture and thus indirectly put pressure on the other rules.[42] Surplus originally was a secondary objective to the largely self-reliant farm. This objective and the concept of surplus changed as farms became more commercial.[43]

By the late 1800s farming had become a business for most. Farmers had either become entrepreneurs or they had gotten out of farming. The *Minnesota Farmer* in 1879 noted that the days when the farmer had limited contact with the outside world were over. "All this is changed now . . . The farmer has become a purchaser — buys all that he wears, buys much that he eats, buys oftentimes his fuel and lights. To meet these demands, he has occasion to study the markets, to find out what people want in exchange for the things he must produce."[44] Adam Rome observes that "farmers knew that the secure yeoman had disappeared with home-spun. They understood that they were now at the mercy of monsoons in India, droughts in Australia, wars in Russia and Turkey, strikes in England, and bread riots in Spain."[45]

News like this affecting agriculture was brought to them by a fast-growing farm press. The farm press promoted commercial agriculture and benefited from it as subsistence farming was replaced by farming oriented to expanding domestic and international markets.[46] In 1877 there were 108 farm papers. During the next fifteen years a new paper was founded every month on average. By the turn of the century, circulation was well over 4,000,000,[47] an impressive figure given the fact that there were but 5,740,000 farms in the country.

Machinery development flourished in the nineteenth century and by the time of the Civil War there were nearly 2000 manufacturing enterprises turning out various farm machines and implements.[48] Scarcely fifteen years after the war, farmers were purchasing nearly 80,000 seeders a year.[49] These and other implements the farmer could see at the local fair.

Various mechanical harvesters reduced the need for hand harvesting. In the grain fields such machines replaced people with scythes and grain cradles.[50] In the process, unique and productive plants — those that here-tofore would have been selected to donate seed — were more likely to go unnoticed. Potential genetic improvements were thus forfeited. Further-more, farmers with large acreage would be disinclined to practice selection or breeding by the old methods. Large acreages required large amounts of seed. For farmer selection to have an impact on next year's crop, a great deal of the seed to be used would have to be identified the old-fashioned way and saved. Surely many farmers began to question whether such a time-consuming practice was worth the effort — particularly when seed could be purchased from other farmers or commercial firms if yields began to fall below acceptable levels.[51]

Seed cleaning machines of increasing efficiency meant that farmers who purchased seed from reputable dealers could get seed free of weed seeds at a fraction of the cost of hand-cleaning. By 1898, engine-powered cleaners could clean 600 bushels of Kentucky blue-grass seed a day, contrasted to 15 to 20 bushels for a person working by hand.[52]

The Patent Office offered patents to secure the marketing foothold of John Deere, McCormick and Wood machines and devoted its annual reports almost exclusively to the topic of increasing agricultural productivity. While concentration in the farm machinery industry cut the number of firms in half by the end of the century, capital investment in the industry rose dramatically with the growing mechanization of the American farm.[53]

To make full use of the machinery and in an attempt to realize as much value in the form of added production from the machinery as possible, farmers purchased more land and brought more land into production. More credit required more cash income and more production to repay the debts. And more production led to lower prices and the beginning of the all-too-familiar boom and bust cycles of American agriculture. Anna Rochester described the situation thusly:

> the market drives the individual farmer to raise the productivity of his labour, by improving his technique. This in turn pushes him to enlarge his scale of operation. Technical change and employment of wage labour react each upon the other and draw the successful farmer nearer and nearer to a completely capitalist form of operation. Both imply increased investment in the process of production.[54]

Tenancy increased in rural America, as did indebtedness. Most farmers expanding their operations were unable to finance this from their own operations and thus had to depend on capital borrowed from nonfarm sources, according to Rochester.[55] Nine million mortgages were outstanding in the 1890s. Half of the farms in Iowa and New Jersey ("The Garden State") were in debt.[56] And mortgages exceeded families in Minnesota, the Dakotas, Kansas, and Nebraska.[57] Many farms held multiple mortgages and were in debt for all they were worth. Loan agents by the hundreds, who worked on commission for private individuals in the East and risked none of their own money, pushed easy credit to the farmers. Some 200 corporations were engaged in the mortgage business in Kansas and Nebraska[58] and agents found that offers of capital from the East exceeded their ability to find borrowers.[59] Land speculation fueled this frenzy and made high mortgage interest tolerable, which only served to increase the amount available. Increases in western land values of hundreds of percent were recorded between 1881 and 1887.[60]

As the nineteenth century came to a close, farm exports had become important as a way of dealing with farm surpluses and a bad national balance of payments problem (a combination which would be repeated in the 1970s with similar results). Faced with low incomes, farmers could choose to fight against the growing power of the monopolies and their abuses (amply documented in popular books by Upton Sinclair and Frank Norris at the turn of the century) or promote agricultural exports. Farm publications chose a hawkish route advocating military protection of markets — even in relation to the British.[61] And the United States did in fact use its power, in Hawaii, Cuba, and the Philippines, to cite but three examples where markets and/or agricultural products and production were significant factors.

Noncommercial and subsistence agriculture had all but died by the turn of the century. Both farms and regions were specialized and cemented into the market economy. Largely self-sufficient at the beginning of the century, the New England states produced only 36 percent of their wheat, 45 percent of their corn, 33 percent of their beef and 27 percent of their pork requirements in 1890. In contrast, the North Central states produced enough wheat to feed four times the population of the region.[62] Seed-saving was still practiced, but by fewer and fewer. (Notable exceptions were grains which were more likely to be saved by farmers because a large quantity of seed was needed and no particular processing was required — one only had to lay aside a portion of the regular harvest. However, significant selection of grains probably decreased with increasing acreage per farm. Farmers continued to save seed, but the lack of improvement in varieties[63] meant that commercial and scientifically bred varieties would ultimately surpass farmer varieties in quality and yield.)

Government free seed had, since 1896, been of a different character. More and more it was seed of standard varieties meant for political patronage, not experimentation.[64] Increasingly this practice was attacked as wasteful spending but, significantly, there seemed to be little protest from farmers claiming that the free seed was still important for purposes of experimentation and adaptation.

The increasing importance of purchased seed can be seen in the development of commercial companies before the turn of the century. For example, D. M. Ferry & Co. (later Ferry-Morse) built a six-story, 300 by 120 foot warehouse in 1887 and another eight-story, 85 by 140 foot warehouse in 1891.[65] Peter Henderson & Co., in its 162-page 1896 catalog, boasted of warehouse capacity in Jersey City of 250,000 bushels constructed in 1888 and 1894.[66]

Farmers involved in commercial agriculture were less and less likely to have the time or economic incentive to breed varieties and (perhaps less so) multiply large quantities of seed. Commercial, market-oriented agriculture encouraged specialization and dependence on the market.

**Table 4.** Home-Grown Seeds as a Percentage of Total Requirement, U.S., by Region, 1918–19.[68]

| Crop | Eastern | Southern | Central | Northern | Far West |
|------|---------|----------|---------|----------|----------|
| Grasses | 5 | 6 | 23 | 69 | 4 |
| Clovers and alfalfa | 6 | 11 | 30 | 18 | 12 |
| Millets | 3 | 12 | 20 | 13 | 7 |
| Forage sorghums | 1 | 36 | 25 | 5 | 16 |
| Small grains | 44 | 45 | 76 | 78 | 59 |

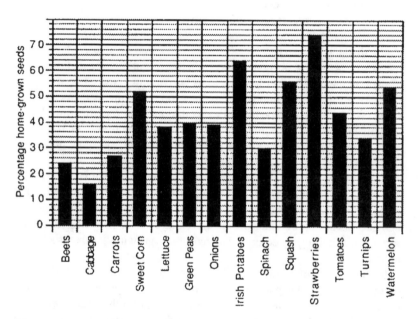

**Figure 1.** Home-Grown Seeds and Plant Materials of Truck Crops as percentage of Total Requirement, U.S. 1918.[69]

Significantly, many (but not all) farmers had already ceased saving their own seeds before scientifically bred plant varieties were widely available.[67] The data available on the number of seed firms and acreage devoted to producing seeds for the commercial market appears to confirm this. Further confirmation is found in data from the USDA's short-lived publication, the *Seed Reporter*, and from a USDA Farmer's Bulletin, as presented in table 4 and figure 1 on previous page. Each draws on a survey from 1918–19.

This data indicates that the transition from farmer seed-saving to dependence on commercial sources was well under way by 1918, though by no means complete. Variations in the percentage of home-grown versus purchased seed are explainable in terms of the difficulty of producing good seed of a crop in a certain region, the difficulty of producing and processing seed of a particular crop (irrespective of the region), and the availability of commercial supplies. (Strawberries and potatoes are rather easy to divide and propagate, for example, whereas carrots require much more care and effort to obtain seeds — one reason for the lower percentage of home-grown seeds.)

The median percentage of home-grown seeds of all truck crops surveyed by the USDA was 40 percent. This substantiates *Seed World's* claim that the industry sells 60% of the garden seed used.[70] For two reasons however, these figures may underrepresent the size and influence of the commercial market in relation to farmer and gardener seed-saving. First, World War I prompted an average 60% rise in seed prices[71] and some crop-specific shortages, thus encouraging home production.[72] Second, many farmers or gardeners may have been intermittent buyers of seeds — buying one year out of three, for example, and thus not really self-reliant in seeds or seed stocks.

Commercial agriculture was gaining in importance. Between 1918–21 and 1932–36, acreage devoted to 15 major vegetable crops for the market rose 80 percent. Per acre labor requirements however, fell by seven percent. Labor requirements dropped even more —19 percent — on those farms most thoroughly commercialized (those growing for the processing industry.)[73]

In the context of a commercializing agriculture where production was oriented towards the marketplace and where low prices are common, there are a number of reasons for farmers giving up their seed saving. A 1921 USDA publication lists them as seen from the farmer's perspective:

> The question has often been asked: 'Why is it that every farmer does not raise and plant his own seeds and thereby save for himself the profit others usually derive in selling him seeds?' Briefly, some of the reasons are as follows: (1) His fields may be foul with noxious weeds; (2) soil, climatic, and other conditions on his farm may be unfavorable for seed production in a given year; (3) altitude, latitude, or rainfall in his locality may preclude the production of a particular kind of seed in any year; (4) he may be able to buy better seeds at a lower cost than can be produced in his locality; (5) he may find it more profitable to grow a crop for hay or forage purposes than for seed production; (6) he may not have the facilities for harvesting,

cleaning, curing, or otherwise preparing his seed for planting purposes; (7) he may need seed of a crop that has not been grown by him for several years, if ever at all; and (8) he may have to replant his fields either with the same kind of seed, his supply of which may have been exhausted with the first planting, or with seed of some catch crop.[74]

New relationships between farmer and seed were clearly becoming visible. Farmers were responsible for having bred virtually all of the varieties in use. These varieties were now beginning to form the basis of commercial ventures. (Public breeding programs did not become important until the twentieth century. In 1898 only three government agricultural experiment stations were listed as being involved in plant breeding.[75])

Fairs and other social agents were promoting a certain standardization (further discussed in the next section) which was not easily met by individual farmers breeding and multiplying seed on their own. The demand for purchased seed was increasing in rural and urban areas. Flower gardening was becoming increasingly popular (the first organized flower show had taken place in Boston in 1829).[76] Even tenants and sharecroppers were encouraged by farm publications to "beautify" their homesteads with flower gardens.[77] By 1919 over 300 companies were specializing in mail-order seeds and mailing out "at least 35,000,000 catalogs annually."[78] Despite the fact that very few scientifically bred vegetable varieties were on the market, the commercial trade now accounts for 60% of all vegetable seed used and claimed it was "now prepared to furnish all the seed supplies needed . . ."[79]

World War I provided some relief for farmers, if war can be called relief. Production increased substantially and for a moment prices rose. In the war's aftermath, however, prices again tumbled and America's overseas allies were in no position to purchase American farm exports. The Depression which was to hit the rest of the country a decade later had already begun in rural America. Many farmers had gone into debt during the war, buying more machinery and land to meet a growing demand in a good market. Now the bills were coming due in a bad market. The answer once again — the only answer an individual farmer could give — was to try to increase production.

Tractors were promoted as a way to do just that. Their numbers increased from 10,000 in 1910 to 1,600,000 in 1939. This decreased the number of horses by half and freed another 50 million acres (no longer needed to raise food for the horses) for commercial production. Not surprisingly, during this same period the only farm category showing a significant increase in numbers was the large farm (over 1000 acres) category, which went from 19 to 29 percent of the total.[80] This increase in large farms necessarily increased the demand for commercial seed as small, self-provisioning farms — farms on which seed saving might have been practical — were replaced or marginalized by large farms where seed-saving would have been a costly and time-consuming nuisance.

As usual, low commodity prices and debt underpinned the need for farmers to produce more, thus solidifying the transformation. The ratio of debt to total farm value rose during this period from 27.3 to 50.2 percent.[81] Foreclosures further consolidated American farmland, widening the gulf between the largest four percent of farms which accounted for a quarter of all production in 1929 and the smallest half, which accounted for 16 percent of production.[82] Likewise, mechanization meant more intensive cultivation of more acres, and this too increased the demand for purchased seed. Thus, as demand increased, potential competition was reduced. There were fewer and fewer farmers wanting or needing access to breeding material.

## SCIENTIFIC PLANT BREEDING

Developments in the understanding of plant reproduction were now rather quickly creating a basis upon which simple mass selection could be superseded by more modern techniques. The genetic material itself was already present.

Sex in plants had long ago been discussed by botanists such as Camerarius and Linné. Camerarius, for example, distinguished male and female reproductive organs in plants as early as 1665. It was not until the beginning of the twentieth century that Darwin's theory of evolution could be combined with Gregor (Johann) Mendel's work on the inheritance of characteristics to form the basis for modern, scientific plant breeding. Working independently, Hugo de Vries in the Netherlands, Karl Correns in Germany and Erich Tschermak von Seysenegg in Austria worked out Mendel's laws. Upon searching the literature for prior discoveries of their work, each found Mendel's material published by Mendel's local natural history society, and each gave credit where credit was due.

Mendel was trained in physics, had a solid mathematical foundation and was demonstrably patient and meticulous by nature. At the time Mendel began his experiments, there was no clear understanding of the inheritance of characteristics. Generally it was believed that offspring represented a "blending" of the parents.

Mendel formulated an elegant and effective experimental design. Utilizing peas, he chose to study the transmission of seven simple and easily identifiable traits, each of which was either dominant or recessive. Seed color was one trait. Mendel worked with varieties which bred true and within the variety always produced either white or gray seeds. In the first generation $(F_1)$ a cross of white and gray seeded varieties yielded only gray seeds. But in the second generation $(F_2)$, Mendel discovered something quite remarkable. The white-coated trait reappeared in a 1:3 ratio. The diagramming of this phenomenon is famous, but still instructive. If "G" designates gray and "w," white, then a gray variety which breeds true becomes "GG" (two G's because it has received the gray characteristic from both parents). A white variety, likewise, is "ww." (Upper and lower cases are used to indicate dominance and recessiveness.)

A crossing of gray and white varieties is therefore:

$$GG \quad X \quad ww$$

This yields four possible combinations:

$$Gw \quad Gw \quad wG \quad wG$$

All will therefore display the gray seed coat trait, because gray is dominant when paired with white. But the white trait has not been lost, as the second generation cross (Gw   X   Gw) reveals:

$$GG \quad Gw \quad wG \quad ww$$

This produces a three to one ratio. Mendel found this ratio repeatedly with all the simply determined traits he studied.

Mendel discovered that repeated crossings did not affect the individual traits: the white seeds were just as white and the gray seeds just as gray as in the beginning. It was also evident in Mendel's experiments that each character was determined independently of the others. Mayr describes the significance of Mendel's discoveries thusly:

> First, all these earlier authors [Darwin, Galton, Weismann and de Vries] postulated the existence of numerous identical determinants for a given unit character in each cell (each nucleus) and speculated, likewise, that many replicas of a single determinant might be transmitted simultaneously to the germ cells. If this were the case, no consistent ratios would be found in crosses. This assumption made the development of a clear-cut genetic theory almost impossible . . . This was Mendel's greatest contribution. Mendel's other significant contribution was the discovery that these particles exist in sets — genes and their alleles, we would now say. Through this assumption it was possible to explain segregation and recombination. His inference that each character is represented in a fertilized egg cell by two, but only two, factors, one derived from the father and the other from the mother, and that these could be different, was the new idea which revolutionized genetics.[83]

Mendel's theories were seemingly neither accepted nor understood when they were published in 1866. Mendel himself doubted that his findings would hold for all species and reserved judgment pending the results of future experiments with other species. Though his paper was cited about a dozen times before 1900,[84] the importance of his work was not realized until it was "rediscovered" by the several scientists mentioned above in 1900. Mendel's experiments confirmed their own. Nevertheless, broader acceptance was not immediate. Scientists debated whether Mendel's theories applied to all species and whether Mendel's explanation — even if correct — was an explanation of one of several or many mechanisms of inheritance. The first decade of the 1900s was, according to Mayr, "preoccupied with evolutionary controversies and with doubts as to the universal validity of Mendelian inheritance."[85]

Historians say that Mendel was rediscovered and confirmed by the three scientists mentioned above. But W. J. Spillman, a wheat breeder at the Washington State Experiment Station, was close on their heels. Spillman's work confirmed that predictable recombinations of parental traits could be found in wheat crosses. Others followed. While "Mendelian genetics" was not immediately accepted (or developed) and was not immediately put to practical use in a crop breeding program, the development of Mendelism was nevertheless rapid and was fueled, Kimmelman asserts, by very practical concerns.[86] A history of Mendelism (beyond the scope of this book) would surely illustrate the social construction of this scientific theory. There is a strong social context to the development and use of Mendelian genetics as we shall see most strikingly in relation to the corn seed business. It is not the case that the "rediscovery" changed dominant ways of thinking, much less "breeding" practices, overnight.[87]

"Natural philosophers" were quickly becoming "scientists," a term suggested by William Whewell to the British Association for the Advancement of Science in Cambridge in 1883. By 1902, the scientists were to have a new name for their new science — "genetics" — coined by William Bateson at the Second International Conference on Plant Breeding and Hybridization in New York in 1906.

Combining Darwin's and Mendel's insights with those of others, selection was meshed with crossing, then called hybridization. For example, a useful variety lacking disease resistance would be crossed with an introduced variety (perhaps unsuitable in many ways except for its disease resistance). The offspring of that crossing displaying resistance would then be "backcrossed" to the original useful variety. Progeny would again be selected for disease resistance. Again these would be backcrossed with the original variety. Eventually, it was learned, one could arrive at the original variety with the added feature of disease resistance, but without any of the deleterious qualities of the other variety. Using such methods, plant breeders could guide and direct evolution! They could look for and incorporate specific traits rather than be content with simply selecting and adapting imported material and accepting what chance and a good eye gave them.

As described above, it may seem as if the rediscovery of Mendel's laws swept away backwardness, ignorance, and superstition and transformed plant breeding overnight. No such thing happened. Mendelism gradually and with some difficulty replaced existing understandings. In the early 1900s, it was not at all clear how this "Mendelism" could be applied. Basic information, in fact, was still missing. At the first meeting of the (Mendelian-inspired) American Breeders Association (the first national membership organization to promote genetics) in 1905, the organizer, Assistant Secretary of Agriculture Willet Hays, lamented that "we do not even well know the pollinating habits of common grains."[88] (At the same conference, Hays revealingly described crop varieties as "vital, changeful, moody things."[89])

The challenge of putting the insights of Mendel into practical use was most impressively taken up by corn breeders. Then as now, wide adaptability and multiple uses helped make corn the most valuable crop in the United States.[90] The work with corn in turn provided an "impetus" and a "key . . . to all scientific breeding."[91]

Early settlers had transformed Indian corn and in the process created some very impressive varieties ("Reid," "Krug," etc.). But for the most part, farmers were still concentrating on the appearance of the ear and were largely ignoring the potential for selection based on both parents. William Beal of the Michigan Agricultural College criticized this practice and recommended that farmers at least detassel plants with bad characteristics to prevent their pollen from fertilizing others. In 1876 he advocated a form of controlled breeding with farmers planting two different strains in alternating rows and detasseling one. This resulted in one row being fertilized by the other and one row being self-fertilized. This was a major step toward a more rational, controlled approach to breeding. Using this method, farmers could repeat their breeding and attempt to "fix" valuable traits. Results were at least somewhat predictable, a potential advantage to commercial firms wanting to establish defined varieties.[92]

Beal's work was important in another regard. While farmers could obtain and use information like this to enhance their own selection techniques, increasingly this information would now come from a new professional elite with more and more skills and knowledge. Following

Beal, Cyril Hopkins of the Illinois Experiment Station advocated use of
the "ear-to-row" method wherein seeds from one ear were all planted in
the same row. This allowed for a comparison of the performance of the
ears. The dean of the Illinois College of Agriculture was prompted to
suggest that corn now be specifically bred and designed for livestock
needs — a portent to a more rationalistic vision which would emerge as
breeding techniques were developed. The Beal and Hopkins methods both
involved variety crossings. Minus Mendelian genetics, neither could go
further and gain insights into which varieties should be crossed or how to
concentrate desired characteristics. Nevertheless, these methods continued to be practiced to some degree into the 1920s.[93]

The next major step was taken by E. M. East at the Connecticut
Experiment Station. East combined the ear-to-row method with varietal
crossing allowing for both repeatable pedigrees and the concentrating of
desired characteristics. East understood from Mendel that inbred lines
would further concentrate characteristics, but it was George Shull at the
Carnegie-backed Station for Experimental Evolution at Cold Spring
Harbor, Long Island, who began crossing inbreds.[94]

On the surface — and certainly to the average farmer — working with
inbreds must have appeared ridiculous. Their yield was substantially
lower than farmer-selected varieties. To the untrained eye, they were
simply inferior. Yet, Shull was on the right track and his experiments
crossing inbred lines revealed hybrid vigor (observed by Darwin in 1871)
and led to further experiments. East resisted the notion of crossing inbreds
and continued to work with varietal crossings. But neither East's varietal
crossings nor Shull's single crosses of inbreds had lived up to early
expectations. Henry Wallace (editor of an influential farm journal, future
founder of the world's largest hybrid seed corn company, son of the
Secretary of Agriculture and future Secretary himself) had given up on
varietal crossings. In the pages of *Wallace's Farmer*, he observed that
"most of our best varieties of corn are the result, not of crossing, but of
selecting . . . "[95] In 1918, in an article directed at boys on the farm, he
offered instruction of how to do varietal crossing using the ear-to-row
method. "Anybody can cross corn," he noted. But he observed that well-
bred corn is better looking but not necessarily better yielding than "scrub"
corn. "Some day someone will learn how to breed corn, but at present we
are very much in the dark. There are many interesting methods of
breeding which can be used, but none absolutely guaranteed to give
results," he lamented.[96] An advertisement placed by Northrup-King Seed
Company in the same issue of the journal began with the statement, "Like
produces Like" — not a slogan for an innovative breeding program

involving inbreds. Eighteen years after the rediscovery of Mendel's laws, breeders were still unable to make full use of them. Indeed Northrup-King's orientation seems in retrospect to have been mired in the past.

Support and vindication for Shull's direction came through the work of Donald Jones (a former student of East's), chief geneticist at the Connecticut station. Jones began double-crossing inbreds using four inbred lines. The technique allowed for greater and more precise manipulation of characters than variety crosses, for example. Hybrid vigor was obtained. And, as Kloppenburg points out, "The crucial difference is that the seed to be used for farm planting is borne on one of the more productive single-cross parents rather than on the weak inbred grandparent, and seed yields per acre are therefore sufficiently large to make the double cross cost-competitive."[97]

As double-cross hybrids required the maintenance of four inbred lines for each double-cross, it was fairly evident that farmers would not play the same role in developing new varieties as in the past.[98] According to Fitzgerald, "Wallace felt that farmers could make a real contribution to the hybrid cause by acting, again, as a corps of independent discoverers of those superior lines," to be used in hybrid breeding.[99] Wallace was now seeing farmers in a new role, as suppliers of *raw materials* to the professional breeder, a dramatic shift in farmers' historic relationship with seed.

The commercial implications of the research were not lost on Jones, who also clearly saw the possibilities of forging a new relationship with farmers — one in which commercial breeders would acquire both physical and legal control over the new seeds:

> The first impression probably gained from the outline of this method of crossing corn is that it is a rather complex proposition. It is somewhat involved, but it is more simple than it seems at first sight. It is not a method that will interest most farmers, but it is something that may easily be taken up by seedsmen; in fact, it is the first time in agricultural history that a seedsman is enabled to gain the full benefit from a desirable origination of his own or something that he has purchased. The man who originates devices to open our boxes of shoe polish or to autograph our camera negatives, is able to patent his product and gain the full reward for his inventiveness. The man who originates a new plant which may be of incalculable benefit to the whole country gets nothing — not even fame — for his pains, as the plants can be propagated by anyone. There is correspondingly less incentive for the production of improved types. The utilization of first generation hybrids enables the originator to keep the parental types and give out only the crossed seeds, which are less valuable for continued propagation.[100]

Jones understood that his double-cross method was effective in producing high-yielding corn. He understood that it was complicated enough that farmers would not try it, but easy enough for professionals to manage it. He realized that the breeder would maintain control over the inbred lines thwarting any attempt by farmers or other breeders to duplicate the breeding. In fact, as Jones observed, it would give the breeder "the same commercial right that an inventor receives from a patented article."[101] And finally, he knew that because hybrids did not "breed true," any attempt to save the seeds of the hybrid for planting the next year would fail. Breeders would gain a proprietary product, protected by nature itself. Farmers would be forced to purchase seed yearly. No more seed saving or simple mass selection.

Jones's work was seized upon by the Department of Agriculture. Henry C. Wallace, Secretary of Agriculture, had his son investigate the department's involvement in corn breeding. Soon thereafter, the department's most vocal skeptic of hybrids was dismissed, according to Fitzgerald, and the USDA threw its full weight behind development of hybrids.[102] In so doing, Fitzgerald notes that it was also dismissing traditional farmer participation in breeding programs in favor of control by scientists of all aspects of crop improvement.[103] By 1924, the annual report of the Office of Experiment Stations "did not even discuss selection as a method of crop improvement . . . "[104,105]

The scientific achievements cited above were not enough in and of themselves to make hybrid corn dominant in the field. Though the hybrids were far superior in yield in the proper setting, they were often ill-adapted to local conditions. Emerging companies like Pioneer Hi-Bred (Wallace's company founded in 1926), DeKalb, Pfister, and Funk, together with the USDA and the agricultural colleges still had the task of producing and marketing adapted hybrids before them.

The first commercial hybrid was Funk's "Pure Line Double Cross no. 250," developed in 1922 and introduced in 1928. It was not adopted on a wide scale. (Only .0013 percent of the corn acreage in Illinois — home of Funk — was in hybrids in 1934.[106]) Supplies were still limited, costs were still high. Farmers who bought the hybrids often tried to save their seed for replanting and the resulting crop failures gave hybrids an undeservedly bad name. Furthermore, unscrupulous seed companies and merchants began marketing fake hybrids.

To explain the specific triumph of hybrid corn — from 0.4 percent of corn acreage in 1933 to 90 percent in 1945[107] — one must begin by citing at least the following factors:

1. Judging standards of corn at agricultural fairs mistakenly gave preference to characteristics which had the effect of depressing yields, which remained flat for the first three decades of the twentieth cen-

tury. Thus, for a number of years, leading farmers had been encouraged to pursue counter-productive breeding avenues.[108] By exercising such a steady influence over the direction of farmer selection, the corn shows also "caused the elimination of many hundreds of varieties," according to Wallace and Brown.[109]

2. The USDA's research funds ceased flowing to corn selection and instead reinforced the move toward hybrids. University researchers were fascinated with Mendelian genetics which helped define for them a "methodological and professional niche that had not existed before."[110] Their development of the science and techniques, including useful statistical tools,[111] provided the scientific foundation for the development of the hybrids.

3. Corn acreage under the Agricultural Adjustment Act of the early 1930s was reduced by 20 to 30 percent. Removing land from production created the obvious incentive to increase production on the remaining acreage. Hybrids were grasped by farmers as an easy way to do this.

4. Yield tests at agricultural fairs and other fora "proved" the hybrids to be superior. In addition to higher yields, hybrid corn generally displayed stiffer stalks and a better root system enabling it to withstand winds.[112] Companies worked hard to develop regionally adapted varieties.

5. Agricultural colleges and companies offered promotions to encourage farmers to try the new hybrids. Funk, for example, offered free hybrid seeds to boys entering yield contests and included promotional hybrid seeds with orders of open-pollinated varieties.[113] Companies advertised their hybrids and farm journals were filled with articles extolling the hybrids.

6. Widespread drought in the mid-1930s caused seed shortages. The shortages forced farmers to use all available seed, making hybrids look even more attractive. More importantly perhaps, it showed advantages of the hybrids.

7. Companies developed the capacity to mass produce large quantities of hybrid seed, reducing the price to the point that increased production more than offset the premium price of hybrid seed. The companies' "army of salesmen converted farmers to hybrid seed in a fraction of the time that it could have been done by ordinary college extension methods," according to Wallace.[114]

The social and scientific development of hybrids came at a time when farmers were already abandoning their own seeds and seed-saving prac-

tices. A new climate was being created — one which emphasized experimentation and innovation by the professional as opposed to what was now
seen as random, haphazard improvement by farmers. Plant breeders were
professionals who possessed technical skills beyond the grasp of the
ordinary farmer. The professional tackled specific problems with a scientific method. With these methods the professional could achieve predictability and uniformity. Breeding results were replicable and the professional held the key allowing control over the breeding process. As the
USDA's 1936 *Yearbook of Agriculture* summarized: "Now the breeder
tends rather to formulate an ideal in his mind and actually create something that meets it as nearly as possible by combining the genes from two
or more organisms."[115]

The forward march of commercialism and scientific plant breeding
during this period is evidence of the increasing rationalization of the seed
breeding and production process. (Indeed it is interesting to note that
packing and dairy companies and large cotton, grain, and fruit growers
were the principal backers of the American Breeders' Association and its
journal.[116]) In telling "The Story of Hybrid Corn" in *Wallace's Farmer*,
Wallace gives an exceptionally clear statement linking the development
of hybrid corn to the larger rationalization process in agriculture:

> Hybrid corn brings to agriculture for the first time the industrial tech-
> nique of standardized parts and mass production. It is based on the fact that
> certain characters can be fixed in a corn plant by inbreeding, that once fixed
> they do not change, and that after that the crossing of these inbreds in a
> certain way will always produce the same result."[117]

This rationalization process, I would contend, reveals itself even in the
names which began to be assigned to the new, scientifically bred varieties
and in the ways in which the breeding process itself was publicly portrayed. At the dawn of scientific plant breeding, the leading corn varieties
normally carried either the name of their originator, a place name, or a
descriptive name. The standard varieties in the Corn Belt in the 1890s
were: Reid's Yellow Dent, Leaming, Boone County White, White Mine,
Riley's Favorite, Golden Eagle, and Champion White Pearl.[118]

In 1917 Funk Seed Company was, according to its general manager H.
H. Miller, interested in giving its new strain of Yellow Dent corn an image
which would indicate Funk's commitment to scientific breeding. The
name "Funk's Utility" was rejected. Miller suggested instead that the
variety be given a number as a name "to signify the experimental work
back of it."[119] The breeder provided Miller with the coded number of the
strain — 176-A — a good choice for a name, Miller thought, because
"that A has selling value."[120] Later Funk's first advertised hybrid would be

designated "Pure Line Double Cross no. 250," a far cry from a "Golden Eagle" or a "Riley's Favorite." (Inbred lines and hybrids originating from the USDA and experiment stations carried similar names, such as US44, the hybrid distributed by the USDA to experiment stations in 1935. Pioneer also used numbers as names.[121]) From the 1920s onward, Funk's catalogs described "in detail the procedures used in hybridizing." They were in Fitzgerald's words "testimonials to scientific experimentation and research."[122] This practice probably helped broaden the perceived distance between farmer and breeder. While companies had access to the genetic materials of farmers for their further breeding work, the reverse was not true.[123]

The story of Pfister Seed Company is even more illustrative of the connection between the new scientific breeding and the naming of plant varieties. The company was founded by Lester Pfister of Illinois. Pfister did not have the formal training many of the others had. He left school for good when he was about 13 to farm. But as a farmer he began his own breeding experiments using the ear-to-row method. In 1932 he came out with his first double-cross hybrid —"Pfister's 4857." Pfister supported public disclosure of hybrid pedigrees (though one wonders what good he thought that might do anyone!). In a 1938 advertisement in *Wallace's Farmer*,[124] Pfister published a photograph showing the four-way cross he had made:


Pfister 159   X   Pfister 187            USDA A   X   USDA HY


          "                    X                    "


Pfister Hybrid 360

**Figure 2.** Pfister hybrid pedigree.


During this period from the early 1900s onwards, the federal government also began to channel germplasm acquired abroad to state experiment stations and agricultural colleges. The nature and purposes of plant collecting changed dramatically. Collection activities were centralized in 1901 in the Section of Seed and Plant Introduction headed by the famous plant explorer, David Fairchild. (Fairchild, the son-in-law of Alexander Graham Bell, was sympathetic with commercial breeding interests. In a 1927 article on his own hybrid breeding experiments, he repeatedly bemoaned the lack of patent protection and speculated about the commercial possibilities of patented varieties.[125])

Collectors were sent forth from the Seed and Plant Introduction Office not so much to find new species or varieties for farmer testing, but to search for specific characteristics which could be deliberately used in formal breeding programs. Writing in 1933, Knowles Ryerson observed:

> In other words *plant exploration is to a large extent becoming a search for genes* [my emphasis]. This is well illustrated by several recent expeditions, including those to New Guinea seeking wild types of sugarcane to develop new, disease-resistant varieties for this country; to Russian Turkestan and Persia, Spain and North Africa for strains of alfalfa to be used in breeding varieties resistant to the bacterial wilt which is now taking heavy toll; and to Mexico and South America for wild and cultivated types of tuber-bearing Solanums for use in breeding disease- and cold-resistant varieties for the different potato districts of the country where losses from disease and from frost are at times disastrous.[126]

Less and less of this exotic material ended up in the hands of actual farmers. What may at first seem to have been a rational decision to direct new germplasm to scientists in fact further reinforced the emerging dominance of scientific plant breeding over farmer selecting. Farmers' were deprived of new breeding materials, not because they were forbidden to use the materials, but because the increasing sophistication of plant breeding was leaving farmers behind. The search for specific, useful characteristics also for the first time gave added potential value to biological materials (species and varieties) which in themselves may have had "little or no intrinsic value," to quote Ryerson, who headed the USDA's Bureau of Plant Industry in 1934.[127] However, this "value" was actually at the gene level — a factor which will become increasingly significant as we shall see in later chapters.

Commercial opposition to competition from the government's program reached back into the nineteenth century. The American Seed Trade Association (ASTA), which was established by 34 seed companies in 1883, opposed the program. Within ten years ASTA had found an advocate in Secretary of Agriculture J. Sterling Morton. Morton, a former farm journal editor, thought the government had no business distributing seeds: ". . . its further continuance is an infringement of the rights of citizens engaged in legitimate trade pursuits."[128] Morton said that the existence of government experiment stations negated the need for seed distribution to farmers, which of course was something quite different.[129] His opposition was joined by farm journals, which had taken up the practice of sending out free seeds as a promotional gimmick with paid subscriptions. The press likewise opposed USDA publication of agricultural reports as undue competition. Morton's efforts on behalf of the seed and farm press industries received no fan mail from Congress. Instead, a resolution was passed ordering Morton to continue seed distribution. Meanwhile, the industry labored under the burden of competing with free seed distributed by the government — a distinct impediment to the establishment of seed as a commodity or the seed industry as a political force. Government distribution, in real competition with industry, increasingly concentrated on tried-and-true varieties of vegetables and flowers instead of just rare or experimental types. But the free seed was popular with the public and with Congress, whose members sent the seeds to constituents with their franking privileges.

In its final years, most seeds in the free seed program were of rather common varieties purchased from seed growers and sent out as patronage by congressmen. This, Galloway claimed (not entirely accurately), had been the case since the years 1889–93 when "practically the entire seed appropriation was expended for standard varieties of vegetable and flower seeds."[130] The practice of giving exotic germplasm to farmers had been cut back to 337,442 packages in 1916.[131] As the head of Seed and Plant Introduction at the USDA put it: ". . . our efforts are in a line quite distinct from that of the Congressional seed distribution . . . Importations are accordingly made, in the great majority of cases, in experimental quantities only, for the use of the experiment stations and private parties having special knowledge and experience in the cultivation of particular crops."[132] In other words, the free seed sent as patronage was of common varieties. The rare seed intended for experimentation was now sent to "professional" breeders, mostly at experiment stations and colleges.

As we have seen, there were many factors behind the rise of the commercial seed industry: the increasing commercialization of American agriculture, the development of scientific breeding, and the cut-off of breeding materials to farmers being some of the major ones. In each of these we can see the conscious efforts of actors working to advance their own interests, working to solve problems that confront them (e.g. the railroad's promotion of agriculture, the private sector's embrace of hybrids, company lobbying against the government's free seed program). Ultimately these actions furthered the development of seeds as a commodity.

The seed industry — both through its trade publications and organizations and presumably individual companies — also directly attacked the practice of farmer seed-saving. In an untitled 1917 editorial in the trade journal *Seed World*, the editors ask, "Are the seedsmen of America going to idly watch the growth of a marketing system that enables farmers to trade among themselves or will the trade take some action to secure at least a portion of this business?"[133] *Seed World* cites efforts to encourage home seed production as part of the war effort, but argues that such seed is (with the exception of corn) not really better adapted. It concludes that "the best advice that can be given to home and market gardeners contemplating seed production is — don't."[134] By 1919 articles with titles such as "Discourage Home Seed Saving" and "Beating the Farmer at His Own Game" were becoming more common. *Seed World* acknowledged that "it is only natural that this condition (seed-saving) has existed and will continue to exist until seedsmen are prepared to offer their farmer patrons better qualities and higher grades than he can grow himself." And the journal observes that "farmers do not, as a general rule, regard the general claims made in catalog advertising matter with much seriousness."[135] Nevertheless, *Seed World* constantly urged companies to educate the public as to the "inferiority" of home-saved seeds and to complain to and educate those who advocated seed-saving. "Seed production is an occupation for which the average farmer or gardener is not fitted . . ." is the remarkable conclusion of one 1919 article.[136] Instead, *Seed World* promoted the idea — and companies claimed — that farmers should trust the seed companies because they were *specialists.* "The world has learned or is fast learning that man does one thing best only when he does nothing else . . ." was the line taken by Mel L. Webster Company in a 1919 advertisement.[137]

## DISCUSSION

Nothing, perhaps, is quite as basic to the agricultural endeavor as the seed. The yearly practice of selecting and saving seed linked farmers to hundreds of generations of their ancestors and to the very origins of agriculture itself. Few changes, therefore, could be so profound as the cessation of farmer seed-saving.

In chapter 1 we found millions of American farmers engaged in experimentation and plant breeding (with government-supplied infusions of genetic diversity), supplying their own seeds. As a commodity form, seeds were almost completely undeveloped. Seed could be owned, of course, but there was no way to own or control it *as breeding material.* Access to this quality (to the use of the genes and reproduction of them in certain combinations as a variety) could not be limited legally. It was free to use, free to multiply and sell. There was also little sense of ownership over "varieties." One might own the seed of a variety, but one did not own the variety itself. In a very real sense, farmers owned and controlled their seed.

The object of chapter 2 is to elucidate the context in which the transition was made from farmers as seed savers to farmers as purchasers of seed. In the process, we uncover the roots of the commercial seed industry and we see the very beginnings of political action from this actor.

Urban expansion and industrialization in nineteenth-century America created growing demand and markets for foodstuffs. Westward expansion fueled by immigration opened rich, new lands for settlement and created the potential for surplus agricultural production to enter the marketplace.

The opening of the Erie Canal in 1825 followed closely by the rapid development of railroads (highlighted by completion of rail connections to the West Coast), linked surplus western agricultural production with eastern markets. Government officials were interested in furthering agriculture as a means of generating private and government wealth. Agriculture was also seen as a way to settle the West and thus expand the influence of government and commerce. Government land grants facilitated the penetration of railway lines westward. Acting out of self-interest to develop a market for their services, railroads initiated educational campaigns designed to increase agricultural production. These campaigns emphasized improved breeds of livestock and varieties of crops. During the second half of the nineteenth century the agricultural fair also flourished. Supported by the railroads, other commercial interests, political figures, and indirectly by the government, the fairs also preached modern agriculture. They educated farmers as to the standards of the marketplace and they helped build a culture which valued the requirements of the marketplace. Crop uniformity replaced diversity and increasingly became a measuring stick of quality in rural culture.[138] As commercial agriculture grew, so did the desire of ambitious farmers for information — a need met by a growing and popular farm press. The interests of the press also were those of modernization and commercial agriculture, for this was where it found advertisers and paying subscribers.

The state was important additionally during this period of internal expansion in land acquisition, promotion of railroads, pacification of Native Americans, and in the restoration of a common currency after the Civil War — all important in facilitating commercial agriculture.

Throughout the second half of the century, marketing and production systems became more rational, organized, and specialized, putting the "household mode of production" with its characteristic self-sufficiency and seed-saving under mounting strain. During this period we witness the rise of a commercial seed industry. It technically begins with the almost incidental marketing of seeds by a Newport, Rhode Island, bookseller in 1763. In a relatively short time it expanded with seed merchants appearing who raised their own seed and focused exclusively on their seed and nursery business.

Further commercialization and production specialization took place with the invention and development of refrigeration. Companies were organized to coordinate shipment of fruits by rail. In major cities, refrigerated warehouses were built to store fruit and serve an eager urban market during the winter months. The middlemen influenced the structure of the market, the terms of sale and even the types of crops grown.[139]

Certain varieties of fruit were found to ship and store better than others. Indeed, development of the winter fruit market in distant cities helped fuel the search for and development of varieties suitable for shipping and storage[140] — a search which continues to this day.

Advances in transportation and expansion of the postal system brought the seedsman to every household through a new marketing device, the illustrated catalog. Catalogs promoted a culture of modernity and improvement, while supplying seeds and empowering the seed industry. Urban gardeners appear to have been the main clientele of the early mail-order seed companies.[141] Under pressures from commercialization, however, farmers begin to use seed companies, merchants, and other farmers as sources of seed to meet a growing portion of their requirements. Significantly, this shift began prior to the development of scientifically bred varieties using Mendelian genetics. Thus, the shift from farmer-saved and -controlled seed to purchased, commoditized seed began to occur not because of a technological imperative, but in the context of a process of rationalization in agriculture.

This process reached into local cultures through such means as agricultural fairs, where farmers learned and were encouraged to adopt certain identifiable standards. In some cases, such as corn, those cosmetic standards were actually linked to factors decreasing production. When scientific advances did begin to facilitate plant breeding some years later, farmer-selected corn seed had been placed at an added disadvantage by adherence to these counter-productive standards and other factors.

Scientific agriculture was furthered by the development of a system of federally supported agricultural colleges, which provided testing sites for scientific plant improvement techniques and training grounds for the first generation of Mendelian plant breeders. Some of the first improved varieties came from these colleges, and the acceptance of these varieties by farmers was enhanced by the status and reputation of the colleges, particularly in relation to the seed industry, which had a spotty reputation.

In this context, the advantages to the farmer of securing seed from outside sources increased. Specialization, market orientation (with its shifting requirements for different species and varieties), and the economic and cultural incorporation of outlying regions further discouraged home seed-saving.

At land-grant (agricultural) colleges and at state experiment stations across the country, breeders were eagerly employing new methods. The complex structures of the chromosome were now being unraveled by a new professional, the scientist. The attention of mathematics was focused on genetics to reveal further the effects of heredity. Rationality was advancing upon plant breeding. Commercial breakthroughs did not quite happen overnight. In the first decade or two of the twentieth century, plant introductions and farmer selections still dominated American agriculture. But their days were numbered as they were being replaced rather quickly. By the 1920s, wheat breeders knew not only about wheat's chromosomes, but also about their number and their genomic relationships. A decade later, the majority of principal wheat varieties — varieties with improved yield and disease resistance — were varieties that had been developed in formal breeding programs.[142]

The science as well as the crop varieties produced by the government were technically in the public domain, but farmers had no direct link giving them authority over the new directions plant breeding was taking. The new technology was helping facilitate social reorganization. Access to germplasm and control over and participation in plant breeding were slipping out of the hands of farmers. Initially this shift appeared innocent enough, if it were noticed at all. Government and university breeders, after all, were skilled and were working "for" the farmer. But a change in the source of a crucial farm input and the relinquishing of the farmers' role in providing it can never be quite so mundane. New actors were rising and power shifts were under way.

As skilled as the intelligent, observant farmer might be in plant selection and simple breeding, there was an incomplete understanding of the mechanisms of genetic inheritance. The development and employment of Mendelian genetics took away the mystery which had heretofore shrouded inheritance. In principle, one could know, understand and master. The world was, in Weber's words, "disenchanted."[143] One therefore could predict and plan.

The advance of genetics created a wall between farmer and scientist which could not easily be scaled. The farmer with a keen eye and unquestioned interest in crops was often an excellent practitioner of mass selection and simple breeding techniques. The difference between farmer and scientist was simply one of degree before the early 1900s. The farmer had used the available germplasm to great advantage, creating thousands of varieties adapted to the various environments in the United States. Now, with the development of genetics, the scientist had tools unavailable to the farmer plus access to the farmers' crop genetic "resources." The farmer could continue to adapt varieties. The major advances, however, and the rapid progress would henceforth be made by scientists armed with genetics, mathematics, and a growing, private and federally supported research establishment. The loss and extinction of farmer-bred crop varieties at the hands of commercial varieties — a largely unintended consequence of the commercialization of agriculture and rise of scientific plant breeding — are discussed in later chapters and in appendix 1.

Scientific advances were made and developed within a context in which commercial firms already existed and farmers were already making the transition from being self-reliant in seeds to being dependent on the yearly procurement of this new commodity. The science of plant breeding could not be separated from the economy of plant breeding and commercial agriculture. Scientific advances could be taken advantage of and used in certain ways because of the context in which they were made and the abilities of certain actors to use them. The most powerful example of this occurred with the development of hybrid corn. Hybrid corn was a proprietary product. Farmers could not know what inbred lines had been used to produce the hybrid, nor did they have access to the privately developed lines. Private breeders could thus "own" the *variety* by controlling the inbreds that constituted it and the knowledge of how the hybrid was produced. As commercial seedsmen discovered, nature's patent in the form of a hybrid was quite similar to a legal patent in effect.

The scientists themselves and their employers were engaged in breeding *programs* — consciously planned efforts to achieve specific results. Compared to farmer plant breeding, which was more informal (and even communal, with neighborhood sharing of plant materials), scientific efforts were more proprietary and highly formalized with objectives, written breeding records and pedigrees, the use of statistics, and reporting. Unlike farmer-breeders, the scientist is not anonymous but is easily identifiable. (The importance of this will become evident in the chapter 3 concerning the Plant Patent Act.)

This situation bears an interesting resemblance to Max Weber's observations on the social development of western music. As Collins explains:

> Another consequence of music being written down in a formal way is that for the first time in history, composers are well known as individuals. Ancient and oriental societies usually had anonymous musicians; compositions might be improvised and then copied by disciples . . . The West, instead, takes a turn toward the composer as a 'creator,' eventually devel-

oping into the cult of musical 'genius' that centered on such figures as
Beethoven and Wagner . . . [144]

The increasing rationalization of plant breeding gave rise to a new set
of possibilities involving more complex forms of organization and coordination of activities, as the rationalization of western music affected the
orchestra, according to Collins. "The new-style composer, competing
with rivals and predecessors to acquire fame by innovations, is a kind of
business entrepreneur in the realm of music,"[145] a situation not unlike that
of the plant breeder in the early part of the twentieth century.

By 1930, profound changes had taken place in U.S. agriculture. Its
structure had changed dramatically over 160 years from subsistence
agriculture to commercial agriculture — a more formal type of agriculture which encourages planning, specialization and rules. An infrastructure had been created involving transportation, communication and marketing systems, research institutions, and commercial enterprises. The
government's free seed program for farmers became a "lost leader"[146] for
the Department of Agriculture and was eventually discontinued under
pressure from an emerging seed industry. Botanical materials imported
for experimentation and development ceased going to farmers and went
instead to scientists. Most importantly, the farmer's relationship to planting materials had changed in the most profound way — one that separated
the farmer from ownership and control (and "creator") of crop varieties.
With hybrids, important qualities of the seeds themselves had changed —
they could no longer be effectively saved for replanting. Farmers had to
buy rather than select and save seeds. This change, of course, implies
others—changes in the culture of agriculture, and changes in relationships
between farmers and the private sector, and between farmers and the
government. These developments set the stage for the struggle to create a
legal structure for the formal ownership of plant varieties.

## NOTES

1. Max Weber quoted in Kirk Kasler, *Max Weber: An Introduction to His Life and Work.*
   Cambridge: Polity Press. 1988: p. 147
2. Collins, Randall, *Max Weber: A Skeleton Key.* Beverly Hills: Sage Publications. 1986: p.
   74ff.
3. McMullen, Neil, *Seeds and World Agricultural Progress.* Washington: National Planning Association. 1987: p. 42ff. Thomas S. Cox, et. al., "The Contribution of Exotic
   Germplasm to American Agriculture," in *Seeds and Sovereignty: The Use and Control of
   Plant Genetic Resources*, edited by Jack Kloppenburg. Durham: Duke University Press.
   1988: p. 118
4. Fogel, R. W., *Railroads and American Economic Growth: Essays in Econometric History.* Baltimore: The Johns Hopkins Press. 1964: p. 17.

5. Hofstadter, Richard, "The Myth of the Happy Yeoman," *American Heritage*, Vol. 7. April, 1956: 43ff.
6. Henretta, James A. "Families and Farms: Mentalité in Pre-Industrial America. *William and Mary Quarterly*. Vol. XXXV, no. 1. January, 1978: p. 17, 30. Henretta points out that surplus was first sold or traded to community members related by kinship or religion before it was taken to a formal, external market.
7. Merrill, M., "Cash is Good to Eat: Self-Sufficiency and Exchange in the Rural Economy of the United States." *Radical History Review*. No. 3. 1977: p. 42–71.
8. North, Douglas C., "International Capital Flows and the Development of the American West," *Journal of Economic History*. Vol. XVI, No. 4. 1956: p. 497.
9. Danhof, Clarence H., *Change in Agriculture: The Northern United States, 1820–1870.* Cambridge, Mass.: Harvard University Press. 1969: p. 27.
10. Henretta, op. cit., p. 24.
11. Schmidt, Louis Bernard. "The Westward Movement of the Wheat Growing Industry in the United States." *Iowa Journal of History and Politics*. Vol. XVIII. July, 1920: p. 404.
12. U.S. Department of Commerce. *Historical Statistics of the United States: Colonial Times to 1970, Part 2.* Bureau of Census. Washington: U.S. Government Printing Office. 1975: p. 732.
13. Pieters, A. J., "Seed Selling, Seed Growing, and Seed Testing," in *Yearbook of Agriculture for 1899.* U.S. Department of Agriculture. Washington: Government Printing Office. 1900: p. 558ff.
14. Gates, Paul Wallace, "The Promotion of Agriculture by the Illinois Central Railroad, 1855–1870." *Agricultural History*. Vol. V, no. 1. January, 1931: p. 58, 67.
15. Smith, Henry Justin, *Chicago's Great Century: 1833–1933.* Chicago: Consolidated Publishers. 1933: p. 36.
16. Stover, J. F., *History of the Illinois Central Railroad.* New York: Macmillan Publishing. 1975: p. 5.
17. Ibid., p. 536–537.
18. Taylor, William A., "The Influence of Refrigeration on the Fruit Industry," *Yearbook of Agriculture, 1900.* Washington: U.S. Government Printing Office/USDA. 1901: p. 577. Taylor details the trails and errors involved in developing refrigerated rail service. He also contends that this development "stimulated" larger plantings which "made possible the loading of cars at single shipping points . . . " p. 576.
19. Stover, op. cit., p. 192, 197, 234.
20. U.S. Department of Commerce, *Historical Statistics*, p. 27.
21. Bryant, Keith L. Jr., *History of the Atchison, Topeka and Santa Fe Railway.* New York: Macmillan. 1974: p. 65.
22. Scott, Roy V. "Railroads and Farmers: Educational Trains in Missouri, 1902–1914." *Agricultural History*. Vo. 36, no. 1. January, 1962: p. 4.
23. Ibid., p. 7.
24. Ibid., p. 12.
25. Jones, C. Clyde, "The Burlington Railroad and Agricultural Policy in the 1920's." *Agricultural History*. Vol. 31, no. 4. October, 1957: p. 71.
26. Ibid., p. 72.
27. Cullinan, G., *The Post Office Department.* New York: Praeger. 1968: p. 54.
28. Long, B. A. W. *Mail by Rail: The Story of the Postal Transportation System.* New York: Simmons-Boardman Publishing. 1951: p. 104.
29. Pieters, op. cit., p. 553.
30. Bishop, W. D. *Report of the Commissioner of Patents for the Year 1859.* 36th Congress, 1st Session, Senate, Ex. Doc. No. 11. Washington: U.S. Government Printing Office. 1860: p. v.
31. Pieters, op. cit., p. 556.
32. Ibid., p. 558–560.
33. Rossiter, Margaret, "Graduate Work in the Agricultural Sciences, 1900–1970." *Agricul-*

*tural History.* Vol. 60, no. 2. Spring, 1986: p. 41.

34. Cleaver, Harry Jr., *The Origins of the Green Revolution.* Ph.D. dissertation, Stanford University. 1975: p. 145ff.
35. True, Alfred Charles, *A History of Agricultural Experimentation and Research in the United States, 1607–1925.* Miscellaneous Publication No. 251, USDA. Washington: U.S. Government Printing Office. 1937: p. 118ff.
36. Brown, Louis Joseph, "The United States Patent Office and the Promotion of Southern Agriculture, 1850–1860." M.A. thesis, Florida State University. 1957: p. 54.
37. Marti, Donald B., *Historical Directory of American Agricultural Fairs.* New York: Greenwood Press. 1986: p. 7.
38. Neely, Wayne Caldwell, *The Agricultural Fair.* New York: Columbia University Press. 1935: p. 21.
39. Ibid., p. 166.
40. Ibid., p. 169.
41. William Parker, cited in Jones, E. L., "Creative Disruptions in American Agriculture 1620–1820." *Agricultural History.* Vol. XLVIII, no. 4. October, 1974: p. 511–12.
42. Danhoff, op. cit., p. 16ff.
43. Ibid., p. 18.
44. Quoted in Rome, Adam Ward. "American Farmers as Entrepreneurs, 1870–1900." *Agricultural History.* Vol. 56, no. 1. January, 1982: p. 38
45. Ibid., p. 38–39
46. Seed companies were big advertisers. As J. H. Collins advised in *Seed World,* "It pays to advertise and the time to advertise is all the time." From "The Food Problem and the Seed Catalogue," *Seed World,* Vol. 3, no. 11, November 5, 1917: p. 596.
47. Rome, op. cit., p. 37–38.
48. From Kennedy, Joseph C. G. (Superintendent of the Census), *Agriculture of the United States in 1860; Compiled from the Original Returns of the 8th Census,* in Rasmussen, Wayne D. (ed.), *Agriculture in the United States: A Documentary History.* Vol. 2. New York: Random House. 1975: p. 918
49. Rosenberg, S. H. (ed.), *Rural America A Century Ago.* St. Joseph, Mich.: American Society of Agricultural Engineers. 1976: p. 12
50. For accounts of early farming practices and the beginnings of a transition to greater mechanization, see *The Best Poor Man's Country: A Geographical Study of Early Southeastern Pennsylvania,* by James T. Lemon. Baltimore: Johns Hopkins Press. 1972. See also Anna Rochester's *Why Farmers Are Poor: The Agricultural Crisis in the United States.* New York: International Press. 1940: p. 81ff. Rochester notes that horse-drawn machines for harvesting grain were most common in the West where labor was scarce. The low price of grain coupled with low to moderate yields forced farmers to cultivate more acreage.
51. As the practice of seed-saving declined, knowledge of how to do it must also have declined. One can imagine that such knowledge was "contextualized," and dependent to a large degree on that context.
52. Pieters, op. cit., p. 566.
53. Mann, Susan A., and James A. Dickinson, "State and Agriculture in Two Eras of American Capitalism," in *The Rural Sociology of the Advanced Societies: Critical Perspectives,* Frederick H. Buttel and Howard Newby (eds.), Montclair, N.J.: Allenheld, Osum. 1980: p. 304
54. Rochester, Anna, *Why Farmers Are Poor: The Agricultural Crisis in the United States.* New York: International Publishers. 1940: p. 76.
55. Ibid., p. 76.
56. Wasserman, Harvey, *Harvey Wasserman's History of the United States.* New York: Harper. 1972: p. 65
57. Hicks, John D., *The Populist Revolt: A History of the Farmers' Alliance and the People's Party.* Minneapolis: University of Minnesota Press. 1931: p. 24. Hicks uses data drawn from the *Eleventh Census* (1890). However, Fred Shannon (*The Farmer's Last Frontier,*

p. 185 — see footnote below) notes that mortgages may have been underreported in the census. It failed to count farms where the farmer was not the sole owner. It also failed to take into account shorter-term and more informal or individual-to-individual loans.

58. Hicks, op. cit., p. 22.

59. Shannon, Fred A., *The Farmer's Last Frontier: Agriculture, 1860–1897*. Vol. V, *The Economic History of the United States*. New York: Farrar & Rinehart. 1945: p. 306.

60. Hicks, op. cit., p. 24–25.

61. Frundt, Henry, *American Agribusiness and U.S. Foreign Agricultural Policy*. Ph.D. dissertation, Rutgers University. 1975: p. 38.

62. Fogel, op. cit., p. 18.

63. Initial adaptation to a new area often produces gains, though that rate of gain is difficult to sustain. This may also have been occuring.

64. Galloway, B. T., "Distribution of Seeds and Plants by the Department of Agriculture." Circular No. 100. Washington: U.S. Department of Agriculture. September, 1912: p. 6. Rare seeds and planting materials did, however, continue to be collected and distributed, but declined in proportion to the "political" seeds, which in the year 1911–12 amounted to 497 tons. The distribution of the experimental seed was more carefully controlled and went to agricultural colleges and bona fide farmer-experimenters.

65. D. M. Ferry & Co. Catalog, Detroit. 1896: p. 2.

66. Peter Henderson & Co. Catalog, New York. 1896: p. 2.

67. An analysis of varieties on agricultural experiment stations' recommended variety lists at the time reveals that an exceptionally low percentage appear to have originated from public or private sector breeding programs. See for example, the list in: "Better Seed Grains and the Seedsman," *Seed World*. Vol 3, no. 6. June 5, 1917: p. 284–285.

68. Edler, George C., "Seed Marketing Hints for the Farmer," Farmers' Bulletin No. 1232, USDA, Washington: Government Printing Office. October, 1921: p. 5. Data for this table came from a USDA Bureau of Markets survey, 1918–19. Data was only available by percentage by state and region, thus no aggregate figures for the U.S. as a whole are possible, as with truck crops.

69. USDA, *Seed Reporter*. U.S. Department of Agriculture, Bureau of Markets. Vol. 2, no. 2. August 10, 1918. Washington. p. 6.

70. Anonymous, "Discourage Home Seed Saving," *Seed World*. Vol. 5, no. 5. April 4, 1919: p. 422.

71. Anonymous, "What the War Has Done for the Seed Trade," *Seed World*. Vol 5, no. 9. June 6, 1919: p. 14.

72. An untitled August 15, 1919, article in *Seed World* (vol. 6, no. 4) notes that home-grown seed amount to half of the total in some communities. "This indicates how extensive home seed saving *has become*." p. 16 [my emphasis] This statement implies an increase in home seed saving, leading one to conclude that the normal market for commercial seed sales was higher than the USDA survey indicated.

73. Hopkins, John A., *Changing Technology and Employment in Agriculture*. Washington: U.S. Government Printing Office/USDA Bureau of Agricultural Economics. May, 1941: p. 134–135.

74. Elder, George C., op. cit., p. 4. Note that the question of "better" seed is only associated with one of the eight reasons given and then only in the context of the seed being better because it is produced in another locality — reminiscent of the earlier view that seed stocks needed to be renewed or "freshened" periodically. On this point, see *The Cottage Garden of America*, by Walter Elder, Philadelphia: Moss & Brother. 1854: p. 170) The pressures of commercialization are clearly evident between the lines of this list, but as of 1921, scientifically bred varieties were not having a commanding effect in the marketplace.

75. Moore, J. N., "Small Fruit Breeding — A Rich Heritage, A Challenging Future." *HortScience*. Vol. 14, no. 3. June, 1979: p. 333

76. Smith, Marvanna (ed.), *Chronological Landmarks in American Agriculture*. Washington: U.S. Department of Agriculture. 1979: p. 10.

77. Fowler, Cary, "The Progressive Farmer." *Southern Changes*. July, 1979.
78. Anonymous, "Pleasing the Mail Order Customer," *Seed World*. Vol 5, no. 2. February 5, 1919: p. 118.
79. Anonymous, "Discourage Home Seed Saving," *Seed World*. Vol. 5, no. 5. April 4, 1919: p. 422.
80. Frundt, op. cit., p. 46. The amount of land in farms from 500–999 acres also increased during this period. The amount of land in farms smaller than 500 acres either stagnated or declined except for tiny, three to nine acre "farms." See *Historical Statistics of the United States: Colonial Times to 1970*, Part 1. Washington: U.S. Government Printing Office. 1975: p. 467.
81. U.S. Department of Agriculture, "Farmers in a Changing World." *The Yearbook of Agriculture, 1940*. Washington: Government Printing Office. 1940: p. 743–744.
82. Frundt, op. cit., p. 49.
83. Mayr, Ernst, *The Growth of Biological Thought: Diversity, Evolution, and Inheritance*. Cambridge: Harvard University Press. 1982: p. 721.
84. Ibid., p. 724.
85. Ibid., p. 731.
86. Kimmelman, Barbara A., "The American Breeders' Association: Genetics and Euginics in an Agricultural Context, 1903–13," *Social Studies of Science*. Vol 12. 1983: p. 177.
87. Mayr also points out that Mendel's theory "was not as complete and therefore not as fully explanatory as had been claimed by geneticists for three quarters of a century." Mayr, op. cit., 1982: p. 725.
88. Hays, Willet M., "Address by Chairman of Organization Committee," *Proceedings of First Meeting of American Breeders' Association held at St. Louis, Mo*. Washington, D.C.: American Breeders' Association. 1905: p. 13.
89. Hays, William M., "Distributing Valuable New Varieties and Breeds," *Proceedings of First Meeting of the American Breeders' Association held at St. Louis, Mo*. Washington, D.C.: American Breeders' Association. 1905: p. 64.
90. According to L. H. Bailey, corn even won a poll for naming of a national flower at the Columbian Exposition in 1893.
91. Sears, E. R., "Genetics and Farming," *Science and Farming: Yearbook of Agriculture, 1943–1947*. U.S. Department of Agriculture. Washington, D.C.: U.S. Government Printing Office. 1947: p. 245.
92. Fitzgerald, Deborah, *The Business of Breeding: Hybrid Corn in Illinois, 1890–1940*. Ithaca: Cornell University Press. 1990: p. 13. Don Duvick (personal communication, 24 June 1992) points out that the uniformity (or lack of it) of the parents would affect the uniformity of the offspring. The major advantage of the method was the ability to produce an intermediate form when such was desired.
93. Fitzgerald, op. cit., p. 23. Fitzgerald says they were widely practiced while Don Duvick (personal communication, 24 June 1992) disputes this. Duvick's point is pursuasive given his long involvement in the corn seed business. He had an extended association with Pioneer Hi-Bred, becoming vice president for research before he retired. Duvick claims that he has never heard those in the industry speak of the use of variety crosses as common.
94. Fitzgerald, op. cit., p. 39.
95. Wallace, Henry (ed.), "Corn Breeding," *Wallace's Farmer*, 26 February 1915, p. 379.
96. Wallace, Henry (ed.), "Corn Breeding Plot," *Wallace's Farmer*, 29 March 1918, p. 578ff
97. Kloppenburg, Jack Ralph Jr., *First the Seed: The Political Economy of Plant Biotechnology, 1492–2000*. Cambridge: Cambridge University Press. 1988: p. 99.
98. In order to establish an inbred line at least five to seven generations are required. At this point characters are fixed and yield has dropped dramatically. Maintaining that line requires that the line always be self-fertilized. Producing a good double-cross hybrid, however, is more involved than crossing any four inbred lines. The trick is in establishing the most advantageous inbreds. Thus it is evident that few farmers would consider the time, trouble, and rather great expense of this new type of corn breeding to be

worthwhile for a production-oriented farm.

99. Fitzgerald, op. cit., p. 55.

100. East, Edward M. and Donald Jones, *Inbreeding and Outbreeding: Their Genetic and Sociological Significance*. Philadelphia: J. B. Lippincott Co. 1919: p. 224.

101. Jones, Donald F., "Selection in Self-Fertilized Lines as the Basis for Corn Improvement." *Journal of the American Society of Agronomy*. Vol. 12, no. 3. March, 1920: p. 87.

102. The USDA even established a federal "field station" on the property of Funk Seed Company in 1918 and picked up the salary of Funk's breeder, who continued with his previous work.

103. Fitzgerald, op. cit., p. 64.

104. Ibid., p. 70.

105. For a more detailed examination of the relationship between the experiment stations and the growth of genetics, see Charles Rosenburg, *No Other Gods: On Science and American Social Thought*. Baltimore: Johns Hopkins University Press. 1976: Part II.

106. Fitzgerald, op. cit., p. 130.

107. Ibid., p. 220.

108. Henry A. Wallace, at age 16, learned this himself by comparing yields of prize-winning seed with those of varieties which had scored poorest in an Iowa corn show. He found that one of the poorest varieties, when planted, outyielded the winners. See *The Hybrid-Corn Makers: Prophets of Plenty* by A. Richard Crabb. New Brunswick: Rutgers University Press. 1947: p. 145ff.

109. Wallace, Henry A., and William L. Brown, *Corn and its Early Fathers*. East Lansing: Michigan State University Press. 1956: p. 121.

110. Fitzgerald, op. cit., p. 72.

111. Wallace states that he had "a lot to do" with founding the Statistical Laboratory at Iowa State College in 1923. Wallace and Brown, op. cit., p. 117. Statistical tools were mostly applied to variety trials. Incidentally, Wallace had harvested corn in such trials as a boy.

112. Fitzgerald, op. cit., p. 195.

113. Ibid., p. 218.

114. Wallace, Henry (ed.), "The Story of Hybrid Corn," *Wallace's Farmer*, 13 August 1938: p. 14 (522).

115. Hambridge, G. and E. N. Bressman, "Forward and Summary," *Yearbook of Agriculture, 1936*. Washington, D.C.: Government Printing Office. 1936: p. 130.

116. Kimmelman, 1983, op. cit., p. 181.

117. Wallace, "The Story of Hybrid Corn," p. 1.

118. Cavanagh, H. M., *Seed, Soil and Science: The Story of Eugene D. Funk*. Chicago: Lakeside Press. 1959: p. 216

119. Fitzgerald, op. cit., p. 148.

120. Ibid., p. 148.

121. Pioneer used a system which based the numerical name of the variety on the year in which it was introduced.

122. Fitzgerald, op. cit., p. 216.

123. While Funk trumpeted the new hybrid techniques, it made clear that the genetic materials themselves, the inbred lines, were strictly private, refusing to share them with other seed companies or farmers. Beyond that, most seed companies (Pfister excepted) even kept their pedigrees secret. Some, however, were using lines developed by the colleges and technically available to the farmer. Doubtless this had something to do with their refusal to divulge pedigrees.

124. Advertisement entitled "Pfister Hybrids Are Different," *Wallace's Farmer*. 13 August 1938: p. 11 (519).

125. "But all these things must remain still 'in the lap of the gods.' The hybrid is made; let it take its course. It shall have to, since the Patent Laws of America will give me no assistance. Were they fair and designed to support invention in other fields than in those of mechanical things, and did they fulfill the objects laid down in the Constitution, matters might be quite otherwise and I might awake some day, as inventors have, to find

myself drawing a royalty from my Actinidia hybrid." (It is interesting to note that it was Fairchild's young son, Graham, who actually performed the pollinating in the absence of his father. Furthermore, it could be pointed out that Fairchild's brother-in-law was Gilbert Grosvenor, president of the National Geographic Society. The society's magazine published an unusual and quite supportive article about plant patenting in 1948.) Quotation above is from "The Fascination of Making a Plant Hybrid," by David Fairchild. *Journal of Heredity*, Vol. XVIII, no. 2, February, 1927: p. 62.

126. Ryerson, Knowles A., "History and Significance of Foreign Plant Introduction Work of the United States Department of Agriculture," *Agricultural History*. Vol. 7, no. 2, April, 1933: p. 124.

127. Ibid., p. 124.

128. Morton, J. Sterling, *Report of the Secretary of Agriculture, 1894*. U.S. Department of Agriculture. Washington: U.S. Government Printing Office. 1894: p. 391.

129. Klose, Norman, *America's Crop Heritage: The History of Foreign Plant Introduction by the Federal Government*. Ames, Iowa: Iowa State College Press. 1950: p. 100.

130. Galloway, B. T., op. cit., p. 5. In the same publication, Galloway gives a later date for the beginnings of distribution of standard varieties under the free seed program — 1896. p. 6.

131. Kloppenburg, op. cit., p. 68.

132. U.S. Department of Agriculture, "Foreign Seeds and Plants: Inventory No. 1." Washington, D.C.: U.S. Government Printing Office. 1899: p. 4.

133. *Seed World*, Vol. 3, no. 4. April 5, 1917, p. 170. The marketing system referred to involves distribution of seeds by government experiment stations.

134. Anonymous, "Good Seed Cannot be Grown by Amateurs," *Seed World*. Vol. 5, no. 3. March 7, 1919: p. 246.

135. Anonymous, "Beating the Farmer at His Own Game," *Seed World*. Vol. 5, no. 6. April 18, 1919. p. 512.

136. Anonymous, "Home Seed Saving Again a Factor," *Seed World*. Vol. 6, no. 4. August 16, 1919. p. 22.

137. Mel L. Webster Co., "Specialists," Advertisement in *Seed World*. Vol. 5, no. 3. March 7, 1919. p. 267. The point here is not so much to dispute the fact that companies are specialists, as to note that the process of rationalization has advanced to the point that specialization is being touted.

138. Don Duvick (personal communication, 24 June 1992) states that "uniformity seems to have been idealized (and idolized) way beyond the needs of the market place," and wonders why this has become so. For explanations, one might explore relationships between cultural and economic factors.

139. See, for example, Lawrence Goodwyn's discussion of the collusion among grain terminals and railroads, and the influence of different shipping rates for farmers and grain elevator companies in *The Populist Moment: A Short History of the Agrarian Revolt in America*. Oxford: Oxford University Press. 1978: p. 70ff.

140. For example, the Elberta peach which originated in the 1800s helped revive the early peach industry of South Carolina and Georgia in the second half of that century. See "The Influence of Refrigeration on the Fruit Industry" by William A. Taylor, in *Yearbook of Agriculture, 1900*. USDA.Washington: U.S. Government Printing Office. 1901: p. 562.

141. The 1899 catalog, "Manual of Everything for the Garden," of Peter Henderson & Co. of New York (which claims to be the largest seed retailer in the country at the time) devotes only three of its 190 pages to "farm" seeds — grasses, grains, and corn.

142. Kloppenburg, op. cit., p. 83.

143. Weber, Max, "Science as a Vocation," in *From Max Weber: Essays in Sociology*, edited by H. H. Gerth and C. Wright Mills, New York: Oxford University Press. 1969: p. 139.

144. Collins, Randall, *Max Weber: A Skeleton Key*. Beverly Hills: Sage Publications. 1986: p. 66.

145. Ibid., p. 67.

146. Rourke, Francis E., *Bureaucracy, Politics, and Public Policy*. 2nd Edition. Boston: Little, Brown & Co. 1976: p. 54.

# PART II: U.S. CONGRESS AND THE COURTS

## The Construction
### of
### Intellectual Property Rights for Plants

CHAPTER **3**

# The Plant Patent Act of 1930

With the Plant Patent Act (PPA) of 1930, commercial nursery interests endeavored to secure exclusive, proprietary rights over plant varieties. The Plant Patent Act provided 17-year patent protection for new varieties of asexually reproduced plants. Asexually reproduced plants are those which are commercially propagated by cuttings or grafts (as opposed to seeds), such as fruit tree varieties and roses.[1]

The Plant Patent Act was historic in that it was the first law to provide legal ownership over plant varieties. We have seen the importance of physical control over plant species and their commercial exploitation in examples involving Kew Gardens. In nineteenth-century America, we saw ownership and control dispersed, for the most part, among farmers who also played an active part in helping create new, adapted plant varieties. During this period there was little sense of anyone having a legally sanctioned, proprietary right over a variety. The rationalization of agriculture, developments in the science and technology of plant breeding, and the rise of the seed and nursery industries provided the larger context for the creation of new forms of ownership as a response to these changing conditions. The PPA was the first plant patenting legislation to be enacted. It was also the beginning of attempts to create a comprehensive system for legal ownership of biological materials encompassing plants, varieties, genes, characteristics, microorganisms, and even animal breeds,[2] which will be explored in later chapters. Therefore, it is important to understand the origins of the act, the context in which it came to be, and the limitations and contradictions in it. In part, these lay the groundwork for future changes and for the expansion of legal forms of ownership, which, as Weber might have noted, are very much a part of the increasing rationalization of this activity.[3]

Given the development of scientific plant breeding in the early twentieth century, it might be assumed that the Plant Patent Act was the successful response of actors attempting to gain legal control over the plant varieties resulting from the new technology. Indeed, it was argued at the time that the PPA was warranted because changes in technology had made inventors out of plant breeders. It would seem, therefore, that the PPA was an example of the efforts of actors trying to change the law in order to utilize better, or benefit more from, the opportunities made

73

possible by powerful new technologies and scientific advances. As Burns
and Ueberhorst correctly point out, sometimes new technologies do not
mesh well with existing legal structures, thus hindering applications of
and benefits from the technology, and encouraging actors to attempt rule
changes.[4]

This insight cannot be applied haphazardly or without substantiation.
While technology is an important part of the context around the Plant
Patent Act, the passage of the act cannot be satisfactorily explained by
referring to advances in plant breeding technologies and resulting "needs"
for changes in the law. In the 1920s there was beginning to be a great deal
of scientifically based plant breeding — principally with sexually reproduced (seed) crops, which were *not* covered by the PPA. Significantly,
very little scientific breeding was being done with asexually reproduced
plants, which *were* covered by the PPA. While changes in technology
provided the backdrop and the public rationale for the passage of a patent
law for plants, it was a law which could not be used by those who were
actually employing the technology cited to justify the law. Thus the bill,
ironically ended up offering patents to a class of plants with which very
little breeding was taking place and rejecting patents on the very plants
undergoing breeding and innovation. It was a powerful refutation of the
old adage that ours is a "nation of laws, not men." How and why, then, did
asexually reproduced plants come to be covered under the act while
sexually reproduced plants were not?

The history of nursery firms roughly parallels that of seed companies.
They got their start in the latter part of the eighteenth and beginning
decades of the nineteenth centuries, benefiting tremendously from the
rationalization and commercialization of agriculture. However, because
of the unique capability of "cloning" fruit trees and many woody
ornamentals, nurseries had a definite advantage in offering distinct, stable
varieties. Once identified, a superior variety could be multiplied in unlimited quantity. Thus, nurseries could establish a business based on the
reputation and the proven performance of uniform, stable varieties. Stark
Brothers, for example, could purchase the rights to the original Delicious
apple tree for a few thousand dollars in 1893, and over the course of the
next 70 years sell over 10,000,000 copies of it, helping them build the
largest nursery in the country.[5]

The ease with which biological duplicates of apple trees, for example,
could be made also presented difficulties to those wanting to gain and
secure economic advantages from exclusive control over particular varieties. There were neither legal structures nor customs offering protection to
those who would wish to own and prevent others from utilizing plant
varieties.

In focusing on the Plant Patent Act of 1930 and on the commercial nursery interests which endeavored to secure exclusive, proprietary rights over plant varieties through this act, we find that the PPA did not arise as the institutionalization of custom or as a simple expression of public opinion.[6] Neither did it come about because it represented the logical unfolding of previous law. Instead the PPA embodied purposes and goals pursued by actors who mobilized and effectively used political power, but within significant constraints. Without these actors, there would have been no law.

Following an examination of the situation of the nursery industry, we turn our attention to the writing of and lobbying for the act. As the act was being passed in 1930, the Empire State Building was under construction, on its way to becoming the world's tallest building. Inventors and innovators Alexander Graham Bell, Thomas Edison, and Henry Ford were household names. Scientific plant breeding was recognized, though perhaps not understood by politicians. Proponents of the PPA worked within this context (and the context of commercialized agriculture already described). The final section of this chapter looks at the law, how it is interpreted and applied, its effects, and the contradictions and problems created by its passage. This will help introduce chapter 4, which concerns the patenting of sexually reproduced plants.

## THE NURSERY INDUSTRY

Most of the larger eastern cities had two or three small nurseries on their outskirts specializing in fruits and flowers by the early nineteenth century. It is estimated that the nurseries occupied not more than 500 acres collectively in 1840.[7] Twenty years later their number had grown to over a thousand and they used between three and four thousand acres.

California's nursery business began in the late 1840s, "indebted," in the words of an emeritus professor of horticulture at the University of California, "to the world's awakening to desirability in new and better plants during the preceding decade."[8] The largest nursery there in the 1850s was in Alameda, where Wilson Flint had 329,000 fruit trees representing 150 varieties. Another had 194,000 trees and plants of over 1,100 varieties (and a production of 4,000 pounds of garden seed).

Nurserymen had to battle prevailing practices to create a market. "Every man his own nurseryman' was a slogan against which the pioneer professional had to contend . . ."[9] But nursery companies proliferated, competition intensified, and prices fell drastically — over 80 percent — between 1856 and 1858, less than a decade after the first named varieties had been imported from the East Coast. "This resulted in one of the earliest fair price codes set by mutual agreement," according to Olmo.[10]

Nurserymen were faced with opportunities and obstacles different from those that had confronted the early seed companies — different to a large extent because of the type of plant materials they handled. Unique fruits produced by a single tree could be more easily identified than a unique wheat or corn plant. Once identified, scion wood (twigs or shoots) could be clipped off the tree and grafted onto rootstock. (It is this scion wood that determines the character of the plant.) In this way thousands of genetically identical plants could be reproduced. This quality of woody plants such as fruit trees and rose bushes, together with the technique of grafting, gave great predictability to and control over commercial reproduction of these plants. Until the development of hybrids in the 1920s and 1930s, seeds could not be "copied" so precisely. But, as illustrated by in the case of nurseries in California described above, it also meant that competitors could quickly flood the market either with exact copies of superior varieties or with complete forgeries. Because fruits take some years before bearing, the forgeries would be undetectable at the time of sale.

Bees pollinating apple blossoms successfully "crossed" thousands of varieties in millions after millions of "breeding experiments." An apple must be pollinated by a different variety in order to produce a fruit. Bees carrying pollen on their legs from one tree unintentionally leave some on flowers of the next tree, thus successfully pollinating the blossoms. Seeds from that apple if planted would produce a tree which was the cross between the tree that bore the apple and the tree that supplied the pollen. This crossing could also be easily accomplished by people, the result being similar to that of variety crossing as described with corn. But such breeding, because it did not utilize stable inbred lines, did not produce particularly predictable or replicable results. The breeding product still appeared to be a matter of chance. More involved breeding — again, due to the nature of most fruit crops — would have involved the expenditure of long periods of time.

Writing in 1921, Folger and Tomson state: "Seed selection and hybridization have been responsible for the improvement of many cultivated plants and for the discovery of many new varieties, but not so for the cultivated fruits. *Practically all varieties of fruit are the result of chance discovery of seedlings.*" [my emphasis][11]

Little "scientific" breeding was taking place. With so many varieties being produced naturally, why would commercial enterprises go to the expense of encouraging even more when the result was so unpredictable?

Significantly, however, nurseries with tens or hundreds of farmer-selected varieties were well situated to notice nature's own breeding experiments (the chance seedlings and naturally occurring bud mutations). And the normal commercial activities of nurseries would bring them into contact with new varieties originating on people's farms. The techniques of deliberately crossing varieties and of reproducing varieties by grafting were within reach of everyone. However, once a significant variety was discovered, the commercial advantage flowed to the commercial nursery-man.

Farmers wanting to grow the best or latest variety could buy one tree, wait for it to reach a sufficient size to begin taking scion wood from it (several years), graft that material, and then wait for the young "whips" to reach profitable bearing age (at least another six years). Or, for the cost of buying a young tree from a nursery (between .50 and $1.50 for trees from reputable dealers in 1930), about three to six years plus some labor and upkeep expenses could be eliminated. Purchased stock was clearly cost-effective. (A tree could yield as much as 12 dollars' worth of apples in a season,[12] so reducing the amount of time until a tree started bearing by purchasing commercial stock could easily pay for the cost of the tree.)

Thus, while many nursery species were easy for farmers to "breed" and multiply, nursery companies expanded because they could provide a unique, visibly differentiated, standardized product at a cost that actually saved the farmer money over a five-year period. Unlike the seedsman, the nurseryman's biggest competition came not from the farmer, but from the competing nurseryman who could legally buy superior or unique stock and set up a large-scale operation to multiply and sell it. Nurseries with unique varieties could only enjoy control — monopoly — for a limited time before others invaded the market with genetically identical plants. (This situation discouraged expenditures for plant breeding and put a premium on rapid multiplication and marketing.) Since fruit trees remain productive for decades, a lost sale was an opportunity lost for a long time. L. H. Bailey's list of plants introduced in 1893 gives some evidence of the trouble certain nurserymen were beginning to have. Each of the corn varieties introduced that year was offered by a single company, whereas most of the rose varieties were offered by multiple "dealers."[13] Large nurseries in particular were thwarted in their attempts to beat the competition by being unable to privatize and control their product.

A number of trade associations were founded as conflicts arose among commercial interests. The American Association of Nurserymen, founded in the 1870s, worked to standardize nomenclature, lower freight rates, rid the industry of dishonest operations, and educate its members about the

latest horticultural and business techniques. The American Pomological
Society was a similar organization; members heard lectures on a wide
range of pomological and business topics at its convention in 1889.
Similar too was the American Seed Trade Association (ASTA) organized
in 1883 to bring order to marketing, lobby against the government's free
seed program, and work for commercial seed interests. The Society of
American Florists, which at its fifth annual convention in 1889 heard a
report from its committee on "exaggerations in illustrated catalogs," acted
to establish a system of certificates for approved catalogs.[14] The Florists'
Protective Association was established for "protection of its members
from the designs of dishonest persons." The National League of Commission Merchants was open only to "houses of known reputation" interested
in divesting the business "of abuses that are said to arise and creep into it
. . ." A Florists' Hail Association was even founded to provide group
insurance for commercial victims of frozen precipitation. In 1889, it
insured over one million square feet of greenhouse glass.

A number of associations centered around specific flowers or fruits
were organized, such as the American Rose Society and the National
Chrysanthemum Society. Such groups typically sought to bring rationality and order to the naming of varieties, a problem reputable nurseries
experienced when dishonest dealers flooded the market with misnamed
varieties as discussed above. Many, including the Chrysanthemum Society, established formal registries of variety names.[15] Regional organizations to deal with the nomenclature problem were also convened. The
Peninsula Horticultural Society (Delaware and Chesapeake peninsula)
empowered a committee to suggest a plan for registration. The committee
reported that "respectable nurserymen" were upset that old varieties were
being sold under new names. "Originators," it said, "seek protection
similar to that afforded by patents."[16]

Stark Brothers Nurseries had become the largest of all U.S. nursery
companies in the early part of the twentieth century.[17] A very brief look at
this nursery is appropriate both because it illustrates well some of the
problems faced by the larger, established nurseries and because it took the
lead in efforts to solve these problems. The situation of Stark Brothers in
the 1920s thus leads us into the events resulting in passage of the Plant
Patent Act in 1930.

Stark Brothers Nurseries was founded in 1816 and incorporated in
Missouri in 1889. The nursery began advertising in newspapers in 1887,
produced its first catalog in 1894, and brought out a color edition in 1896.
The Stark family had large landholdings, business relationships with
railroads, and very powerful political contacts on the state and national
levels.[18]

Despite the fact that it was the country's leading nursery, its involvement in breeding was practically nil. According to Terry, a sympathetic historian of the company, "chance seedlings and bud sports have been the main sources of Stark's famous varieties of apples and other fruits . . ."[19] And Clay Logan, current president of Stark Brothers, states that the company has "never" done any breeding work.[20] An examination of the Stark Brothers' catalog for 1930 illustrates this point. The cover features the "Starking Double-Red Delicious" apple, which was discovered as a bud mutation on a Delicious apple tree growing in New Jersey. Stark purchased the tree for $6000 and promptly erected a fence around it to prevent others from obtaining grafting wood. According to the catalog, it was "the greatest red apple of all time." (The "original" Delicious apple was a chance seedling discovered by Jesse Hiatt on his Iowa farm in 1868. Hiatt named it "Hawkeye."[21] Stark Brothers bought it and changed the name to "Stark Red Delicious.") The second apple featured was the "Staymared Stark Double-Red Stayman Winesap." Two pages are devoted to this bud sport discovered in Virginia and again purchased by Stark Brothers. "Stark's Golden Delicious" receives eight pages of attention. It was discovered in Virginia and purchased for $5000. Of the eight apples prominently displayed in the catalog, only one possibly appears to have been the result of intentional crossing, the "Stark King David" — a simple cross between two well-known apples, Jonathan and Winesap.[22] Interestingly, unlike the variety names of the hybrid corns emerging during this period, Stark's fruit varieties, appropriately, do not bear names touting a scientific plant breeding origin. Instead, the names remain very traditional.

Stark Brothers marketed some varieties produced by Luther Burbank. Burbank, who died in 1926, was known as the "plant wizard" and "had tremendous influence on fruit improvement and popularized plant breeding worldwide."[23] It is unclear, however, just how much Burbank's varieties were the result of intentional breeding. One of his first plums, the "Burbank plum," for example, was actually one he imported from Japan in 1885 and renamed after himself.[24] Stark Brothers paid Burbank for the rights to market his varieties and in turn Burbank endorsed Stark varieties and bequeathed his "treasure box" of seeds to Stark when he died.

Stark's business was based on varieties, not breeding. It rested on the ability of Stark to purchase new, desirable varieties as they arose and mass-market them. It did not depend on Stark's breeding new varieties which it could not keep out of the hands of eager competitors. Stark enjoyed economies of scale and a reputation for selling quality stock and varieties which were true-to-name. But Stark's fruit varieties, like most

nursery species, were particularly vulnerable to others acquiring, multiplying, and selling them. Stark's attempts to gain exclusive control over
the marketing of its varieties by having its customers sign contracts
(printed on the catalog order form) saying they would not propagate and
offer Stark's varieties for sale was not successful.[25] Once a variety "es-
caped" from a single customer, it could be propagated legally and with
impunity by others with whom Stark had no contractual relationship. If
Stark Brothers could obtain and enforce exclusive control over its varieties and prevent others from selling them, it could dramatically expand its
sales.

Not surprisingly, some of the earliest suggestions of patent or trademark protection for plant varieties (1870s) came from the nursery industry.[26] For decades there was no consensus on what form this should take,
however. Prominent horticulturalists such as Luther Burbank and Liberty
Hyde Bailey found a number of the proposals deficient. Though the idea
of protection was regularly discussed at nursery association meetings (in
contrast to seed association meetings), little action was taken.

W. M. Hays, an assistant secretary of agriculture and one of the leading
organizers of the American Breeders' Association (ABA) took up the
cause, timidly. At the first meeting of the association in 1905, Hays
remarked that "possibly laws or business practices can be devised which
will give private individuals, animal breeders, seed firms and nursery
firms practically a patent right or a royalty on new blood lines."[27] But even
a suggestion from such a prominent person as Hays was not enough to
pass a law and the ABA was hardly the organization to shepherd legislation through Congress. Its membership was small and diverse, including
intellectuals, scientists, and farmers. It was concerned mainly with developing Mendelian genetics, yet was split by various interests, among them
plant breeding and eugenics. It had no full-time staff. And it suffered
serious financial difficulties in even publishing a journal, as well as
internal political tensions, according to Kimmelman.[28] Hays himself was
busy with his job at the USDA and with trying to keep the ABA afloat
while promoting the "Country Life" movement.

Such recommendations and Stark's own difficulties in controlling its
varieties, led to the 1906 tabling of "A Bill to amend the laws of the
United States relating to patents in the interest of the originators of
horticultural products," introduced by Congressman Champ Clark, who
represented Stark Nurseries' district and was a friend of the family's. The
bill would have allowed the registration of the name of a new variety as a
trademark. But some congressmen were worried that the bill would
regulate state as well as interstate commerce. And one congressman noted

that "protests have reached the committee from great nurserymen against the passage of the bill." The split in nursery operators' ranks occurred along commercial/propagator lines, with purely commercial companies opposing the legislation.[29] No serious lobbying effort was mounted and the bill was never approved by committee. More bills were introduced in 1907, 1908 and 1910. None was passed. In Europe similar measures were being proposed, especially loudly in France among fruit growers, but none were successful.[30]

The failure to pass patenting legislation covering plant varieties can be explained by a number of factors. First, it is unclear how active seed companies were, individually or collectively, in attempts to pass such legislation. Nurseries, with the possible exception of Stark's, were not particularly active either and were unorganized for the effort. The record seems to indicate that patenting bills were not actively promoted. It must be remembered that seed companies faced bigger problems than securing their exclusive rights over particular varieties. First and foremost was the struggle simply to commoditize seeds. The fight to eliminate government competition from the free seed program did not come to an end until 1924. Furthermore, seed companies had to contend with state seed laws, the first of which was passed in 1897. These laws were primarily aimed at protecting farmers by regulating germination standards, weed seed content, labeling, and nomenclature practices. In general these laws were ultimately helpful to large, established seed businesses, but the immediate effects on and reception by the seed trade were not uniformly positive.

The long years of competing with farmer seed-saving and free government seed had produced its share of dishonest practices and dishonest seedsmen and had weakened the entire industry.[31] Adulterated and mislabeled seed was common, as were exaggerated claims. These created a public relations and political problem. In the words of an official of the Association of Official Seed Analysts at an ASTA convention, the situation in the seed business was "caveat emptor with a vengeance . . . "[32] The USDA even published lists of seedsmen known to sell adulterated seed.[33] But this did not seem to solve the problem. State seed laws were often a response to this situation. As the president of the Association of Official Seed Analysts put it in 1930:

> If neither his regard for the prosperity of the farmer, or the permanence of his own business could induce such a dealer to cease his undesirable selling practices, it was apparent that pressure from outside must be brought and this pressure must be of a type to be effective. Efforts were made by the better class of seedsmen to eliminate this menace to their own interests, but without avail. Apparently, the only alternative was a resort to

law. For a time this seemed like "jumping from the frying pan into the fire," for much of the legislation enacted was extremely undesirable in character.[34]

Consequently, such laws were often viewed by industry officials as "ill considered and unenforceable." Ten states passed state seed laws in the 1920s. But by the late twenties, states were beginning to reconsider their legislation — a potentially threatening situation — prompting various seed trade organizations to turn their attention to drafting and promoting uniform state laws and federal seed legislation.[35]

It would appear that seed industry groups were distracted by other concerns of more immediate importance to their members than the issue of legal protection of varieties. Furthermore, many seed companies could not point to genuinely new varieties needing or deserving patent protection. And those that could — or were about to — were often involved in producing hybrids which offered a form of biological protection that made patents redundant. Absent significant numbers of distinct new varieties being produced by seed companies, variety protection through something like a patent law would hardly have been considered a business necessity. The American Seed Trade Association was, after all, an association of seed *traders* as its name implies. Members typically referred to themselves either as "traders" or "growers" of seed, rarely if ever calling themselves "breeders." Significantly, the pages of the seed trade journals are filled with articles about many problems — shipping rates, the inadequacy of the postal system, dishonest seedsmen, the free seed program, exports, merchandizing difficulties — but the issue of variety protection is missing.

Finally, seed companies faced mounting financial problems after 1925. In the next 9 years, the annual volume of seed sales fell by half reflecting farmers' attempts to economize in the face of the Depression.[36]

Despite their legislative impotence, nursery companies, Hays, and others had begun to introduce the notion that the plant breeder was like the industrial inventor and as such was deserving of similar incentives and rewards.[37] David Fairchild, a prominent scientist, took up this point in the pages of the *Journal of Heredity*.[38] And in the pages of the Stark Brothers Catalog, photos of Burbank — the great plant inventor — were shown with those of the other great inventors of the day, Thomas Edison and Henry Ford. Never mind that "invention" (as opposed to discovery) had little to do with Stark's catalog offerings![39]

The American Association of Nurserymen (AAN) turned to the issue of varietal protection in earnest in 1923, appointing a committee (which included Lloyd Stark) to work on the problem. Soon thereafter, Paul Stark of Stark Brothers Nurseries was named chair of the committee. He arranged for the committee to meet with high-ranking USDA officials (including some, such as David Fairchild, who were already sympathetic to their concerns). Meetings with allied associations such as ASTA and the Society of American Florists were held in 1926.[40] Discussions did not immediately center on patenting as a solution to the nurserymen's problems — the alternative of varietal registration was also discussed, and eventually rejected. Several sources credit a Washington patent attorney, Harry C. Robb, Sr., with first having the idea of introducing a patent bill.[41] It is obvious from the short history already given that the idea had circulated for some time. But it is likely that Stark and his committee used Robb to draft the legislation.[42] Robb's initial interest had been piqued when he unsuccessfully tried to obtain a trademark on a new plum variety some years earlier.

In order to sidestep expected opposition to plant patenting, Paul Stark's bill omitted coverage for sexually (seed) reproducing plants such as grains and vegetables. Stark had convinced ASTA to "drop their efforts" earlier in 1930.[43] According to ASTA records, Stark observed:

> It seemed to be the wise thing to get established the principle that Congress recognized the rights of the plant breeder and originator. Then, in the light of experience, effort could be made to get protection also for seed propagated plants which would be much easier after this fundamental principle was established.[44]

Practically, the bill would cover only fruits and some flowers, like roses. Potatoes and Jerusalem artichokes were also omitted. The report from the Committee on Patents to the House of Representatives explained the omission this way: "This exception is made because this group alone, among asexually reproduced plants, is propagated by the same part of the plant that is sold as food."[45] It could also have been said that farmers used this part as planting material. The omission would ease the concerns of those who would be troubled that the bill would deprive farmers of the right to use the products of their fields as they saw fit.

The bill was formally introduced by Republican Senator John Townsend of Delaware and Republican Representative Fred Purnell of Indiana. Townsend, it should be noted, owned thousands of acres of apple and peach orchards.[46] He owned several canning and processing companies. For a time he operated a string of 23 strawberry processing plants stretching from Tennessee to Delaware, possibly including operations involved in strawberry breeding or propagation.[47] He was involved in diversified large-scale farming operations, had banking and timber inter-

ests, and had business relationships with the railroad industry as a supplier
of timber and a former employee of the Pennsylvania Railroad.[48]

Stark and his committee spent "six months' steady activity in Washington" rounding up support.[49] They obtained the predictable endorsement of
several industry groups. More importantly they garnered official support
from the Commissioner of Patents,[50] the secretaries of Commerce and
Agriculture, the Grange (which had close government ties and had supported the government's plan to end the free seed program) and the Farm
Bureau (with its historic ties to the Country Life movement, "scientific
agriculture," and commercial interests).

Proponents saw in the bill their best opportunity in years to acquire
patent rights for plants. Reeling from the crash of 1929, the Administration was eager to "do something" for agriculture.

By anyone's standards — even Washington's — the claims made for
the bill were extravagant. The Patent Committee's report to the House
spoke of the history of men who had developed new plants of "inestimable
value to humanity and have died in poverty." It implied that the bill would
help researchers develop cold-hardy apples, substitutes for rubber, and
new classes of plants, and that it would be "of incalculable value in
maintaining public health and prosperity, and in promoting public safety
and the national defense. Finally plant patents will mean better agricultural products that will give the public more actual value for its dollar."[51]

More realistically, proponents saw the plant patenting bill as an opportunity to gain legal control over varieties *as varieties*, and to begin to
move the government out of the breeding business and to secure that
activity for private interests. "To-day," the Committee on Patents report
stated, "plant breeding and research is dependent, in large part, upon
Government funds to Government experiment stations, or the limited
endeavors of the amateur breeder. It is hoped that the bill will afford a
sound basis for investing capital in plant breeding and consequently
stimulate plant development through private funds."[52]

The assistance of Thomas Edison, the most famous inventor of the day,
was solicited by Stark. Edison was trying to breed goldenrod to produce a
rubber substitute and thus approached the subject of plant breeding with
sympathy. He sent a telegram to Congress saying, in part: "Nothing that
Congress could do to help farming would be of greater value and perma-
nence than to give to the plant breeder the same status as the mechanical
and chemical inventors now have through the patent law. There are but
few plant breeders. This will, I feel sure, give us many Burbanks."[53]

Luther Burbank, a friend of Edison's, had died four years earlier.
Burbank had become the country's most famous horticulturalist and plant

breeder, his name a household word.[54] Burbank was also a promoter. His Luther Burbank Society included among its life members his friend Thomas Edison, Phoebe Hearst, John Muir, and Hugo de Vries. Burbank had cooperated with Stark Brothers from 1893 to the 1920s. Paul Stark's father, Clarence, had journeyed to Burbank's California plant-breeding station in 1893 and cemented a business relationship with him that would result in Stark's marketing many of the varieties developed by Burbank. Burbank was unquestionably prolific, developing, discovering or improving some 800 varieties of trees, vegetables, fruits and flowers. Ironically, his most successful "invention" was the Burbank potato, developed when he was a market gardener in 1872, a crop which would not have been covered by the bill in question.

Burbank had early on voiced his opposition to patents. In a pamphlet entitled, *How to Judge Novelties*, published in 1911, he stated:

> No patent can be obtained on any improvement of plants, and for one I am glad that it is so. The reward is in the joy of having done good work, and the impotent envy and jealousy of those who know nothing of the labor and sacrifices necessary, and who are by nature and cultivation, kickers rather than lifters.

> Happening however to be endowed with a fair business capacity I have so far never been stranded as have most others who have attempted similar work, even on an almost infinitely smaller scale."[55]

Furthermore, Burbank's standing in the scientific community had deteriorated by the time of his death. Biographer Peter Dreyer recounts that Burbank's friend (and a life member of the Burbank Society) John Burroughs "had, like most scientists, come to associate the name of Burbank with the worst kind of horticultural quackery."[56]

Neither Burbank's initial opposition to plant patenting nor the tarnishing of his scientific reputation dulled his usefulness to patent proponents in the political setting. Burbank's final statement on patenting had been in support of the concept. It was used most effectively. Various accounts (Terry, Doyle) have incorrectly credited Burbank's statement with immediately changing the tide of the debate and virtually forcing the patent opposition to concede.

According to these accounts, on May 5, 1930, Congressman Fiorello LaGuardia (a future mayor of New York and future supporter of the National Sharecroppers Fund which would launch opposition to seed patenting in the 1970s) stood in the well of the U.S. House of Representatives and railed against the plant patenting bill. Cosponsor, Congressman Purnell asked LaGuardia what he thought of Burbank, to which

LaGuardia replied, "I think he is one of the greatest Americans that ever lived." Purnell then read into the record excerpts from a letter Burbank had sent to Stark shortly before his death.

A man can patent a mouse trap or copyright a nasty song, but if he gives to the world a new fruit that will add millions to the value of earth's annual harvests he will be fortunate if he is rewarded by so much as having his name connected with the result. Though the surface of plant experimentation has thus far been only scratched and there is so much immeasurably important work waiting to be done in this line I would hesitate to advise a young man, no matter how gifted or devoted, to adopt plant breeding as a life work until America takes some action to protect his unquestioned rights to some benefit from his achievements.

Bested by the clever debating strategy, according to Terry, LaGuardia "immediately took the floor and said: 'I withdraw my objection to this bill and move its adoption.'"[57] LaGuardia, however, never made such a statement. In fact he persisted with his opposition to the bill, saying that he did "not believe it possible to protect him (the plant breeder) by patent rights." Rather than debate ending with victory for the bill, it was tabled for two weeks.[58] What if LaGuardia had known of Burbank's anti-patent statement and could have used that in the debate? What if he had been familiar with Burbank's controversial standing in the scientific community? Apparently he was not. Possessing political power, he nevertheless was not an expert in this rather technical field.

Wavering politicians were targeted. New York's Democratic Senator Royal S. Copeland, for example, acknowledged getting letters from constituents opposing the bill and asked for more time to study the objections. Within three days he had received stacks of mail from nurserymen. Copeland forthwith rose in the Senate to observe:

The Stark Delicious apple to my mind is one of the most delicious apples I have ever tasted. It is well named. It required years of effort in Missouri before the apple was developed. They now sell it under a bond that no one who has the trees may sell or give away any of the grafts. I have 100 of them on my farm. I think it is such a remarkable product that I feel extremely thankful that somebody had the energy to work out the development of the plant . . . For my part, I am very happy to join in support of the bill.[59]

No small amount of confusion and misunderstanding is evidenced in the debate. Senator Copeland in the above statement refers to the years of effort required to develop the Delicious apple (effort worthy of rewarding and encouraging by patents), an apple simply discovered by a farmer on his Iowa farm. And the committee report on the bill states that the bill will provide "an incentive to asexually reproduce new varieties," as if there were another way to reproduce a fruit variety at the time.[60] Lack of knowledge on the part of those in Congress markedly affected the quality of the deliberations.

The particulars of the debate, while interesting, will not be furthered explored here. The history shows a sustained effort on the part of identifiable actors to legislate. Their actions were creative — they made choices. But they also made compromises due to the specific context and games in which they found themselves, and the limitations of their own powers and knowledge. In summary, several representatives raised questions about the practicality and constitutionality of the bill. Others evidenced concern about patenting food plants. The debate was spirited at times, but not sustained. Whether representatives had "better things to do," or became convinced of the merits of the bill and their own prior misconceptions of it as Terry suggests, cannot be conclusively determined. The bill had no organized opposition, and proponents made skillful use of House and Senate rules to guide the bill through both houses of Congress without a recorded vote[61] — beginning a string of plant patent laws, all passed without recorded votes.

The bill quickly made its way to President Hoover's desk where it was signed as the Plant Patent Act of 1930 (PPA). Stark's committee had spent $12,000 on lawyers' fees and other expenses — a controversial amount within the AAN.[62] But a landmark bill, the first ever to grant patent protection to plant varieties, had been passed. Within the coming months, six of the first eighteen patents issued would go to Stark Brothers for varieties developed by Burbank[63] — not much incentive for further research on his part, but reward enough, perhaps.

## THE SUBSTANCE AND PRACTICE OF THE LAW

While a great deal was made politically of the desirability and appropriateness of granting to plant breeders rights equivalent to those enjoyed by mechanical inventors, the crux of the problem faced by companies such as Stark was not so much to protect the inventor as it was to capture economic and legal control over the variety, regardless of whether it was invented or not. The Plant Patent Act as drafted by Stark and Robb and signed by Hoover offered rights to anyone who "has invented *or discovered* and asexually reproduced any distinct and new variety of plant, other than a tuber-propagated plant . . ." [my emphasis].

The original draft had included protection for "mere finds," a phrase which some Administration and congressional sources had found objectionable. The Commissioner of Patents stated rather disparagingly that the bill mostly seemed intended to "encourage our citizens generally to be on the lookout for varieties produced by natural processes; that is, by nature's accidental cross pollination . . ." His concern however was to encourage *"plant breeders*, nurserymen, and horticulturalists" (emphasis in original).[64] Given the rarity of actual "breeding" in the nursery business at the time, Stark's committee must have been concerned with how to protect the patentability of "nature's accidental cross pollination" while meeting the commissioner's concern. The compromise struck allowed for protection of a discovery as long as it was not a completely wild plant or one growing in wild, uncultivated circumstances. The compromise was insignificant in its effect on the industry. For example, if a valuable "sport" were discovered on a wild apple tree, the PPA would not cover the patenting of the sport. However, if someone cut the limb off the tree and took it back to the nursery, it would cover the variety "created" by propagating the sport. As patent attorney and sympathetic PPA historian Robert Starr Allyn asserted, it was clear that "no one is entitled to a patent unless he is the author or discoverer of the invention."[65] *Discoverer* of an *invention*? Who then is the inventor? Presumably the plant itself, for it seems that plants often do what would qualify as invention under the criteria of this Act, by themselves. Such ambiguity was officially sanctioned in a section added to the Act before passage, which stated that "No *plant* patent shall be declared invalid on the ground of noncompliance . . . if the description is made as complete as reasonably possible" (emphasis in original). In other words, the Patent Office could determine the degree of specificity required, the standards having been legally lowered for plants.

In attempting to define what an invention was under the PPA, Allyn concluded that "The only adequate test we know of is — in the first instance, does it appeal to the Patent Office Examiner as worthy of the grant of a patent? In the second instance, does the Court think that the inventor is entitled to a reward?"[66] In analyzing the first plant patents granted, Allyn found a number of questionable interpretations. Claims were made and granted for fruit and nut varieties though the claims had been made for their blossoms, fruits, and nuts. A Burbank plum was patented based on the uniqueness of "the early ripening period of the fruit, as shown." A drawing was attached, but one wonders how well it really showed the early ripening period. Patent 71 was granted for the "Howard Strawberry" even though it had been developed in 1907, distributed, discussed in print, and offered for sale for some years. And a freesia (patent 17) won a medal in a flower show in 1928, three years before an application was filed for patent protection.[67]

Allyn concluded (not surprisingly, given the Commissioner of Patents' concerns) that "the Patent Office draws some sort of distinction between new varieties of plants which may be found or discovered by professional plant breeders and those that may be discovered by the non-professionals."[68] The law, however, was being administered by the Patent Office and had been turned over for interpretation and implementation to Division I, "Closure Operators; Fences; Gates; Tillage; Handling Implements." Robert Cook, editor of the *Journal of Heredity* at the time, charged that the chief examiner was "completely innocent of even the rudiments of botanical or horticultural knowledge." Without such knowledge, he observed, "absurdities will continue."[69] If the Patent Office was erring, however, it was erring on the side of issuing patents[70] and thus providing companies with the legal tool for which they had lobbied.

Interpretations of the Act by the Patent Office actually had the effect of creating an interesting distinction between the "inventor" (or discoverer) and the grantee of the patent. Patent 11, for example, recognizes "joint inventors"— one person who discovered a bud-mutation on a rose, and a second who did nothing but propagate it. Another fascinating example is that of Lenton Newman, who at age 14 when he was known as "Spud" on his parents' Texas farm, noticed a rose bloom without a thorn. Spud and his father took cuttings and planted them and eventually sold all of the thornless rose bushes he had invented to a leading southern rose grower for $250. The rose grower applied for and received a patent. Two years later after selling nearly 300,000 thornless "Festival" roses, the company sold the rights to the variety for $10,000.[71] The distinction between discoverer and propagator and the decision by the Patent Office to accept both as "co-inventors" thus facilitated new relationships wherein the inventor/discoverer (narrowly defined) would not necessarily receive all the credit. Legitimate rights could be claimed by the propagator — the company.[72]

In allowing discoveries, and in recognizing those who simply propagated as inventors, the Plant Patent Act was arguably not focused on the protection and encouragement of breeding. Protection was concentrated at the varietal level regardless of whether any mental act of invention had taken place in producing it. In fact, varietal rights were given to people for stumbling across what plants did on their own. And in the case of propagators, stumbling was not even necessary. The PPA did not recognize the individual inventor or the creative act as much as it recognized and rewarded the *system* that produced the new variety, whether by luck or design.

Several other features of the act are worth noting. First, it specified that the new variety must be "distinct," but failed to define this term. Congress (in agreement with industry) declined to require that the variety represent any improvement — an irony, given industry's argument that the bill would encourage the production of better varieties.

Secondly, it eliminated the standard industrial patent requirement that the invention be described sufficiently well to enable someone skilled in the art to reproduce it. This was a major concession to the patent applicant and a loss for society given the traditional trade involved in patents, namely that knowledge is given to society in exchange for a government-granted, limited-term monopoly. This will be discussed in more depth later.

Thirdly, the law protected the plant only, not its fruit or flowers, and in so doing determined at what level royalties would be charged. The patent would cover the plant as an instrument of reproduction.

Finally, the law excluded  from coverage broad categories of plants, opening the way for future battles. Not only were sexually reproducing plants excluded, but tuber-propagated plants such as potatoes and Jerusalem artichokes were also excluded. Stark's cautions to the seed trade had been well founded. Congress was apparently not willing to allow patents to be placed on food. According to the report to the House Committee as quoted earlier, "This exception is made because this group alone, among asexually reproduced plants, is propagated by the same part of the plant that is sold as food."[73] This interpretation is confirmed by the fact that early patents were granted for *nonfood* tuber-propagated plants despite the fact that the Act expressly excluded such plants.[74] In other words, it was not the "tuber propagating" characteristic that troubled the politicians, but the fact that the patent might cover the very item sold and consumed as food.[75] An amendment (H.R. 1490) to the act to provide for the grant of patents on cereals, offered in the 73rd Congress, was not even given a committee hearing.

As we shall soon see, each of these points will again become controversial in the context of future debates on patent coverage for plants, genes and microorganisms. Stark was remarkably prescient in his view that the Plant Patent Act would open the door for extensions of protection. But he could scarcely have foreseen that so many of the points in his experimental law would still be hotly debated over 60 years later.

Of the main objective, the securing of control over and a legal mechanism of reward for new varieties, Stark would have little to complain about in the coming years. The PPA has helped Stark Brothers become the biggest retail nursery in the country. Thirty percent of all apple patents, 15 percent of plum patents and 10 percent of peach patents have gone to the company. Jackson & Perkins and Hill Brothers dominate rose patents.

Concentration levels by crop are high — never have the top ten companies accounted for fewer than a third of the more than 5000 patents granted since passage of the act.[76] More importantly, the law achieved what Stark had predicted and what the seed trade had wanted — a precedent for the future establishment of patent protection for sexually reproducing plants.

## DISCUSSION

The material in this chapter demonstrates the importance of viewing events, such as the passage of a law, in the richness of the societal (and biological) context. The approval of the Plant Patent Act of 1930 becomes much more understandable when we place it within the context of the gradual separation of the farmer from control of the seed and the creation of seed as a commodity form (and the relationship of these to the development of seed and nursery industries). These processes in turn were the creation of numerous actors, from railroad companies acting to create business for themselves to agricultural associations promoting ideal, standardized plant varieties and even clever, enterprising farmers themselves who established early commercial enterprises.

While "scientific" plant breeding was revolutionizing the corn seed business, making it possible for plant breeders to plan and direct the evolution of this crop, nursery businesses still relied upon farmer selections and the fortuitous discovery of chance mutations to provide them with new varieties. Fruit tree breeding — more time-consuming and costly than breeding of seed-producing annuals — was not being practiced by nursery companies.

Woody plants such as fruits, berries and roses could be cloned — this technique was well understood. Utilizing cuttings, nurseries could make exact copies of varieties of these plants. Nursery companies taking advantage of this needed only to identify and obtain superior varieties (perhaps arising as a chance mutation or discovery in a farmer's field), in order to establish a business based on particular, identifiable, stable varieties. The commercial drawback was that once marketed, these varieties were accessible to all and could be easily multiplied and sold by competitors. Attempts by the leading nursery company, Stark Brothers, to maintain control over its varieties by erecting fences around the original tree of a variety, and by contracting with buyers of their trees not to multiply them further and sell them, proved ineffective.

As we have seen, the struggle to control plants is an old one. In an era of commercialized agriculture, however, it became centered not on species, but on particular varieties possessing unique and valuable traits. Experiencing the inadequacy of existing mechanisms of control, specific social actors (in this case, nursery companies) contested ownership and control questions in a new arena, engaging in a sustained and conscious attempt to legislate. The context within which this was done both constrained and facilitated their actions. The constraints eventually forced compromises narrowing the scope of the law. But the efforts to establish a legal system of varietal ownership were facilitated by the milieu of innovation which existed. Lawmakers were aware and appreciative but not particularly knowledgeable of the efforts of plant breeders. In lobbying for the PPA, proponents equated plant breeding with mechanical invention. Plant breeders became inventors.

Skillful organizing, coalition building, lobbying and negotiation took place. This activity repelled a number of potential threats to the legislation — even those arising from within industry circles (from the ASTA, which would have welcomed a law covering seeds, and from nursery "propagators" whose business would be restricted by the PPA). The real "experts" were not those who actually passed the law, but were the companies. The congressional battle was fought on their terms and boiled down to whether it was feasible to employ patents. The bigger questions — whether it was desirable, or whether there was any innovation taking place to justify the traditional rationale behind the granting of patents — were never asked.[77]

Burns and Ueberhorst have noted that the introduction of new technology involves social reorganizing and that new technologies sometimes do not "fit" with existing legal structures.[78] On the surface, this would seem to be such a case. With the development of plant breeding tools allowing for the science of breeding to replace the magic of evolution and selection, it might have seemed logical that laws be formulated to protect this new class of inventors. Indeed, this argument was made. But it was made by and for actors who were not engaged in typically inventive activity. Nursery companies were not breeding new varieties, but were only taking newly discovered varieties and commercializing them. So while new technologies provided part of the context of the 1930 act and were used as a political tool in efforts to get the law enacted, current and anticipated use of the new technology was not the immediate impetus behind these efforts. The nursery companies, in other words, were not constructing laws to facilitate their use of the technology or help make its use more profitable. But they did take political advantage of the breeding work being undertaken to argue that patent rights should be provided to plant breeders — just not those "plant breeders" actually engaged in plant breeding (those working with sexually reproducing corps).

Clearly, the patent rewarded not the individual innovator, for in this case it would be the tree or bush producing the valuable mutation or the bee that cross-pollinated two existing varieties to produce a new combination. In practice, the law even seemed to bypass the new variety's human discoverer, typically a lucky farmer, or as in the case of the first thornless rose, an observant 14-year-old boy. Instead, the PPA serves to reward the *system* which propagates the discovery, takes it to the patent office, and utilizes the patent to exclude others from reproducing and selling the patented discovery. It is this power of property (the variety) to exclude and prevent others from certain uses of it that gives advantages to the owner.[79]

Farmers may engage in a broader range of activities (originating, selecting, discovering, propagating) than nursery professionals. But it is not the farmer that is in a position to utilize the power and authority granted by the patent — further evidence that it is the system that is being reward for system-characteristics as opposed to the individual inventor for a creative act. The PPA thereby specified new relationships[80] aiding in institutionalizing the "power and status, resource control, and future strategic action capabilities" of the victorious actors.[81] The bulk of the initial patents accrued to the company that led the effort to secure the new law.

In the initial application of the law is revealed the difference between the law as advocated for and written, and the law as practiced. Due both to the biological nature of the material to be covered and political constraints, social agents failed in their attempts simply to amend the utility patent statutes to include plants. Instead, a *sui generis* statute was created, one which allowed lax descriptions of the invention, a liberal policy regarding discoveries, and no clear indication that the new plant variety constituted an improvement over existing ones. These "adjustments" allowed for considerable and opportune interpretations of the law, helping facilitate the coverage of varieties which might have been excluded under more stringent rules. Still, as Allyn, Cook and others observe, many questionable patents were granted.

Finally, while the Plant Patent Act of 1930 represented a remarkable and radical change in the rules regarding ownership of plant materials, inconsistencies and deficiencies were immediately noticed. Joseph Rossman, an examiner for the Patent Office observed less than a year after passage of the PPA that:

> after the law in its present form, or as modified, has begun to function smoothly, justice demands that it be extended to cover sexually reproduced varieties. In the last analysis, this is the field most needing patent protec-

tion for no sexually reproduced variety can possibly be the result of casual hybridization, or a chance find, as are many varieties in the field covered by the present law.[82]

Remarkably, patent lawyer Allyn jokingly anticipated more radical applications. "Who," he asked, "will say that a patent may not be granted for a bread and milk plant produced by crossing a bread fruit tree with a milkweed by the dark of the moon?"[83] Paul Stark may have been right in advising the seed industry to forego the battle over PPA and allow the nursery industry to establish in the PPA a precedent for patent rights for plant breeders. But, as we shall again see in the next chapter, precedents by themselves do not create law.

## NOTES

1. Apple trees, for example, produce seed from which new trees can be obtained. But commercially, apple trees are reproduced by people using grafting techniques. A twig from a tree of the desired variety is physically joined (grafted) to an appropriate root-stock. The above-ground portion of the tree will be a clone (an "identical" copy) of the tree from that the grafted twig was taken. Had seed been used, the resulting tree would be a genetic combination of the tree from which the seed was taken and the tree which provided the pollen to fertilize it. In other words, it would not be an exact copy or a duplicate of the desired variety, as trees of the same variety cannot generally fertilize each other.

2. Of course, at this point there was no intention that we know of any actor to create such a comprehensive system involving all of these items. There was, as we shall see, a desire among some to see that sexually reproduced species be covered.

3. Weber, Max, *The Theory of Social and Economic Organization.* Edited by Talcott Parsons. New York: Oxford University Press. 1947: 328ff.

4. Burns, Tom R. and Reinhard Ueberhorst, *Creative Democracy: Systematic Conflict Resolution and Policymaking in a World of High Science and Technology.* New York: Praeger. 1988: p. 23.

5. Terry, Dickson, *The Stark Story: Stark Nurseries 150th Anniversary.* St. Louis: Missouri Historical Society. 1966: p. 40.

6. Chambliss, William, and Robert Seidman, *Law, Order and Power.* 2nd Edition. Reading, Mass.: Addison-Wesley. 1982: p. 63, 140.

7. Wickson, Edward J., *California Nurserymen and the Plant Industry: 1850–1910.* Los Angeles: California Association of Nurserymen. 1921: p. 18.

8. Ibid., p. 19.

9. Ibid., p. 21.

10. Olmo, H. P., "California," in *History of Fruit Growing and Handling in United States of America and Canada,* edited by W. H. Upshall. University Park, Penn.: American Pomological Society. 1976: p. 17.

11. Folger, J. C., and S. M. Thomson, *The Commercial Apple Industry of North America.* New York: Macmillan Co. 1921: p. 389.

12. This figure may be overstated somewhat as the data involved comes from claims made about yields and prices from "Golden Delicious" apple trees as related in the 1930 Stark Brothers Nursery Yearbook (catalog), p. 11.

13. Bailey, Liberty H., *Annals of Horticulture in North America for the Year 1893.* New York: Orange Judd Co. 1894: p. 127ff.

14. Bailey, Liberty H., *Annals of Horticulture in North America for the Year 1889*. New York: Rural Publishing Co. 1890: p. 88.

15. Information is sparse on the precise work and tactics of the associations, though Constitutions and conference agendas can sometimes be found. Most information is of a general reporting nature and can be found in books such as L. H. Bailey's *Annals of Horticulture* during the 1880s and 1890s.

16. Committee on Registration of the Peninsula Horticultural Society, "Registration of New Fruits," in *The American Garden*, Vol. XII, no. 6. June, 1891: p. 338.

17. It was four times larger than any other nursery in capitalization according to information made public in a congressional hearing on HR 13570, "Authorizing the Registration of the Names of Horticultural Products and to Protect the Same." Hearings, U.S. House Committee on Patents. 59th Congress, March 28, 1906. Washington: Government Printing Office. 1906: p. 15.

18. Terry, op. cit. For example, Speaker of the U.S. House of Representatives, Champ Clark, was a friend of the Starks and an early teacher of Lloyd Stark's. (Clark had been city attorney in Louisiana, Missouri, hometown of Stark's Nurseries.) Clark engineered a visit of President Teddy Roosevelt to the nursery and appointed Lloyd Stark to Annapolis. Lloyd would later become a Republican governor of Missouri.

19. Ibid., p. 71.

20. Telephone interview with Clay Logan, President, Stark Brothers Nurseries, Louisiana, Mo., April 24, 1992.

21. Nichols, Harry E., "Iowa," in *History of Fruit Growing and Handling in United States of America*, edited by W. H. Upshall. University Park, Penn.: American Pomological Society. 1976: p. 55.

22. Stark Brothers Nursery, *Stark Yearbook, 1930*. Louisiana, Missouri: Stark Brothers Nursery. 1930: p. 21.

23. Olmo, op. cit., p. 19.

24. Ibid., p. 19.

25. Barbee, David Rankin, "Bill Before Hoover Grants Plant Patents," *Washington Post*, May 25, 1930: p. 1. (Barbee addressed the specific failure of Stark Brothers' contracts.) Robb, Harry C., "Plant Patents." *Journal of the Patent Office Society*. Vol. XV, no. 10, October, 1933: p. 762. Harry Robb, addressed the conditions in the industry as a whole, stating that without patents the threat of "piracy" amounted to a "100% certainty."

26. White, Richard P., *A Century of Service: A History of the Nursery Industry Associations of the United States*. Washington: American Association of Nurserymen. 1975: p. 128ff.

27. Hays, W. H., "Distributing Valuable New Varieties and Breeds." *Proceedings of the First Meeting of the American Breeders' Association held in St. Louis, Mo*. Washington: American Breeders' Association. 1905: p. 62.

28. Kimmelman, op. cit., p. 181. Interestingly, Hays sought financing from large commercial agriculture concerns, including fruit growers. These were the basis of financing the ABA's *American Breeders' Magazine*.

29. U.S. House of Representatives Committee on Patents, 59th Congress, Hearings on HR 13570 "Authorizing the Registration of the Names of Horticultural Products and to Protect the Same." Washington: Government Printing Office. March 28,1906: p. 15.

30. Heitz, Andre, "History of the UPOV Convention and the Rationale for Plant Breeders' Rights, in *Proceedings, UPOV Seminar on the Nature of and Rationale for the Protection of Plant Varieties under the UPOV Convention*. Geneva: Union for the Protection of New Varieties of Plants. 1990: p. 2.

31. The nursery industry was not as weakened by government distribution of nursery stocks. By the 1920s, the government was mostly distributing reforesting and erosion-control species. This affected businesses such as Stark's only marginally.

32. American Seed Trade Association, *Proceedings of the American Seed Trade Association, 1909*. Hartford, Conn.: Hartford Press. 1909: p. 58.

33. Brown, E., "How Seed Testing Helps the Farmer," *Yearbook of Agriculture, 1915.* Washington: Government Printing Office. 1916: p. 315.
34. Stone, A. L., "20 Years of State Seed Laws," in *Seed World.* Vol. 27, No. 6. March 21, 1930: p. 28.
35. Ibid. See also "Seed Legislation" by Curtis Nye Smith (counsel to ASTA) in *Seed World,* Vol. 5, no. 9, June 6, 1919: p. 24.
36. Kloppenburg, 1988, op. cit., p. 81–82.
37. In the presentation to the ABA cited above, Hays remarks: "Inventors who create new values, and creative breeders who add to the transmitting efficiency of plants and animals, are alike in that they too often do not secure for themselves reasonable remuneration. It is to the interest of the manufacturer, the grower of pedigreed seeds or pedigreed animals, and the general public that a liberal share of the new values go to the inventor and to the creative breeder." p. 58.
38. Fairchild, David, "The Fascination of Making a Plant Hybrid." *Journal of Heredity.* Vol. XVIII, no. 2. February, 1927: p. 62.
39. It should be noted here that the Patent Act of 1790 itemized eligible subject matter. As amended in 1793, it covered "any art, machine, manufacture, or composition of matter, or any new and useful improvement." Before 1930, it was assumed that a "product of nature" could not fit into the patentable categories. See Beier, F. K. and J. Straus, "Patents in a Time of Rapid Scientific and Technological Change: Inventions in Biotechnology" in *Biotechnology and Patent Protection* by F. K. Beier, R. S. Crespi and J. Straus. Paris: Organisation for Economic Co-operation and Development. 1985: p. 25.
40. White, Richard, op. cit., p. 131.
41. Kneen, Orville H., "Patent Plants Enrich Our World," *National Geographic Magazine,* March 1948: p. 364ff.
42. Regarding the origin of the bill, it should be noted that Rep. Fred Purnell, the chief sponsor in the House, acknowledged in the hearings that he had "not had a great deal to do with the preparation of it . . . " In a telephone interview with Frank B. Robb, Harry Robb's nephew and himself a partner in the law firm of Robb and Robb (which was founded by Harry Robb and Frank Robb's father, John, Frank Robb stated that Robb and Stark worked together on the bill. He believes Harry Robb drafted the bill utilizing Stark's knowledge of plants. Harry Robb was an admirer of Burbank, according to Frank Robb, and perhaps was "encouraged" in part by a desire to see his work rewarded. Frank Robb could not say with certainty whether Harry Robb was formally employed by Stark Brothers or the AAN while he was working on the plant patent bill, however, it is known that the AAN incurred "legal expenses" during the effort to pass the legislation. (On this point, see Richard White, cited in this chapter.) After passage of the Act, Harry Robb handled most of Stark Brothers patent applications and Robb and Robb became the chief firm in the country handling plant patent applications according to both Frank Robb and Clay Logan, current president of Stark Brothers and a member of the Stark family. Interview conducted with Frank B. Robb, Willoughby, Ohio, April 28, 1992.
43. Kloppenburg, op. cit. p. 261.
44. American Seed Trade Association, 1930, op. cit., p. 66.
45. U.S. House of Representatives Committee on Patents, Report to Accompany H.R. 11372. Report No. 1129. April 30, 1930: p. 6.
46. Doyle, Jack, *Altered Harvest: Agriculture, Genetics and the Fate of the World's Food Supply.* New York: Viking. 1985: p. 51.
47. An article in *Business Week,* August 26, 1931, entitled "Patenting of Plants Promises Big Profits — and Big Problems," notes (p. 29) the possible interest of E. W. Townsend & Son of Salisbury, Maryland in using the Plant Patent Act to protect strawberry varieties. Senator Townsend is thought to have had strawberry companies operating in Maryland, though it cannot be determined for certain that there is a connection.
48. James White & Co. *The National Cyclopedia of American Biography.* Clifton, N.J.: James T. White & Co. 1982: p. 213–14

49. Terry, op. cit., p. 85.
50. This support came after a compromise, which will be discussed below involving what types of materials would be covered.
51. U.S. House of Representatives Committee on Patents, op. cit., p. 3.
52. Ibid., p. 2.
53. Ibid., p. 3.
54. Dreyer, Peter, *A Gardener Touched with Genius*. New York: Coward, McCarn & Geoghegan. 1975.
55. Luther Burbank, quoted in Dreyer, op. cit., p. 237.
56. Ibid., p. 280.
57. Terry, op. cit., p. 86. Curiously, Terry, who had access to Stark Brothers' files, shows the original Burbank statement to have been in the form of a letter addressed to Paul Stark, "Chairman, National Committee for Plant Patents." four years earlier. However, in the Congressional debate it was used as having come in an unsolicited telegram from his widow and having been a statement from a "manuscript." Stark obviously knew of the existence of the statement, but did not use it himself. Did he ask Burbank's widow to telegram for dramatic effect the statement he had received himself in a letter four years earlier?
58. *Congressional Record*, U.S. House of Representatives, May 5, 1930: p. 8392.
59. *Congressional Record*, U.S. Senate, April 17, 1930: p. 7200.
60. U.S. Senate Committee on Patents, "Report from the Committee on Patents on S. 4015. Report 315, 71st Congress, 2nd Session. April 2, 1930: p. 4.
61. After passage in the House, a motion to reconsider was defeated, evidence of some lingering but insufficient opposition.
62. White, Richard, op. cit., p. 132.
63. Anonymous, "Plant Patents with Common Names." Washington: American Association of Nurserymen. 1963: p. 1.
64. Robertson, Thomas E., "Memorandum for Secretary of Commerce R. P. Lamont," March 8, 1930.
65. Allyn, Robert Starr, *The First Plant Patents: A Discussion of the New Law and Patent Office Practice*. Brooklyn: Educational Foundations, Inc. 1934: p. 44.
66. Ibid., p. 30.
67. Ibid., p. 31ff, 39, 40.
68. Ibid., p. 31.
69. Cook, Robert, "Other Plant Patents," *Journal of Heredity*. Vol. XXIV, no. 2. February, 1933: p. 53.
70. Allyn, op. cit., p. 57.
71. Kneen, op. cit., p. 361ff.
72. This distinction is not offered here as a primarily legal one, as the original inventor could always sell the rights to someone else as in the case of "Spud" Newman. This distinction merely confirms and reinforces both the emphasis on variety production as opposed to actual breeding and invention, and the role of the propagator, which is almost always held by a company or institution.
73. U.S. Committee on Patents, op.cit., p. 6.
74. Patents Nos. 17, 19, 32, 36, 43, 44, 77 and 98 cover tuber (bulb and corm) propagated flowers — freesia, gladiolus, dahlia.
75. Rossman, Joseph, "Plant Patents," *Journal of the Patent Office*, Vol. XIII, no. 1, January 1931: p. 16.
76. Mooney, Pat Roy, "The Law of the Seed." *Development Dialogue*. No. 1-2. Uppsala: Dag Hammarskjöld Foundation. 1983: p. 160.
77. Rourke notes that political controversies typically are transformed by powerful actors into technical problems. See Rourke, Francis E., *Bureaucracy, Politics and Public Policy*. Boston: Little, Brown & Co. 1976: p. 74.
78. Burns and Ueberhorst, op. cit., p. 299.

098 Unnatural Selection

79. Chambliss and Seidman, op. cit., p. 91.
80. Ibid., p. 35.
81. Burns, Tom R., and Helena Flam, *The Shaping of Social Organization: Social Rule System Theory with Applications.* London: Sage Publications. 1987: p. 18.
82. Rossman, op. cit., p. 25. In fact, Rossman shows that he is unfamiliar with sexually reproduced plants. They can, of course, simply be found or be the result of casual crossing. The main point in the quote, however, is Rossman's correct observation that the PPA created an imbalance between the legal protection offered for different categories of plants.
83. Allyn, Robert Starr, "Plant Patent Queries: A Patent Attorney's Views on the Law," *The Journal of Heredity.* Vol. 24, no. 2. February, 1933: p. 58.

# CHAPTER 4

# The Plant Variety Protection Act of 1970

Were law simply the result of the logical, step-by-step unfolding of legal ideas, we might be able to write a system of equations to simulate it. But law is revealed and developed through social relationships.[1] It is made by actors who act in a certain context and who face constraints and opportunities as they endeavor to create new laws and alter existing social relationships. Indeed, new property laws indicate new relationships,[2] in this case between small and large seed companies, seed companies and farmers, and private and public sector plant breeders.

The passage of the Plant Patent Act (PPA) was followed by the adoption of similar laws in other countries: Germany in 1933; Austria in 1938; the Netherlands in 1941. But these laws did not expand upon the concept that limited patenting to asexually reproduced plants.

Forty years elapsed between the passage of the Plant Patent Act and the Plant Variety Protection Act of 1970. During this period, it is not the "logic" of plant variety protection that is revealed. In fact, one could argue that if the PPA were passed to protect plant breeders, it would more logically have excluded the species it covered and covered the species it excluded, for little breeding activity was occurring in asexually reproducing (nursery) crops in comparison with sexually reproducing crops in 1930. What has taken place in the intervening forty years is not so much the revealing of the wisdom of variety protection for seed-producing crops as a number of other more concrete and social factors.

The commercialization of agriculture and decline of farmer seed-saving had helped facilitate the further development of a commercial seed industry, though the persistence of seed-saving of some crops meant that further commercial opportunities remained untapped. Scientific plant breeding methods became more practical, not the least because the economic context increasingly favored their use. But, as we saw in the 1930 PPA, it is not the "discovery" of a new technology that alone provides the compelling stimulus for the passage of the new law. Significantly, we saw — particularly within the private seed industry — the organizing and strengthening of political expertise and power. Among other actors — farmers and the public sector — we find a weakening of power at least as it affects activity in the area under investigation.

99

Much of the relevant history, the broad context surrounding the passage of the Plant Variety Protection Act, is explored in the two preceding chapters and the reader is strongly urged to keep this in mind, for this context is crucial to the understanding of the developments discussed here. The present chapter adds detail to this context, and explores efforts to obtain intellectual property rights protection for new varieties of sexually reproducing plants. Themes involving rationalization and the interrelationships between law, technology and politics will once again be visited. In particular, however, this chapter focuses on the purposeful, innovative and sustained political activities of actors involved in the development and passage of the PVPA.

Thousands of "farmer varieties" existed by the 1930s. The USDA has documented literally hundreds of varieties each of wheat, oats, tomatoes, beans, etc. that farmers were using in the last century.[3] As we have seen, biological differences between these sexually reproduced plants and asexually reproduced plants (such as apples)  had an impact on the commercialization of planting materials by the seed and nursery industries. In asexually reproduced plants the nursery industry had built-in uniformity and the potential for easy name identification and protection. But in the 1930s, breeding for uniformity in seed crops was still a "tedious and expensive process," according to W. H. Nixon of the Ferry-Morse Seed Company.[4] Furthermore, inbreeding and re-crossing of most crops was still "in the experiment stage," as Nixon put it. Under such conditions, one can imagine that neither the desire for patent protection nor the capability of meeting uniformity standards under patent laws was very high in the seed business. (In fact, there was no agreement on what constituted a distinct variety at this time.[5]) As an Asgrow Seed Company advertisement put it in 1942, "one of the plant-breeder's major tasks is to maintain old varieties at their best . . . "[6] The day when plant breeders focused on creating new, distinct and uniform varieties had not yet come. Seed companies were still typically dealing in the varieties bequeathed them from earlier days by farmers and market gardeners.[7]

Through the 1940s, seed company officials had greater problems than the lack of variety protection on their minds. Unscrupulous practices still plagued both reputable companies and farmers. During the spring of 1947, 44 percent of the companies reviewed by the USDA were sent warning letters for apparent violations of the Federal Seed Act's prohibition against giving misleading impressions about the history or quality of seed in their catalogs.[8] Regulation of the industry flourished, manifesting itself in the founding of an organization of professional regulators — the Association of American Seed Control Officials (AASCO) — in 1955.

The original Federal Seed Law had been passed in 1912 and amended and expanded in 1916 and 1926. A new Federal Seed Act was passed in 1939 and amended in 1956 and 1958. These laws provided the basis for inspections of interstate shipments of seeds. In addition, all states now had state seed laws on the books, many influenced by the USDA's model uniform state seed law.

Seed company executives were understandably growing alarmed at calls for more regulation coming from seed control officials. Most disturbing was their call for "compulsory registration" of varieties. Compulsory registration meant that the government would be able to require that varieties sold in interstate commerce be discernibly different and perhaps better than those already being sold. The choice of what could be marketed would be taken from the seed company and placed in the hands of government officials.

Earl Page of Corneli Seed Company complained in the pages of the journal *Seed World* that "years of labor and thousands of dollars of expense to bring about a subtle but important improvement would be wasted if the government official ruled that the improvement was indistinguishable."[9] The AASCO favored compulsory registration at least in part as a means of giving officials greater control and clearer criteria. The association's president acknowledged that officials "promulgate rules and regulations setting forth details and clarifications as to the interpretations that they, as enforcement officers, will place on the requirement of their laws." And in a few states where no written rules existed, "enforcement practices are left to the judgment of the enforcement official."[10]

Large, reputable seed companies faced what must have been considered an uncomfortable dilemma. On the one hand, "seed control" by the government could help clean up the industry, ridding it of "bad elements." On the other, it threatened to restrict company practices and lessen what little control companies had over "their" varieties.

The ability of the "handful of seedmen who do breeding and stock seed maintenance" to exercise control over their product and profit from it was thwarted by "the financial strain of subsidizing the price cutting parasites," seedmen who took the varieties, multiplied them, and sold them at cut rates.[11] "With the increased production, [the leveling-effect of] certification, and usage of named, publicly-developed varieties, many seedsmen found themselves in competition with each other on the same items," according to Robert Kalton, the research director of Rudy-Patrick Seed Company.[12] This led to price-cutting.[13] And, Kalton claimed, it led to some companies going out of business and others beginning research programs.[14,15] As one executive put it, "we are a sick industry . . . The only valid answer is that prices have to go up."[16]

Partially as a result of these pressures plus the progressive development and availability of practical breeding techniques, and the "requiring" of new varieties of fresh vegetables (such as beans, cucumbers, tomatoes, beets, carrots, radishes and others) "tailored to suit the [mechanical harvesting] machine,"[17,18] companies began to develop more extensive in-house breeding *programs*.

In their new, focused breeding programs, companies were first interested in following the example of the corn seed industry by pursuing hybrids. Breeding of open-pollinated vegetables through major, costly and sophisticated multicrop breeding programs was not the dominant form in the seed industry in the 1950s or early 1960s though the foundations of such programs were now clearly visible. Plant breeding was ceasing to be a haphazard, individual effort and becoming a rational, planned, goal-oriented activity with a basis in science situated in commercial enterprises. The implications of this development were significant as they marked or announced a new set of possibilities, opportunities and obstacles which could affect seed as a commodity form, as a resource, and as a raw material. Similarly, these developments, while rooted in changed social relationships and influenced by scientific developments, were also part of the context in which further changes in these areas would be likely to take place.

Associated with the trends noted above was the replacement of the local market gardener with the produce/shipper and canning industries. These large growers and processors were "appreciative of minute improvements," according to Ed Weimortz, then a vice president with Ferry-Morse Seed Company. And Weimortz claims that they often displayed considerable loyalty to companies engaged in breeding. He claims that bean canners in the early 1960s might refuse to buy seed from the "pirates" even though the seed was essentially identical to that offered by the breeder and the cost was only half as much.[19] Thus, while the seed industry faced obstacles in reaping profits from its varietal development, modest breeding (or perhaps more accurately "improvement") programs were a rational and profitable tool for large seed companies wishing to address the economic pressures of the day.

There were still other more crop-specific reasons for increased private sector breeding activity. Most notable is the case of soybeans, which in the early 1950s were on their way to becoming the second most valuable crop in the country (after corn) and the principal high-protein livestock feed. Between 1950 and 1970, acreage planted to soybeans increased by almost 27,000,000 acres — 172 percent.[20] Northrup-King set up its soybean breeding program in 1969 based on the expectation that some form of variety protection was imminent.[21] Due to harvesting and handling peculiarities for soybean seed, the crop lent itself to being commercialized. But, in the absence of variety protection laws, this valuable seed also lent itself to being acquired, multiplied and sold by nonbreeding seed companies. Wheat, on the other hand, showed promise as a candidate for hybridization and several breeding programs were initiated with this in mind. By the late 1960s, however, there was some concern among industry people that wheat could not be profitably hybridized. Biological protection of wheat through hybridization was therefore in some doubt.

Initially, private sector breeding programs were largely staffed by scientists recruited from the public sector.[22] Northrup-King was involved in vegetable breeding on a fairly large scale by the early 1950s and Ferry-Morse, Burpee, and Asgrow were also engaged in breeding work.[23] During this period, seed companies gradually made the transition out of the simple selecting and "strain" development work which had characterized the early days and begin to engage in more rigorous, scientific varietal development, particularly with hybrids, as noted above.[24] By the 1960s, companies were releasing an increasing number of varieties, which they themselves had developed in breeding programs costing upwards of a total of $100,000, excluding capital outlays and equipment.[25]

Robert Kalton noted in 1963 that the sale of proprietary varieties would demand that research produce high quality seed with "assured genetic identity . . ."[26] And Harold Loden, then president of the Southern Seedsmen's Association, observed that "we have seen major expansions in private research programs within the past few years . . . Likewise, the competitive developments within the seed industry have magnified the importance of proprietary varieties in all crops."[27] While companies may have seen the advantages of engaging in research to produce "proprietary varieties" as a response to competition, low prices, and the growing market for machine-harvestable varieties, *no law existed sanctioning the proprietary status of these "proprietary varieties."*

Despite the growing importance of proprietary varieties to at least one segment of the seed industry and the absence of legal protection of those varieties, it was not immediately evident that there was anything close to a consensus regarding the desirability of new laws. In Europe, variety protection had begun to take shape in the form of laws. But at least in the minds of American seedsmen, these laws were linked with the strict compulsory registration systems found in much of Europe and abhorrent to American seedsmen. As the president of ASTA put it in 1963, European laws establishing patent-like control over new sexually reproduced plant varieties were "an integral part of a larger program which in total excludes entirely from sale any seeds which are not on the official list of approved varieties and which are not certified."[28] "Breeders' rights," he argued, entailed a loss in "breeders' freedoms."

Representatives of six European nations had gotten together in 1961 to create the Union for the Protection of New Varieties of Plants (UPOV). The creation of UPOV had been set in motion by three organizations, one of commercial plant breeders to promote plant variety protection, one organization which existed to promote industrial patents, and the International Chamber of Commerce. France hosted a preparatory meeting in 1957. Twelve countries, all from western Europe, were invited to participate in the process. Six ended up as founders of UPOV.

The issue was the establishment of proprietary rights, the securing of a tool that could be used for marketing purposes. This would not be how all attendees described their goals. French Under-Secretary of State for Agriculture Kleber Loustau talked of equity and referred to the principles that had been established by the U.S. Plant Patent Act and more generally to the United Nations' Universal Declaration of Human Rights.[29] Answering anticipated concerns about the creation of monopolies, Loustau cited the "pressing need to promote research in all its forms . . ."[30]

UPOV's achievement was the crafting of a delicate consensus on the question of how plant varieties should be protected. The result was a convention signed in 1961 which would go into effect in 1968 and would encourage the adoption of *sui generis* laws for protecting new plant varieties. The UPOV approach was to take plant variety protection out of the realm of patent law by creating its own distinct system.

Events in Europe did not go unnoticed. The larger companies in the United States were already becoming international in their outlook, a reflection of the internationalization of the business. As Allenby White of Northrup King and Co. observed in 1963: "If something happens to a crop in Fresno, California, or in Salem, Oregon, the odds are it will be known and felt in Copenhagen, Bologna, and Rotterdam by the next day. A new tariff, a new law, either here or abroad sends reverberations throughout the *international seed trade*"[31] [my emphasis].

The concept of a *sui generis* form of protection like that proposed by UPOV was not new to the U.S. seed industry, even if patents were apparently its first choice. A small British booklet on what the Europeans now called "Plant Breeders' Rights," became a "best seller among plant breeders everywhere."[32] Allenby White (who headed the international division and research for Northrup-King) and several USDA officials attended the 1961 UPOV meeting in Paris. White returned determined to bring some form of protection to American shores.

Various sectors of the seed industry were already interested in protecting their varieties. Executives of private cotton breeding operations had been discussing the matter for some time in Texas and had had meetings with experiment station officials to discuss the stations' use of privately developed cotton varieties. They had also promoted changes in certification rules to provide a degree of protection and control for breeders over their varieties.[33] At the time only a small percentage of the seed used was certified or purchased from the original developer.[34] The effort among these companies led to the formation of the National Council of Commercial Plant Breeders, which drew its membership from companies interested in a wide range of crops in addition to cotton.[35]

Already various companies and trade organizations were experimenting with different means of protection in the absence of laws. Of course many companies were trying to develop hybrid breeding programs to obviate the need for other forms of protection. Some were experimenting with breeder-grower contracts whereby the grower acknowledged ownership of the variety by the breeder and agreed to provide royalties. These agreements also dealt with the question of what happens when the grower discovers a valuable mutation in a variety "owned," according to the contract, by the breeder. This was a sensitive issue around which was much animosity. Essentially it was a fight between the breeder who does not discover and the discoverer who does not breed. Both desired to claim ownership over something for which they were only marginally responsible. Most contracts called for a split in royalties in such situations. An executive of one seed company claimed that such arrangements made further government interference unnecessary, but admitted that these nonlegislative measures were not easy to enforce.[36] Enforcement of these or industry codes of conduct faced the prospect that industry sanctions against transgressors would most likely run afoul of antitrust laws.[37] Suggestions that variety names be protected were met with the reply that that would not protect the germplasm.

Attempts to broaden the Plant Patent Act, however, might subject that act to a court challenge which could prove disastrous. At the time, the Supreme Court was regularly striking down patents for lack of invention — a point on which plant breeders would be particularly weak. One justice had remarked that the only valid patent was one that had not yet appeared in a case before the Court.[38] Industry officials were reluctant to subject themselves to the criteria and interpretations being given the patent law by the courts.[39] Furthermore, attempts to find protection under the patent umbrella might prove difficult politically. Would Congress now sanction the patenting of "food?" A 1959 attempt by potato industry interests to obtain coverage under the Plant Patent Act had failed on this basis.[40] Another unsuccessful attempt had been made in 1960.

A four-hour symposium (sponsored by a number of professional and trade organizations) attended by 600 private and public sector officials in Colorado in 1963 showed considerable differences of opinion on what to do. Few speakers seemed to have a clear idea even of what breeders' rights were. Several felt that this was an insidious attempt to institute compulsory registration of varieties with government testing and approved (and *disapproved*) varieties. One contended that "germ plasm control is in reality breeder control."[41] Seed companies wanted no part of a system which might have the government allowing access to the market only to varieties deemed by the government to be an improvement over existing ones.[42]

Addressing the symposium, Allenby White listed what he saw as the advantages and disadvantages of plant breeders' rights. The disadvantages: (1) cost of administration/testing; (2) release of varieties would be delayed; and (3) seed prices would be higher. The advantages: (1) the public would know that a new variety was distinct; (2) there would be stimulation of plant breeding in open, self-pollinated crops, but regulation might discourage it in hybrids.[43]

In a consensus statement, the symposium concluded: "Crops specialists participating in the symposium enumerated more disadvantages than advantages for a system of breeders' rights such as prescribed by the Paris Convention."[44]

The growing involvement of the American Seed Trade Association's (ASTA) in legislative matters had been facilitated by the 1960 move of its headquarters from Chicago to Washington and by increasing pressure from member companies to get more involved in politics at the national and international level.[45] This pressure resulted in a series of by-law amendments approved by a vote of the members to facilitate this "new tack." ASTA decided that its staff should relate more with the USDA, other agencies and Congress, and that the "top employed officer . . . should become a skilled and resourceful, two-way interpreter between government and industry representatives."[46]

Concurrent with ASTA's increasing politicization, it established in 1963 a committee whose driving force became Allenby White, to study developments in the field of variety protection.[47] (The committee included Harold Loden, who had been active in the efforts of Texas cotton breeders which finally resulted in the passage of state legislation offering some varietal protection through certification procedures.) Talks had been under way with the public sector for a decade over public/private relations and over the questions of protection, seed certification, and registration. Most seed companies probably wanted some form of protection, but without the burden of proving or having certified that their varieties were better or represented improvements over old varieties. However, the industry was split rather predictably. Grass and forage crop companies desperately wanted protection because of the ease of saving and multiplying such seed. (Interestingly, Allenby White's professional background was as a forage crop breeder and Northrup-King, his employer, was largely a forage seed company in those days.[48]) Companies whose main activities were in hybrids could afford to sit on the sidelines knowing that legal protection would give them little if anything that they did not already have through the biological protection of hybrids. Small companies initially perceived variety protection as a threat which would restrict their ability to sell the varieties of their choice. Still, the latter group was not as energetic in their opposition as proponents were in their advocacy. ASTA officials such as John Sutherland began meeting with company officials, in an attempt to convince small companies, for example, that variety protection would encourage research resulting in new varieties which they could obtain through contracts or integration with the large companies.

At the same time that White chaired ASTA's Breeders' Rights Committee, Dale Porter, a top lawyer for Pioneer Hi-Bred, headed up ASTA's legislative committee. This committee was primarily concerned with the Federal Seed Act and the threat of compulsory registration. Given the linkage between plant breeders' rights and registration in Europe, it was natural that White and Porter join forces. Porter, who was employed by a company primarily engaged in hybrid corn, did not see a strong corporate self-interest in promoting breeders' rights, per se, though it was recognized that variety protection would allow Pioneer to get into soybean breeding. But he and Pioneer were more interested in insuring that compulsory registration not be a part of whatever system was finally established. As he acknowledges, it was primarily a "defensive" position.[49]

ASTA's attention was apparently still focused on patents when in 1967 it proposed a simple amendment to the Plant Patent Act.[50] Where the PPA spoke of "asexually reproducing plants" the amendment would simply add "or sexually," and would have the effect of expanding the act to include all plants. This simple proposal was killed in the U.S. Senate Judiciary Committee rather simply by substantial opposition from the public breeders and the U.S. Department of Agriculture. The USDA said that enforcement would be difficult, "free interchange of information and genetic materials would be inhibited," and "it would be harmful to the small commercial breeders and seed producers."[51] Significantly, horticulturalists were unsympathetic, feeling that the inclusion of sexually reproducing seed into their act might ultimately prove to be a liability if not a threat to the act itself — a realistic view given the fact that a presidential commission on the patent system looked into the issue and stated that it did not regard the patent system to be "the proper vehicle" for protecting *either* sexually or asexually reproducing plants.[52] Even the Farm Bureau voiced its opposition. ASTA officials now began to question whether patents were the proper vehicle, because of both political difficulties and the desire to avoid legal controversies sure to arise from adding sexually reproducing plants to the patent act (as outlined above). Out of the defeated proposal came a series of meetings between the private and public sector for further discussions.

The USDA remained hostile apparently because officials felt that sexually reproducing plants could not be kept pure enough to make protection workable. And, they feared that patents would restrict the traditional free flow of information and breeding materials among scientists. Secretary of Agriculture Freeman released a strongly worded statement to Congress stressing both points. Unstated was the influence inside the USDA of certain interests such as seed control officials, who perceived the pressures of the seed industry as a threat. Nevertheless, USDA's internal study group concluded that "with the increased role of industry in developing new varieties, some sort of protection system is *inevitable*"[53] [my emphasis].

Soon thereafter a Federal-State Variety Protection Working Group was formed. In late 1968 and early 1969, four study groups held meetings around the country involving public agency officials. The American Seed Trade Association participated in these meetings. At the first two meetings, ASTA described four alternatives — three involving amendments to the Plant Patent Act (which the Judiciary Committee had already turned down) and a fourth involving amendments to the Federal Seed Act.

The Plant Variety Protection Act (PVPA) was "drafted by ASTA during early January 1969," according to Martin Weiss of the USDA. By mid-January, ASTA had decided to drop the other alternatives and go with PVPA.[54] John Sutherland, ASTA's top staff person, sat down over a weekend with a copy of the 1930 Plant Patent Act, pulled sections out and fashioned a crude draft. Loden recalls that ASTA employed a Chicago attorney, Louis Robertson (since deceased), who did the major part of the drafting and legal work on the bill.[55] In any case, both Robertson and Sutherland, of course, were well aware of the UPOV model and it was helpful too; but for reasons previously outlined, ASTA proceeded to fashion its own bill.[56] The Sutherland draft was worked on intensively for three days by Sutherland, Porter of Pioneer Hi-Bred, and White of Northrup-King at Northrup-King's headquarters in Minneapolis. Robertson continued to provide valuable legal advice.[57]

In brief, the Plant Variety Protection Act would grant a 17-year "patent-like" certificate for new varieties of sexually reproducing plants. It would not cover hybrids. But the breeder of a new, open-pollinated variety of corn, for example, could obtain a certificate if the government accepted the breeder's application attesting that the variety was new, distinct, uniform and stable. Enforcement of the act was left to the certificate-holder, through the civil courts. Finally, in apparent recognition of the fact that it is not just law but the administration of law that is important, the bill as drafted by ASTA called for the establishment of a PVP office and a commissioner of PVP. According to a future president of ASTA, James Chaney, "The important point here is that this office will be totally separated from the USDA's Consumer and Marketing Service, which is the agency charged with enforcement of our Federal Seed Act. This separation of powers is considered important by our industry."[58] As Chaney and others in the industry understood, it was important to insure that the Act would be administered by people more sympathetic than the seed control officials, whom industry could not trust.

Sutherland, White, Loden, and others held numerous meetings with the seed trade and with farmers' groups around the country to mobilize support for variety protection. As Loden put it, "Any time we heard of a pocket of opposition we would go and sit down and talk to them."[59] They attended state seed association meetings and pressed the case that the bill would not harm small-scale seed traders. Among these meetings was one with the Texas Seedsmen's Association. Congressman Poage of Texas was then the powerful chairman of the House Committee on Agriculture and as it turned out Representative Eligio "Kika" de la Garza of Texas chaired the subcommittee to which the bill would be referred, thus Sutherland felt it was important to mobilize support in Texas. Sutherland asked for Loden's help and Loden turned to the "legislative man" at Anderson Clayton, the parent company of Paymaster (Loden's employer). George Hall, who was a friend of Congressman Graham Purcell's, agreed to approach him to sponsor the bill. Purcell consented.[60]

The elections in the fall of 1968 brought a new party and a new president into power. Richard Nixon appointed Clifford Hardin as Secretary of Agriculture. Clifford Hardin appointed Richard Lyng to be one of his assistant secretaries. (Lyng was on the way up. By the end of his professional career in the 1980s, Lyng had been a state director of agriculture in California under Governor Ronald Reagan, and a Secretary of Agriculture under President Ronald Reagan.) Of interest at this point is the fact that he and his family had owned and operated a seed business which they sold to Northrup-King.[61] The seed industry would have had the ear of the new assistant secretary.

Officials from a number of seed trade and breeding organizations, including ASTA, met with staff of Lyng's department and others from USDA. A meeting in March, 1969, ended without agreement. But progress had been made. According to Weiss, "interchanges of viewpoints continued until all major differences relating to the systems and extent of variety protection were reconciled."[62]

Prior to the negotiations both White and the USDA committee had described the establishment of some type of protection system as "inevitable." White's goal was to bring the USDA "on board." At the political level the USDA was now potentially sympathetic to ASTA's position. The final key to this support was J. Phil Campbell. Campbell, then under secretary of agriculture, had been Georgia's commissioner of agriculture for some years and was a close personal friend of Harold Loden's. Campbell had helped write and pass a strong Georgia state seed law. In a meeting with Loden, Campbell insisted that ASTA's bill explicitly provide for farmers being allowed to save their own seed and sell some of this seed to neighbors. Without this provision, he indicated that the USDA would oppose the bill. Loden doubts that Campbell had "a single person" pressure him to take this stance. According to Loden, it simply grew out of Campbell's experiences in Georgia and his personal opinions.[63] Thus it does not appear that the provision securing farmers' rights to save and (to a limited extent) trade in seeds of protected varieties — a major provision in PVPA defining relationships between farmers, companies, and seed — owes its existence to either direct farmer or public breeder lobbying.[64]

As the PVPA would not establish plant *patents*, strictly speaking, proponents were successful in getting hearings scheduled in the Agriculture Committee, a friendlier forum than the House Judiciary Subcommittee on Patents, chaired by Representative Robert Kastenmeier, a foe of the proposal.

As congressional representatives considered the bill, they needed only to glance at their morning newspapers to learn of the crisis in which American farmers and the seed industry found themselves — a crisis that appeared to require a plant breeding solution. It seems that virtually every hybrid seed corn company — and public program — was using the same source of cytoplasmic male sterility (CMS), a device that reduces the cost of producing the hybrids. Agronomists in the Philippines had warned of a disease blight in 1961. Subsequent reports linking the blight to this trait failed to result in any changes in the way companies produced their hybrids. In the spring of 1970 the blight took hold in Florida and began racing northward. By the time cold weather stopped it that fall, it had marched through most of the South. Half of some southern states' corn crop was destroyed. Nationwide, the harvest loss was put at 15 percent — more than a billion bushels.[65]

Allenby White, in the position generally accorded the most important person supporting the dominant viewpoint, led the list of those testifying in Representative Eligio "Kika" de la Garza's Subcommittee on Departmental Operations of the House Committee on Agriculture. Gone were the concerns White had expressed to the symposium seven years earlier: the cost of administration and testing, the delay of new varieties, and higher seed prices. Other concerns were simply turned into positives. Addressing the threat of plant breeders' rights to public plant breeding, White told the subcommittee that the bill would "*allow* our Government agricultural experiment stations to increase their efforts on needed basic research" [my emphasis]. He noted that "it would permit public expenditures for applied plant breeding to be deviated to important areas which industry may not pursue" (a clear reference to the coming division of labor between public and private sector, and attempts to remove the public sector as a competitor to commercial plant breeders). White asserted that the act "will give farmers and gardeners more choice, and varieties which are better in yield or in quality, and so forth," while rejecting any notion of registration or quality testing by the government to verify such claims as a requirement for coverage under PVPA.

White reviewed the process of consultations with government officials that had taken place during the drafting of the legislation. He described the March, 1969, meeting with USDA officials saying that many "significant amendments" had been made concerning the public interest, "especially that of the farmer," who, it should be noted, was not represented at the meeting by any organization. The resulting bill, according to White, represented "a real testimonial to the efficacy of sincere Government-industry dialog."

White briefly reviewed objections, seemingly unaware of a major one that was about to drop. Of the concern over higher seed prices, he observed, curiously, that "the purchaser may choose the price he is willing to pay." Of the concern over the restriction of germplasm, he claimed:

"Whether this happens or not will be determined by the policy of the individual experiment station." Nothing was said about exchanges between companies. Objections raised by the Washington (State) Wheat Commission regarding insuring of baking qualities of wheat were dismissed with the observation that state laws could be passed regulating quality, if necessary. And finally, White claimed that the act would be "essentially self-financed."[66]

A string of corporate executives followed White, some making claims quite similar to those made for the 1930 act. Harold Loden of ACCO Seed (and a future president and employee of ASTA) observed that the act would "aid in our Nation's commitments to aid in feeding and clothing the underdeveloped nations of the world."[67] After a great deal of persuasion, Paul Stark of Stark Brothers, the principal architect behind the 1930 Plant Patent Act, appeared to support the PVPA and warned, as he had forty years earlier, that it should not be made part of the Plant Patent Act.[68]

The surprises of the day came from two unexpected sources. Andrew Klein, a patent lawyer and chairman of the committee of the American Bar Association formed to investigate this bill, appeared saying he had found out about the hearings only the day before, "by accident." He stated that the majority on his committee disapproved of the PVPA. Klein argued — strangely and erroneously — that the PVPA would invalidate the Plant Patent Act.[69]

A few minutes later Eldrow Reeve of Campbell Soup Company took his seat at the witness table. Reeve charged that the PVPA would "severely impede progress in the development of new varieties of plants." It would delay the release of new varieties and restrict access to germplasm. In recent years leading up to this bill, Reeve claimed, "there has been a perceptible reluctance among plant breeders to exchange genetical material. We believe enactment of HR 13634 would essentially eliminate exchange of valuable germ plasm and severely curtail the development of new varieties." Reeve ended by adding that administration of the act would be difficult and costly and that the present system "encourages creativity and affords seed certification and development of F1 hybrids."[70] Reeve offered no compromises publicly. Privately, representatives of Campbell's and Heinz stated that they wanted all vegetables and fungi explicitly deleted from the bill. Negotiations with seed industry officials indicated that Campbell's and Heinz would not endorse the PVPA without concessions. Ultimately they stated that they could live with the act if it excluded three vegetables, but they quickly amended the offer to add three more.[71]

Hearings in the Senate the following day were a repeat of the first day's hearings. There were no new surprises. The American Bar Association's and Campbell's opposition were not enough to stop the bill. It passed both committees. Remarkably, in the House Committee's report on the bill to the full House, almost two pages of Allenby White's testimony were lifted and used verbatim, without attribution, as the official findings of the committee.[72]

The Senate Committee on the Judiciary was also looking at the bill. Senator Eastland of Mississippi, using his prerogative as chairman of the Senate Judiciary Committee, had asked that the bill be sent to his committee. While Eastland was regarded as close to the National Cotton Council, he had other countervailing pressures causing him to be concerned about the bill. Campbell's was considering the construction of a large processing plant in his state. According to Loden, Campbell's told the senator it would pull out of Mississippi if the PVPA were passed. Eastland in turn let it be known that the bill was dead unless Campbell's could be placated[73] and offered the assistance of his staff in arranging a compromise. In the late fall of 1970, after the hearings, a meeting in Denver, Colorado, involving ASTA (mostly garden seed companies) and the Cotton Council resolved to try to settle the dispute by agreeing to delete the six vegetables from the act. Significantly, at this meeting ASTA pledged to the affected companies to work to end the exemption "at the earliest possible moment."[74] (ASTA's attempt to do so is the focus of the next chapter.)

In the three months that passed between the hearings in June and the release of the Judiciary Committee's report in September, 1970, an accommodation had been reached with Campbell Soup Company on the extent of coverage of the act.[75] The Committee reported the bill favorably having added an amendment that the act would not apply to carrots, celery, cucumbers, okra, peppers, and tomatoes!

The Committee explained its action saying:

> One significant segment of the industry, which is engaged in the processing of vegetables, conducts its own research and development programs aimed at developing new varieties which best fit its requirements. In order to utilize the benefits of mass production techniques, it is essential that this segment of the industry have high quality varieties which are ideally suited to the soils and climate in different production areas and which are also susceptible to rapid mechanical harvesting. This segment of the industry is not engaged in research designed to develop new varieties for sale in commercial seed channels. Since they do not produce new varieties for sale as such and their business is not related thereto, no useful purpose would be gained by having the provisions of this bill apply to them.[76]

The explanation obviously does not tell the full story. Companies like Campbell's were not the only ones engaged in the breeding of these crops.[77] Seed companies and public sector breeders were also involved.

The "logic" of excluding these vegetables would be equally valid when applied to many other species. So the claim that the act would serve no useful purpose in covering these vegetables clearly ignores the fact that some other problem must have been foreseen — a problem the report avoids mentioning, perhaps because this problem would also apply to all of the species covered by the act, or perhaps because the problem was political and the solution would involve accommodation of one or two private companies. The problem, in fact, as seen by Campbell's was that raised in its testimony: the restriction on exchanges of germplasm, the delays in issuance of new varieties, and the point not raised — the desire of Campbell's, Heinz, and others to avoid higher seed prices and royalty payments. The USDA could have seconded several of Campbell's concerns. They realized that protection requirements and the application process itself would inevitably hold up releases of new varieties and they anticipated a "flood of applications" from companies that had been sitting on varieties in anticipation of the enactment of the PVPA.[78] These would be issues of concern to food processors and firms, like Campbell's, whose in-house breeders had traditionally benefited from access to public and private sector germplasm and finished varieties. Campbell's wanted to be sure that there were tomato varieties available that precisely suited their processing needs, thus they engaged in breeding. Could they be assured of this in the future without unrestricted access to germplasm?

Apparently the seed industry elected not to fight the issue of exempting the six vegetables and risk defeat of the bill. Better to achieve protection for all species but six than none at all.

Meanwhile in Congress, some supporters of the PVPA invoked scenes of the corn blight to encourage colleagues to support the seed industry in finding a solution to this terrible problem — even though it was commercial concentration on hybrids (and the use of uniform CMS) that had precipitated the problem. In any event, the act would not encourage solutions for the blight or research in the corn business. Hybrids (which dominated the marketplace) were ineligible for coverage under the PVPA and the industry was already well on its way to replacing the CMS which produced vulnerability to the blight.

Little debate took place when the bill reached the floor of the House. The Campbell's challenge had been accommodated. The seed industry was in no mood to fight Campbell's. They had waited forty years. The "foot in the door" which they hoped the PPA would be was just that — just a foot in the door. The seed industry would get its PVPA. But coverage would not extend to the six vegetables of most concern to Campbell's.

The bill proposed protection for all new sexually reproducing plant varieties that met certain requirements of distinctness, uniformity, and stability. The period of protection was 17 years. Reflecting the seed industry's suspicions of variety testing and compulsory registration, the bill established its own Plant Variety Protection Office to administer the Act, removing and separating it from several seemingly appropriate USDA agencies which industry officials feared might have a tendency to be unfriendly.

In addition to the Campbell's Soup compromise, the final PVPA bill contained major concessions for farmers and to those concerned about tying up breeding materials. Farmers would specifically be allowed to save their own seed for replanting and could even sell PVPA-protected seeds to neighbors if that were not their principal business. (Even Allenby White testified that he viewed this as a "right" held by farmers.[79]) PVPA-protected varieties could also be used as breeding material for the creation of new, protectable varieties without any form of licensing or royalties. For public sector breeders and seed control officials who had resisted the concept of breeders' rights for some years, H. R. Fortmann of the Northeast Association of Agricultural Experiment Stations stated simply: "There really isn't much more to say. We have seen; we have considered; we have compromised . . ."[80] As John Sutherland of ASTA saw it, "Let's take 98 percent of our cake and we can come back later" for the rest.[81]

Jack Doyle recounts the process under which the PVPA was formally approved:

> When Congress finally moved to "consider" the Plant Variety Protection Act for final passage, it was under the worst of circumstances: a pre-holiday, end-of-Congress, lame-duck session in December 1970, with mountains of left-over business to attend to . . . Final House approval of the bill occurred under a suspension of the rules, and the measure was passed on a voice vote.[82,83]

It is safe to say that few representatives understood what the bill was about. Only seven spoke. Kastenmeier, whose committee had been avoided for the main hearings, complained about possible costs to the farmer and about the potential for restricting of information and breeding materials. But there was no organized opposition.

The next day the Senate passed the bill and it was on its way to Richard Nixon's desk. But something funny happened on the way to this forum.

As was the custom in the White House, a memo was prepared outlining the pros and cons of the bill. This memo would normally contain a recommendation to the president as to whether he should sign or veto the bill. Nine agencies were involved in the review process for this bill. Two recommended a veto, two recommended signing, and five expressed no opinion or at least voiced no objection. On the surface the contest pitted the opposition of the Office of Management and Budget (OMB) and the president's special assistant for consumer affairs (Virginia Knauer) against the bill's supporters, the USDA and the U.S. Civil Service Commission.

The Justice Department's Richard Kleindienst noted that protection did not seem to be needed in order to produce fine, new varieties and offered the example of Norman Borlaug, who earlier that month had received the Nobel Peace Prize for his work in Mexico breeding new wheats. John Sutherland, ASTA's chief lobbyist for the bill, recalls that the Justice Department, not the OMB, was the chief obstacle. Loden confirms Sutherland's view. The Justice Department was simply against the grant of "exclusive rights" in any field, and in this instance particularly one involving food production. Asked to recount how the department's opposition was overcome, Sutherland replied, "I can tell you a lot of things that were happening, but I'm not going to." He said his bosses at ASTA left him alone and didn't tell him how to get the job done. He "didn't do anything illegal," but the story, if told, would embarrass some people.[84] In a subsequent interview, Sutherland stated that he was never aware of exactly who within the Justice Department opposed the PVPA, though he knew it was a high-ranking official. He went on to say that Attorney General John Mitchell interceded to reverse the opposition of his own department. Sutherland claims to have had "direct" access to Mitchell.[85] Sutherland also acknowledged that J. Phil Campbell, an under secretary of agriculture, was quite helpful (though the implication in the interview was that Campbell did not actually help with this particular problem).[86]

The OMB and the USDA had an initial meeting to air their differences. Richard Lyng participated actively, arguing that the industry had to have this bill. But the OMB, perhaps acting as surrogate or messenger for the Justice Department, was unconvinced. Two days before the president had to act (a bill is "pocket vetoed" if it is not signed within ten days), a memo was prepared recommending a veto, complete with a proposed statement announcing the veto. The statement said that no convincing case had been made for the bill and cited the likelihood of higher seed prices to farmers, "deleterious effect(s)" on free exchange, and the difficulties of enforcement.

According to Doyle, the veto message was stopped by OMB director, George Shultz (later to become Reagan's secretary of state). Shultz ordered his assistant director to change the memo to recommend approval. As an agency, OMB "clears and coordinates departmental advice on proposed legislation and makes recommendations about presidential action on legislative enactments."[87] Thus, OMB's action could have come about as a result either of a reversal of the Justice Department's opposition, or the convincing of the OMB itself of the merits of the bill despite the opinion of the Justice Department, or both. A case can be made that both took place.

Loden cites Richard Lyng (assistant secretary of agriculture, whose family had sold their seed business to Northrup-King) as being instrumental.[88] Some years later over lunch, Loden recalls that Lyng said he had to go to a friend in the Office of Management and Budget and solicit his help. Lyng was well connected at OMB, being a personal friend of Casper Weinberger, who was then deputy director.[89] But it was Associate Director Arnold Weber, whom Lyng remembers having to convince. Weber called Lyng saying that he wanted to talk to him about the PVPA which he described as a "terrible" piece of legislation. Lyng met with Weber and as he describes it, "I don't know whether the wisdom of my argument prevailed, or if these were just friends of mine."[90] Lyng recalls having spoken to both Harold Loden and Allenby White ("a good friend") about the legislation, but denies that he was a expert on this bill. The discussion at OMB, according to Lyng, did not center on the technical aspects of the bill as much as on Lyng's general philosophical support for the bill. It was through this personal contact, according to Loden, that the opposition was quickly reversed.[91]

It was now December 24, 1970. A hasty, unenthusiastic rewrite of the memo was made. Compare the concluding paragraph of the memo recommending a veto (on the left), with the rewritten memo recommending support (on the right):

**Table 5.** Veto Becomes Approval, PVPA, 1970

| Recommendation for Veto | Recommendation for Approval |
| --- | --- |
| "On balance, we believe the extension of a monopoly right to this type of food and textile producing plant varieties has not been justified by a clearly demonstrated need. In addition, there are other practical and administrative problems which would benefit from further study. Accordingly, we recommend disapproval of the bill and have prepared the attached draft memorandum of disapproval for your consideration." | "In summary, protection of food and textile producing plant varieties of this type has not, in our view, been justified by a clearly demonstrated need. In addition, there are other practical and administrative problems which would benefit from further study. Accordingly, we think that more extensive consideration of this proposal by the congressional committes concerned would have been desirable. However, we do not believe that these concerns warrant your disapproaval of the bill." |

"Some retired USDA officials who were involved in the USDA/BOB review of the patent bill say that the seed industry had a contact in the White House who helped persuade BOB and the President of the merits of the Act," according to Doyle.[92] That could well have been Lyng's contacts at OMB itself, for Shultz as OMB director had been moved into the White House, had regular access to the president and served essentially as a "White House Special Assistant," thus blurring "the distinction between personal and institutional staff responsibilities . . . ."[93]

Later on December 24, 1970, taking OMB's recommendation, Nixon signed the bill. On the night before Christmas, industry had its long-awaited prize.

## DISCUSSION

Between 1930 and 1970, growth of the seed industry proceeded with the further commercialization of agriculture and commodification of seed. Farmers had been and the public sector (to a lesser extent) was being removed as obstacles to the privatization of seed. The Plant Variety Protection Act was seen by many within both the private and public sectors as a tool that would facilitate a further division of labor between the two sectors, decreasing public sector involvement in varietal breeding and release of crops also bred by private companies. A number of factors were at work here including the role of research, the low price of farm commodities, and the emphasis on production. The seed industry support-ed many of these developments and became a major beneficiary of them.

Not only had the seed-saving farmer disappeared, but we now know that much of the seed farmers had been saving had also disappeared (see appendix 1). The explosion of diversity which had been ignited by seed collecting and distribution programs and by immigration was wiped out as farmers ceased saving their own seed. Irrespective of the quality of these varieties relative to purchased seed, the farmer lost a measure of self-reliance in the process. And some portion of the germplasm itself, with all of its adaptation to different American environments, pests, diseases, and cultures became extinct, never again to be seen or used by a farmer or professional plant breeder. This loss of control of seeds and subsequent dependence on purchased seed is highlighted in table 12 in appendix 1 which compares the number of varieties in use from the 1800s to 1903 as cataloged by the USDA, with the number of these same varieties that could be found in U.S. government collections in the 1980s. This table indicates a significant, progressive reduction in germplasm available to U.S. farmers and it dramatically shows the degree to which farmer-bred varieties in the United States came to be replaced. (See chapter 6 for a further discussion of the importance of farmer-bred varieties in international politics.)

While Mendel's laws of heredity had been known for seventy years by 1970, their use in commercial plant breeding programs was still being articulated and developed, demonstrating clearly the importance of social factors to the employment of science and technology. Discoveries in and of themselves are not enough to insure use. Deployment and effects of deployment are contextually bound in social reality. In this case are specifically illustrated the importance, first, of commercial developments to the use of scientific innovations, and second, the way in which these scientific and commercial developments influenced the making of law — law which according to some actors would reward and encourage research.

In the context of commercial developments and the concentration of seed production into the hands of a few, advances in science and plant breeding techniques helped cast a new light and a new value on genes. "Genetic erosion," the loss of genetic diversity through extinction, has been an unintended consequence of modern plant breeding. To the extent that a breeder produces a successful variety, it can displace genetic material needed for future breeding programs. The loss of genetic diversity was realized by some to be the loss of valuable genes. The transformation of a once abundant resource into a rare one was the beginning of a new twist to an old problem: how to guarantee access to this shrinking resource and how to exercise control over it. The question of control and ownership thus expanded, slowly and subtley, from plant varieties to the genes themselves. This issue was not faced directly by 1970 but during the 1970s and early 1980s the conditions were being created for it to surface and some of the actors were beginning to see some of the dimensions of this problem — a problem we shall explore in later chapters.

"Qualitative shifts and new orders of magnitude" in problems of control, management and organization have often been associated with major changes in technology.[94] Scientific and technological advances and commercial developments created the possibility of privatizing the breeding and marketing of one very valuable crop (corn) without the need of formal legal protection which had been sought since the 1800s. However, with open-pollinated crops, the technology presented the opportunity of separating farmers from seed development *without* necessarily facilitating the control of new varieties by individual actors. The technology may have been too complicated or inaccessible for farmers, but there were private firms willing and able to use the technology to thwart attempts by

individual breeders to control their new varieties. Though there was
nothing strictly or legally preventing the use of Mendelian genetics, lack
of enforceable rules over the ownership and control of the results of
genetic work was seen by certain seed companies engaged in breeding
work as a deterrent to their receiving full or adequate benefits (thereby
reducing the incentive for further research and development). In this
sense, the law was viewed as inadequate in helping secure these benefits
in light of new scientific and technological developments and the commercial opportunities they presented.

While the scientific developments described thus far were important,
one cannot fail to appreciate the importance of the political and economic
conditions and the development of the capability of exploiting these
developments. The "causal lines," as Weber notes, run back and forth
between technical, economic and political factors. "There is no resting
point."[95] Interestingly, just as the development of systematized, written
music in the West made it possible to assign "credit" to individual
composers, according to Weber,[96] certain advances in plant breeding
made possible (but not inevitable) recognition and assignment of value to
the contributions of individual, professional plant breeders. The passage
of the 1970 PVPA cannot, however, be explained by asserting that the
economic system or the new plant breeding technologies simply called
forth or generated the legislation. Even if one were to claim that systems
and technologies have needs — a dubious proposition — the existence of
such needs would not guarantee or explain their fulfillment. Nor can we
explain the PVPA as the inevitable result of extending the legal logic
embodied in the 1930 Plant Patent Act. (Considerable effort was to be
expended just in getting grudging and qualified endorsement of the PVPA
by the main supporter of the PPA.) I have tried here to explain the passage
of the PVPA by identifying specific actors and examining their goal-
oriented action within a context which, as described, at times both
constrained and facilitated that action. These actors made a sustained
effort to legislate, particularly intensive from the early 1960s onward. The
result of these endeavors was change, socially conditioned.

In the founding of UPOV were clear indications that the seed industry
was becoming an international one. The regulations and legal protection
advanced by UPOV crossed borders. In the United States, however, a
powerful segment of the seed industry had its sights set on domestic
protection for "its" varieties. In the fight for PVPA, that segment showed
flexibility and the beginnings of political power. An ability to organize
and overcome divisions within the industry was also demonstrated by the
large companies engaged in breeding of certain crops, as witnessed in the

efforts of Allenby White and Harold Loden, who successfully assuaged the fears of small companies.

A new administration in Washington demonstrated that the public sector could be divided, with some offices less enthusiastic about PVPA than others. Public officials did not necessarily support the interests of the public sector as then organized. They joined forces with industry to help restructure public breeding and research efforts along lines more "complementary" to private sector activities. Public plant breeders sought to mitigate the effects of what they realized was the "inevitable" introduction of some form of protection for private plant breeders. Their influence over the process was quite real (and may account for the research exemption and public breeders' eligibility for PVPA certificates), but by the time the PVPA bill was introduced into Congress their choices were well constrained.

While the arena in which the PVPA was won was a public one, the debate was handled as quietly as possible, with as few participants as possible. (This, however, is not meant to imply conspiracy.) At this stage, the policy system had no public input. Important decisions could be made without the need or bother of involving the public. The crucial events in the "public" debate were not public at all: the initial meetings between the industry and the USDA, the drafting of the bill, the accommodation with Campbell's Soup Company, and the final, last-minute lobbying in the White House. In this respect, the legislative history of the PVPA conforms to Ripley and Franklin's description of the workings of a "subgovernment," typically composed of some elected officials, a few bureaucrats and representatives of private groups involved in the particular issue.[97] One may be more likely to find this subgovernment formation operating on reasonably noncontroversial matters, where there is a possibility as well as an incentive and tendency to reach agreement within such a circle and avoid enlarging the group creating a more public situation. Indeed, while one might argue that the PVPA was quite important in that it defined and reformulated property relations, it nonetheless was not an issue that actively involved more than a tiny handful of the hundreds of representatives and senators in the U.S. Congress. None attempted to take advantage of the issue politically with the general public. It could be argued that few, if any, were fully educated about the subject addressed by the act.

ASTA's drafting of the PVPA was, therefore, not simply an example of an ordinary, garden-variety interest group at work. It indicates that ASTA was gaining and using political power — that it had the stature, standing, and credibility to presume to draft its own legislation and, with the help of contacts in influential positions, push it through Congress. ASTA's insistence on establishing a PVPA office removed from seed control agencies demonstrates an awareness of the importance not just of achieving the law but of controlling its administration and influencing the regulatory process. By the time the PVPA was passed, ASTA was an actor of growing political sophistication and power, far improved over the days prior to the passage of the PPA in 1930 when it could do little to keep from being dealt out of that legislation.

The property rights established by the PVPA are property rights over *varieties* of plants, in biological terms over certain *combinations* of genes. In this respect the act defines new relationships between the owners of these rights and other actors, particularly those companies that previously multiplied and resold varieties bred by others. This practice was made illegal under PVPA and civil remedies backed by the enforcement of the state were provided for under the act. This gave legitimacy to the notion of ownership of varieties (thus formalizing the illegitimacy of "piracy") and changed the nature of marketing, the securing of market position, and enforcement of rights. It also replaced the "gentlemen's agreements" that heretofore had discouraged "piracy."

The 1970 PVPA also overcame a seemingly major political obstacle always faced before that time — the resistance to the patenting of "food." This resistance was overcome through the efforts of new actors with sufficient power to change rule systems regarding plant variety ownership. The passage of PVPA thus indicated a shift in power, control, and access over plant genetic resources from farmers and the government to the private sector.

The exclusion of six vegetables from the act reveals the limits of the power of the seed industry and the constraints imposed by the power of opposing actors with different and conflicting desires.

This was not a test of industry versus anti-industry forces, but a challenge posed by different segments within the broader seed industry. Companies (such as processors) engaged in breeding for their own purposes have little use for proprietary varieties. They are more concerned that patent-like laws may deter the full and free exchange of germplasm used in their breeding programs. Other companies engaged in breeding for commercial sales to farmers and competing with other companies for that market are more interested in protecting their varieties and securing their position in the market. Understandably, they may be reluctant to exchange germplasm, if that resource may end up benefiting a competitor. The interests of these two types of companies, a Campbell's Soup and a

Northrup-King, for example, clashed in 1970. The effect was a law that looks strangely illogical if one does not understand the context of the legislative struggle.

Finally, in the PVPA we see the seeds of a future battle. Specifically they are tomato, celery, pepper, okra, carrot and cucumber seeds — the crops specifically excluded from coverage under the PVPA. When the next battle was fought over these six crops, the world would have changed almost as dramatically as it did between 1930 and 1970. The fight for six vegetables was very different than history might lead us to suspect.

## NOTES

1. Milovanovic, Dragan, *Weberian and Marxian Analysis of Law: Development and Functions of Law in a Capitalist Mode of Production.* Aldershot, U.K.: Avebury. 1989: p. 24.
2. Chambliss, William, and Robert Seidman, *Law, Order and Power.* Second Edition. Reading, Mass.: Addison-Wesley. 1982: p. 35.
3. USDA data indicate over 500 varieties of garden beans, over 500 varieties of cabbage and nearly 500 varieties of lettuce and radish, for example. See Tracy, W. W., Jr., *American Varieties of Vegetables for the Years 1901 and 1902.* Bureau of Plant Industry, Bulletin No. 21, U.S. Department of Agriculture. Washington, D.C.: Government Printing Office. 1907.
4. Nixon, W.H., "Vegetable Breeding Is Important," *Seed World.* Vol. 32, No. 1. July 8, 1932: p. 12.
5. Hastings, Donald M., "Vegetable Seed Novelties and New Important Seed Strains," *Seed World.* Vol 32, no. 2. July 22, 1932: p. 12.
6. Associated Seed Growers, "Old Favorites Can Be Well Bred Too!" *Seed World.* Vol. 51, no. 5. March 6, 1942: p. 6.
7. Nixon, op. cit., p. 12.
8. Anonymous, "Editorial." *Seed World.* Vol. 61, no. 18. September 19, 1947: p. 7.
9. Page, Earl M., "Compulsory Registration of Varieties," *Seed World.* Vol 90, no. 3. February 9, 1962: p. 19.
10. Midyette, J. W., Jr., "Compulsory Registration of Varieties," *Seed World.* Vol. 90, no. 8. April 27, 1962: p. 14.
11. Carter, William B., "Speaking Out on Vegetable Seed Prices," *Seed World.* Vol. 90, no. 7. April 13, 1962: p. 1. Note that the seedsmen referred to here were not those dealing with hybrids. Hybrids do not reproduce true to the variety. Thus competitors were not able to reproduce hybrid seed and compete with the original breeder.
12. Kalton, Robert R., "The Impact of Commercial Research Programs on Field Seeds," *Seed World.* Vol. 92, no. 7. April 12, 1963: p. 6.
13. Prices were stable or declined during the 1950s and early 1960s according to Neil McMullin, *Seeds and World Agricultural Progress.* Washington: National Planning Association. 1987: p. 91.
14. Kalton, op. cit., p. 6.
15. Dr. Ed Weimortz, vice president of the international division of Ferry-Morse Seed Company during this period, reinforced in a telephone interview (Woodland, Calif., June 15, 1992) that the effects of competition compelled the large seed companies to devote more resources to varietal development despite the risk of pirating. Development of new varieties established the company with the consumer and large companies with efficient marketing systems could still reap a profit despite the effects of pirating.

16. Carter, op. cit., p. 1.
17. Page, Earl M., "Garden Seed Breeding And Production in the United States," *Seed World*. Vol. 92, no. 10. May 24, 1963: p. 10.
18. In 1973, Jim Hightower identified "without making any deliberate effort," mechanization projects involving 25 different crops at various agricultural colleges in the U.S. See Jim Hightower, *Hard Tomatoes, Hard Times*. Cambridge, Mass.: Schenkman Publishing. 1973. (Mechanization of some crops such as cotton, was already well advanced. See George Tindall's *The Emergence of the New South, 1913–1945*. Baton Rouge:Louisiana University Press. 1948.)
19. Interview with Dr. Ed Weimortz. As large growers, produce/shippers stood to gain from varietal improvements made by seed companies. Given that seed constituted a relatively small part of overall costs of production, even tiny improvements in yield might more than offset the increased cost of supporting the seed breeder by foregoing the cheaper, "pirated" seed.
20. Schaub, James, W. C. McArthur, et. al., *The U.S. Soybean Industry*. U.S. Department of Agriculture, Economic Research Service, Agricultural Economic Report No. 588. Washington: U.S. Government Printing Office. May, 1988: p. 4.
21. Telephone interview with Dr. Robert Romig, ice president for research, Northrup-King, Minneapolis, Minn., June 15, 1992.
22. Kalton, Robert, op. cit., p. 6.
23. Interview with Don Duvick (retired vice president for research for Pioneer Hi-Bred), Des Moines, Iowa, May 21, 1992. (Duvick visited Northrup-King in 1952 and saw their breeding programs.)
24. Interview with Dr. Ed Weimortz.
25. Kalton, op. cit., p. 6.
26. Ibid., p. 10.
27. Loden, Harold D., "Speaking Out On Research In The Seed Industry," *Seed World*. Vol. 93, no. 10. November 22, 1963: p. 2.
28. Clark, A. Bryan, "Breeders' Rights and Breeders' Freedom," *Seed World*. Vol. 93, no. 12. December 27, 1963: p. 15.
29. Heitz, Andre, "History of the UPOV Convention and the Rationale for Plant Breeders's Rights," in *Proceedings, UPOV Seminar on the Nature of and Rationale for the Protection of Plant Varieties under the UPOV Convention*. Geneva: Union for the Protection of New Varieties of Plants. 1990: p. 18.
30. Ibid., p. 19.
31. White, Allenby L., "The Effect of Breeders' Rights on the Seed Trade," in *Plant Breeder's Rights*, ASA Special Publication Number 3, edited by H. L. Hamilton. Denver: Crop Science Society of America in cooperation with the American Society for Horticultural Science, the American Seed Trade Association, the International Crop Improvement Association and the National Council of Commercial Plant Breeders. March, 1964: p. 67.
32. Page, op. cit., p. 11.
33. See Dr. Harold D. Loden's "Statement" on House Bill 294 Before the Senate Agriculture Committee at Austin, Texas, March 18, 1969; his "Statement" to the House Interim Agriculture Committee Hearing, Lubbock, Texas, July 26, 1966; and Loden's "Report on Developments of Breeder's Rights for Commercially Developed Cotton Varieties Through Certification and Patent System," Annual Meeting, Texas Certified Seed Producers, Inc. in Dallas, Texas. January 9, 1967.
34. Later, in hearings on PVPA (House of Representatives, Committee on Agriculture, Subcommittee on Departmental Operations, Ninety-First Congress, Second Session, June 10, 1970.) J. Ritchie Smith, assistant director of research for the National Cotton Council, stated that the ten big cotton firms felt that passage of PVPA would result in a doubling of their research expenditures (p. 40). Interestingly, Smith also volunteered that the bill would allow any farmer "the right to reproduce seed for his own planting" (p. 40).

Apparently, the firms were more concerned with commercial pirating of their varieties than with farmers planting saved seed.

35. Telephone interview with Dr. Harold Loden (former president of Paymaster and former President of ASTA), Athens, Ga., July 9, 1992.
36. Miller, Cloy. "Germ Plasm Control As It Would Affect Variety Improvement and Researse of Asexually Produced Crops," in *Plant Breeder's Rights*, edited by H.L. Hamilton, op.cit., p. 56.
37. Dorsey, John G., "U.S. Laws and Regulations on Protection of Varieties and Juridical Requirements for Breeders' Rights." in *Plant Breeders' Rights*, edited by H. L. Hamilton, op. cit., p. 29.
38. Ibid., p. 22.
39. Telephone interview with John Sutherland, Jackson Hole, Wyo., June 15, 1992. Sutherland went to work for the American Seed Trade Association in its Washington office in mid-1960 and became its top staff official (executive vice president) in 1965, a post he held until 1972.
40. White, Richard P., *A Century of Service: A History of the Nursery Industry Associations of the United States*. Washington: American Association of Nurserymen. 1975: p. 257.
41. Carew, John, "Germ Plasm Control as it Would Affect Variety Improvement and Release of Vegetables and Flowers," in *Plant Breeder's Rights*, edited by H. L. Hamilton, op. cit., p. 36.
42. In the early 1960s this was a dominant theme in discussions within the seed industry and was constantly referred to in my interviews with participants and in articles in seed trade publications. Many people apparently could not easily envisage a system that would provide variety protection without the interference of government testing and registration, which might have the effect of dictating to a company what it could or could not sell, under what name, etc. Indeed, American "seed control officials" favored stricter and mandatory registration, and compulsory registration and breeders' rights were linked in Europe. Thus, initial scepticism towards breeders' rights in the U.S. was due in part to antipathy toward compulsory registration.
43. White, Allenby, op.cit., p. 77.
44. Quoted in *Plant Breeder's Rights*, edited by H. L. Hamilton, op.cit., p. 77.
45. Clark, A. Bryan, "Shall The ASTA Take A New Tack?" *Seed World*. Vol. 94, no. 11, June 12, 1964: p. 16ff. (Clark was president of ASTA at the time.)
46. Ibid., p. 18.
47. According to Dr. Harold Loden, Ken Christiansen of ASTA's international committee suggested the formation of the Breeders' Rights Study Committee, though obviously the creation of the committee was due to more than the proposal of an individual.
48. Telephone interview with Dr. Robert Romig, vice president for research, Northrup-King, Minneapolis, Minn., June 15, 1992.
49. Personal interview with Dale Porter in Des Moines, Iowa, May 21, 1992.
50. While focused on patents, ASTA was apparently open to considering other forms of protection. Harold Loden, then president of ASTA, remarked that "I do not want to leave the impression that any segment of the industry feels that amendment of the Plant Patent Act provides the only acceptable basis of breeders' rights protection. In fact, the reverse is true. It is the position of ASTA that breeders' rights could be afforded through several systems, operating simultaneously . . ." Quote from "Breeders' Rights, Plant Patents and Variety Protection," by Dr. Harold Loden, *Seedsmen's Digest*. January, 1969: p. 24.
51. Weiss, Martin G., "Public-Industry Position on Plant Variety Protection." *HortScience*. Vol 4, no. 2. Summer, 1969: p. 84.
52. Ibid., p. 84. (Significantly, however, the committee after hearing testimony from Loden and White agreed that the seed industry did need some form of protection.)
53. Ibid., p. 84.
54. Ibid., p. 85.

55. Interview with Harold Loden.
56. It should also be noted that the original bill did not contain provisions for "reciprocity." The sticking point was that under European legislation the grant of rights was contingent on government tests of the variety whereas in the U.S. companies did not want the government involved in testing — instead they wanted to be able to submit their own tests in support of their applications.
57. Interview with John Sutherland. After leaving ASTA in 1972, Sutherland joined Northrup-King as vice president for personnel and special projects.
58. Chaney, James W., "A National Plant Variety Protection System." Seed World, Vol. 106, no. 1, January 9, 1970: p. 11. At the time, Chaney was vice-president of Keystone Seed Company, which was soon acquired by Union Carbide.
59. Interview with Harold Loden.
60. Ibid.
61. The Lyng family seed company also had ties with Pfister (PAG), distributing hybrid corn for them before being bought out by Northrup-King.
62. Weiss, op. cit., p. 85.
63. Interview with Harold Loden.
64. According to John Sutherland of ASTA, the principal concession to farmers which gave them the right to save seed of protected varieties without paying royalties to the original variety owner had been insisted on by Senator Bellmon of Oklahoma, who believed that the entire bill would be politically threatened without this provision. This account differs from that of Loden who attributes this provision to J. Phil Campbell. Loden remembers a meeting with Campbell in Campbell's office during which Campbell said the exemption would have to be inserted if the USDA were to support the bill. It is possible that Bellmon was endorsing but not initiating this point. It is important to note that Campbell has given testimony in court regarding the "intent" of Congress in approving this "farmers' exemption" from his self-acknowledged status as the originator of the idea of this exemption. Both Loden's and Sutherland's accounts appear plausible, though Loden's is more specific and firsthand. This exemption was the last significant change made to the PVPA bill before passage, according to Loden. None of the other principals interviewed had knowledge of this piece of the history.
65. Doyle, Jack, Altered Harvest: Agriculture, Genetics and the Fate of the World's Food Supply. New York: Viking. 1985: p. 1–8.
66. White, Allenby, "Statement" (as chairman of the Breeders' Rights Study Committee, American Seed Trade Association) to the Subcommittee on Departmental Operations, Committee on Agriculture, U.S. House of Representatives. Hearings on the proposed Plant Variety Protection Act. June 10, 1970. p. 8ff.
67. Loden, Harold, "Statement" (as director of research ACCO Seed, Anderson, Clayton) to the Subcommittee on Departmental Operations, Committee on Agriculture, U.S. House of Representatives. Hearings on the proposed Plant Variety Protection Act. June 10, 1970. p. 28.
68. Stark, Paul. "Statement" (as senior vice president, Stark Brothers Nurseries) to the Subcommittee on Departmental Operations, Committee on Agriculture, U.S. House of Representatives. Hearings on the proposed Plant Variety Protection Act. June 10, 1970. p. 32. According to Loden, Stark had appeared uninvited at a seed industry meeting in Kansas City where government officials were present and had strongly criticized the bill. Both Loden (who became personal friends with Stark and visited his family, etc.) and Sutherland state that considerable effort was expended in convincing Stark to support the bill and testify. Loden says that a Stark Senate contact was important in helping move the bill through Congress.
69. Klein, Andrew, "Statement" (Synnestvedt and Lechner, Patent Lawyers/ABA) to the Subcommittee on Departmental Operations, Committee on Agriculture, U.S. House of Representatives. Hearings on proposed Plant Variety Protection Act. June 10, 1970. p. 39ff.

70. Reeve, Eldrow, "Statement" (Campbell Soup Co.) to the Subcommittee on Departmental Operations, Committee on Agriculture, U.S. House of Representatives. Hearings on the proposed Plant Variety Protection Act. June 10, 1970. p. 57.

71. Telephone interview with John Sutherland, June 15, 1992. Sutherland was a key figure in these negotiations.

72. U.S. House of Representatives Committee on Agriculture, "Report to Accompany S. 3070." Report no. 91-1605, 91st Congress, 2nd Session. October 13, 1970: p. 1–3.

73. Interview with Harold Loden.

74. Interview with Harold Loden.

75. Although only Campbell's presented formal testimony, they apparently did so with the support of Heinz. Representatives of Heinz played an important and strong role in the negotiations. The accommodation was worked out and sealed through the office of Senator Eastland of Mississippi, according to John Sutherland. Sutherland says that Heinz and Campbell's "had his ear," through their production/processing operations in his state.

76. U.S. Senate Committee on the Judiciary. Plant Variety Protection Act, Report to Accompany S. 3070. Washington: U.S. Government Printing Office. September 29, 1970: p. 2.

77. According to Sutherland, Campbell's actually wanted to be able to purchase commercially bred seed, save and multiply it, and distribute it to their growers in following years without any royalty obligations to the breeders. Sutherland — obviously not a neutral source on this point — claims that this was an untenable position to argue in the negotiations.

78. Letter from C. R. Edwards, acting chief, Seed Branch, USDA Consumer and Marketing Service to Paul Kulp, Planning and Evaluation Staff, USDA, December 18, 1970.

79. White, Allenby, "Statement." op. cit., p. 17.

80. Fortmann, H. R., "Plant Variety Protection Legislation: The State-Federal Viewpoint," Seed World. Vol. 105, no. 8, November 28, 1969: p. 5.

81. Interview with John Sutherland.

82. Doyle, op. cit., p. 62–63.

83. Sutherland states that the bill was thirty-fourth in line for consideration at a time in the session when it was thought that fewer than five bills would be considered before adjournment. Sutherland says that he mobilized political pressure quickly and had the bill moved from thirty-fourth to second on the list.

84. Interview with John Sutherland.

85. Telephone interview with John Sutherland, July 26, 1992. When asked why Mitchell would be interested in this bill, the following exchange took place: Sutherland: What state's Mitchell from? C. F.: Illinois? Sutherland: And is Illinois a big agricultural state? C. F.: Yes. Sutherland: Does that answer your question? In fact, Mitchell is not from Illinois. His professional career prior to the Justice Department was as a New York lawyer specializing in public finance and bonds particularly regarding public housing. There is no hint of a rural or agricultural connection in biographies of either Mitchell or his flamboyant wife, Martha. This exchange may simply have been Sutherland's way of explaining that Mitchell had old contacts with agricultural interests (perhaps through personal friendships rather than business dealings). In any case, Mitchell's interest in the legislation and the nature of Sutherland's contact with him remain a mystery.

86. Jim Hightower describes Campbell as a proponent of corporate integration, or "vertical coordination," in Campbell's words. See various references to Campbell in Hightower's Eat Your Heart Out: Food Profiteering in America. New York: Crown. 1975.

87. Shafritz, Jay M., The Dorsey Dictionary of American Government and Politics. Chicago: Dorsey Press. 1988: p. 385.

88. Sutherland, however, denies that Lyng was involved so crucially and points instead to his own lobbying work with Mitchell.

89. Lyng and Weinberger had served together on the California Republican Central Committee and were both senior officials in Governor Ronald Reagan's administration in California. Lyng describes Weinberger as a "good friend."

90. Telephone interview with Richard Lyng, Modesto, Calif., July 26, 1992.
91. Interview with Harold Loden.
92. Doyle, op. cit., p. 65. The Bureau of Budget (BOB) was in the midst of changing its name to the Office of Management and Budget (OMB).
93. Berman, Larry, *The Office of Management and Budget and the Presidency, 1921–1979*. Princeton: Princeton University Press. 1979: p. 117.
94. Burns and Flam, op. cit., p. 299.
95. Max Weber as quoted in Milovanovic, op. cit., 1989: p. 16.
96. Collins, Randall, *Max Weber: A Skeleton Key*. Beverly Hills: Sage Publications. 1986: p. 70ff.
97. Ripley, Randall B., and Grace A. Franklin, *Congress, the Bureaucracy, and Public Policy*. Homewood, Ill.: Dorsey Press. 1976: p. 6.

# CHAPTER 5

# Congress and the Courts Extend Property Rights, 1980

The 1970 Plant Variety Protection Act provided for patent-like protection for most sexually reproducing plants. As a result of pressure from certain corporate interests, however, Congress refused to extend this protection to six specific vegetables. But, as described, laws are time and context bound and do not simply build upon precedent. In the decade between the 1970 act and its expansion in 1980, their context changed considerably.

The seed industry grew and matured. With significant takeover activity from transnational corporations, it experienced restructuring and gained political power and experience, particularly through its trade association. For certain types of seed companies, markets were no longer seen in terms of states or regions; these companies searched the world for suitable markets. The exclusion of the six vegetables in 1970 grew from an annoyance to an impediment — an obstacle for U.S. participation in a treaty guaranteeing reciprocal patent rights abroad. If U.S.-based companies were to benefit from guaranteed protection in their biggest export markets, the U.S. law had to be changed. What might appear to the casual observer as the logical extension of the 1970 Act (and what congressional supporters dubbed a "minor piece of housekeeping legislation") is understood in a different way when analyzed in context.

This chapter is about much more than just the passage of a law. As law, the 1970 act was more important because it established the basis for new types of property relationships and it provided legitimacy for private ownership of sexually reproducing plant varieties. By 1980, new and very different actors had emerged with sufficient power to threaten passage of the proposed amendment. Opponents from the 1970 battle had either become supporters or they had become quiet. And levels of skills and access to resources were strikingly different among the actors involved.

This chapter also concerns the emergence of these new actors, the way in which issues were created and reshaped, the arenas used, and how relationships among actors changed. It is about a context profoundly altered. The 1980 law was not passed to give consistency to the 1970 law. Indeed by 1980, the importance of the 1970 law had changed. Were the 1970 law to have been passed in 1980, it would have been passed for rather different reasons. The motivations behind plant variety protection changed between the late 1960s and the late 1970s. Thus, the 1980 act must be interpreted and understood in different terms.

The 1980 act does not really "settle" the issue of property rights over biological material even though it appeared to by extending patent-like coverage to all crops. Shifts in power, changes in technology, and new economic opportunities are among factors that can lead to challenges of existing law and interpretations of that law. Property rights can be formalized through the interpretation and enforcement of laws as well as by the passage of laws. The two processes are not completely separate, as one can form part of the context in which social agents pursue the other.

It has not been my objective in this book to present a linear history of scientific and legal developments concerning plant breeding. It has been convenient to group these developments around legislation passed in 1930, 1970 and 1980, but at this point it becomes obvious that certain roads intersect and each has its origin prior to 1980. I have waited until now to discuss them because thematically they are more important to events after 1980.

In the remainder of chapter 5, I look at the remarkable developments in science and technology which preceded creation of the biotechnology industry. This industry is heavily involved in and actually dependent upon research as a revenue-producing activity. The ability to raise funds for research is tied to securing patent protection. Thus, I examine the importance of patent protection to the new industry. The real problem faced by the industry is how to extend patent protection quickly to new classes of living material. The answer is not through the legislative process. Alternatives chosen by two companies illustrate the deficiencies of both old and new strategies and point to problems that actors will soon try to solve in yet different ways. Significantly this chapter is the last dealing with "solutions" that can be obtained nationally. The technology, the problems, the opportunities, the new actors, and the solutions are leading to international arenas.

Less than a year after the passage of the Plant Variety Protection Act of 1970, grain farmers in the Soviet Union settled in for the winter confident that their fields had been seeded with the best, high-yielding variety known in their country, Besostaja. Winter temperatures slid lower and lower. When the spring rains failed to materialize, a few experts watching both locally and in the U.S. via satellite knew that the Soviets were in big trouble. Indeed they were. Besostaja, a fine wheat for fine times, was neither cold-hardy nor drought-tolerant. The government elected to buy its way out of disaster.

The Canadian Wheat Board was among the first to realize the extent of the problem and the shrewd deals it made in the spring of 1972 are still talked about. The USDA was a little slower. Once it determined that the Soviets would be big buyers, it helped facilitate loans to the USSR in order to encourage large grain purchases from American corporations. The USDA officials who secretly negotiated the deals ended up as top executives of several of these grain companies. Meanwhile, the companies bought wheat cheaply from the farmers, before anyone knew there was a crisis. When word of the crisis was made public, grain prices shot up. By this time, the farmers had already sold their grain. Only the companies had any for sale. On the Rotterdam market, wheat rose from $65 to $90 a metric ton.

In the Sahel, the drought was beginning to take its toll on crops, livestock and people. Americans watched Africans die of starvation on their television sets. Aid agencies entered the market and purchased more grain. American politicians were quick to see the silver lining. Hubert Humphrey had long ago observed:

> I have heard that people may become dependent on us for food. I know that is not supposed to be good news. To me that is good news, because before people can do anything they have got to eat. And if you are looking for a way to get people to lean on you, in terms of their cooperation with you, it seems to me that food dependence would be a great thing."[1]

On the American prairies, farmers were ecstatic over high grain prices which looked as though they could only go higher. Government officials did nothing to moderate the enthusiasm. Secretary of Agriculture Earl Butz advised farmers to prepare for the big export boom by planting "fence row to fence row," and warned them in the same breath that they would have to "get big or get out" of farming. Farmers raced into debt, buying more land, plowing more under, and buying more machinery, fertilizers, and seeds. Over 40 million additional acres were put into production in the first half of the decade,[2] but with consequences that were not foreseen.

The combination of increased production and high prices can be a tonic for many ills. In this case, farm exports helped to offset a disastrous balance of payments deficit stemming from the costs of the Vietnam War. Both the war and its costs were escalating. The trade deficit of $7 billion in 1972 was being compared to the deficit of $2 billion a year earlier.

Nixon's special trade representative to Europe and Japan, William Eberle (President of Boise Cascade), said: "As far as the U.S. is concerned, progress in agriculture is the *sine qua non* of progress in normaliz-

ing the international economic situation and improving our trade relations."[3] Agricultural exports jumped from $5.7 billion in 1969 to $11.1
billion in 1973. By then, they were accounting for 30 percent of all
harvested cropland in the United States.[4] In crops such as corn and
soybeans, the figure was much higher. Farm exports now far exceeded
those of chemical products and American consumer goods in value.

Aided by a booming export market, a "mature" domestic market, tax
breaks and other government incentives, the American food industry
began to focus its attention on foreign sales. Expansion abroad, what the
Wall Street Journal called "the parade to foreign lands," was already well
under way when the "Russian Grain Deal" came to be felt.[5] Furthermore,
profit rates for general business abroad were far higher than domestic
rates for American transnationals.[6]

In most of the food processing sectors, companies expanded abroad by
acquiring foreign companies. The most notable exception to this practice
was in the agricultural chemicals sector, where the more common practice
was to form a new subsidiary,[7] an indication perhaps of the newness of
capital intensive agriculture and the lack of indigenous infrastructures and
companies.

In the efforts to amend and expand the 1970 Plant Variety Protection
Act, it is evident that many large seed companies now participated in the
international economy; they had joined the parade. Takeovers in the
industry had become commonplace. Whereas in 1961 the USDA could
claim in its Yearbook of Agriculture that big business was nowhere to be
found in the seed trade, scarcely more than a decade later big business was
everywhere. Very big business: ITT, Monsanto, Shell, ICI, Upjohn, and
many others. Large transnationals, many involved in sales of petrochem-
icals and other agricultural inputs, were adding seeds to their product
lines. Seeds, in many cases, could be sold through the same distribution
channels they were already establishing, both in the United States and
abroad.

There were other reasons as well. Some of the large transnationals were
flush with the cash that flowed through the petroleum industry in the
1970s. Some wanted to "move closer to the consumer" in uncertain
economic times.[8] Low interest rates at the beginning of the decade,
coupled with inheritance taxes facing the heirs of many successful seed
companies founded early in the century facilitated the acquisitions.[9] Drug
and petrochemical companies found that seed companies fitted well into
their corporate structures — they could feel comfortable with the need for
research, testing and such. Finally, the attention being focused on the need
to increase food production drew constant attention to the seed industry.

Any production increases would almost inevitably call for more or better seed from the seed industry. All of these factors, plus an attractive rate of return within the seed industry, encouraged takeovers.

The takeovers propelled once local and regionally oriented seed companies into the international market. Ciba-Geigy did not buy Funk Seeds in order to sell seeds in a few midwestern and southern states only. Funk Seeds was on its way to becoming Funk Seeds International with sales in Europe and other markets.

The prospectus to a report (sold for $25,000 a copy) on the seed industry produced by a consulting firm headed by a former seed company owner, stated that "for multinational corporations, seed lends itself to world-wide commercialization . . . the global seed trade is one of the fastest-growing, most profitable industries in the food chain."[10]

Concurrent with the internationalization of the seed industry was the growth of concern about the loss of genetic diversity in agricultural crops. The two are not unconnected, as has been noted. Among scientists, this concern had its roots in the work of N.I. Vavilov in the 1920s. Vavilov was a friend of Harry Harlan, an American barley expert. Harlan, it will be recalled, was the first to warn in writing of the threat posed by the loss of genetic diversity. But it was his son Jack who, as much as anyone, ignited concern in the scientific community with his respected work and passionate writings.

Famine in Africa,  the emerging dominance of transnationals in the food business, rising food prices, and bankrupt farmers helped give rise to a nonfarmer-based, activist "food movement" in North America in the 1970s. Various advocacy and aid-oriented organizations sprang up: the Agribusiness Accountability Project, Oxfam, Bread for the World, Church World Service (sponsors of CROP walks), etc. Many of these groups were founded or led by activists who had been involved in the civil rights and antiwar movements of the 1960s and 1970s. These people came to the topic with a willingness to be critical of existing structures, a certain international perspective, and a flexibility in their approach to "political work."

Throughout the 1970s a small but steady stream of critical analyses of American agriculture and the "world food crisis" were published — by Jim Hightower, Al Krebs, Susan DeMarco and Susan Sechler with the Agribusiness Accountability Project, by Susan George with the Institute for Policy Studies in Washington, and by Frances Moore Lappé, Joseph Collins and myself with the newly formed Institute for Food and Development Policy in New York and San Francisco.

Events seemed to be propelling both industry and activist organizations to look beyond American borders. When, in 1979, the American Seed Trade Association drew up and had introduced "minor housekeeping legislation" to pull the six previously deleted vegetables into the Plant Variety Protection Act, industry and activists collided.

Part of my work with Lappé and Collins on the book, *Food First*, had been to research the social and economic impacts of the Green Revolution. In the process, I stumbled upon two articles written by Dr. Jack Harlan in the early 1970s : "The Genetics of Disaster" and "Our Vanishing Crop Genetic Resources." Harlan was asking if we would wake up to this crisis only after it was too late:

> Who would survive if wheat, rice or maize were to be destroyed? To suggest such a possibility would have seemed absurd a few years ago. It is not absurd now. How real are the dangers? What is the potential magnitude of the disaster? One might as well ask how serious is atomic warfare. The consequences of failure of one of our major food plants are beyond imagination."[11]

The articles by Harlan made a deep impression but there was no obvious context within which a nonscientist could act. Following the publication of *Food First*, I was invited to give a number of lectures in the United States and Canada. On occasion I would mention the problem posed by the loss of genetic diversity. It was, as you might say in show business, not a crowd-pleaser. Few who had come to hear about hunger and politics wanted to hear about genetics and seeds. One who did was Pat Mooney, a Canadian. Mooney had dropped out of high school in frustration, in part due to the system's inability to stimulate or educate a bright student who happened to be legally blind. Mooney's interests were international[12] and his concern was for the Third World. He originated the "CROP walks" in Canada and was instrumental in founding a number of organizations — still in existence today — to conduct development and development education projects.

Pat Mooney's challenge was to "do something." But what? Soon, he learned that Canada was introducing "plant breeders' rights" legislation. Wondering if and suspecting that this might have a connection with genetic diversity issues, we called Erna Bennett at the International Board for Plant Genetic Resources in Rome. A noted scientist and a radical, Irish political activist Bennett used forceful language to claim that the legislation would have a negative impact on plant genetic diversity. With this encouragement, Mooney began to speak out against the Canadian legislation. In late 1979, a collection of pieces he had written about genetic erosion, the seed trade, patenting, and the "gene rich" and the "gene poor" dimensions of North-South relations, was published by Inter Pares for the Canadian Council for International Cooperation and the International Coalition for Development Action (ICDA) under the title, *Seeds of the Earth: A Private or Public Resource?*

After completion of *Food First*, I moved back to North Carolina, founded the Agricultural Resources Center and then joined the staff of the National Sharecroppers Fund/Rural Advancement Fund (an advocacy group established in 1937), and proceeded to write a directory for farmers and gardeners to sources of "old-fashioned" vegetable seeds and fruit and nut varieties (an earlier draft of which had been written for and distributed by the Agricultural Resources Center).[13] An essay in the back of the NSF/ RAF directory served to educate the reader about the loss of genetic diversity. Some attention was paid to patenting. *The Graham Center Seed Directory* was very successful. Perhaps 5000 had been ordered through the mail when I learned, almost by accident, of the proposed amendment to the PVPA in the United States.

On July 4, 1979, a three-page letter over my signature was mailed to those who had purchased the Seed Directory. It listed a number of concerns with the proposed amendments to the PVPA: loss of genetic diversity, consolidation in the seed industry, difficulty of enforcing the law, increasing seed prices for farmers, the proposed joining of UPOV, and the spectre of illegal vegetable varieties. Recipients were asked to write to their representatives in Congress and those on the two committees considering the legislation. They were also asked to send a copy of these letters back to the National Sharecroppers Fund, publisher of the directory.[14]

At the time, the PVPA amendment was viewed as noncontroversial and scheduled for a one-hour proforma hearing followed by "mark-up," meaning routine referral to the full House for approval.

Between learning of the amendment and the first hearing, I had traveled to Washington for meetings with various organizations to enlist their help in fighting the legislation. Several were receptive, but none had any background on the topic. Jack Doyle, coming off of a fight over rural, high-transmission electric power lines, proved to be very helpful as he had experience "on the Hill." Doyle was employed by the Environmental Policy Center (which has since merged with and taken the name of Friends of the Earth).

Quickly, an informal coalition was formed which included environmental organizations, the National Farmers Union, gardening groups, and church organizations. What these groups lacked in scientific or legal expertise, they made up for with an ability to reach the public, and the press. Hundreds of letters began to flood Congress — most coming not from the traditional "protesters" but from small towns and rural areas, from people who had purchased Seed Directories in hopes of finding an old variety from their childhood.

Seed industry officials involved in the effort were surprised and rattled by the unexpected opposition.[15] An issue which they assumed had been defused since passage of the PVPA in 1970 was suddenly afire. This time the Department of Agriculture was supportive of the amendment, but they could see Congressional support slipping. Representative George Brown of California, a cosponsor of the bill, wrote Representative Kika de la Garza, chairman of the Subcommittee on Department Investigations, Oversight and Research, on November 8, 1979, to say that he was "uncomfortable moving this legislation." Brown pointed out: "I have been surprised at the outpouring of opinion directed at H.R. 999, the bill to amend the Plant Variety Protection Act of 1970. I have received more mail on this issue than on any other agriculture issue in recent memory. I was even approached on this issue at the U.N. Conference on Science and Technology in Geneva, which I attended in August."[16]

Brown's letter effectively put a temporary halt to the bill and gave proponents and opponents time to regroup. Opponents took the offensive by going to the press and in short order articles appeared around the country. These articles reflected the various interests of the opponents. A number of opponents, myself included, saw the PVPA debate as an opportunity to educate the public and policy makers about the loss of genetic diversity. Plant patenting was bad, we thought. Genetic erosion was worse. None of us had any detailed knowledge of the history of the seed industry, and its earlier attempts to pass legislation. We were unaware of the hearings on the PVPA in 1970. Such information might have been useful. Nor did we have any knowledge of the technological advances underway in plant breeding, or any suspicion of how these might affect the PVPA in the future. Finally, none of us really expected the battle to last long. We anticipated early defeat. Long-term research, planning, and strategizing were never properly undertaken for what was perceived to be a short-term project.

The seed industry tried various approaches to deal with what one farm reporter called a "tempest in a peapod." It attempted to discredit opponents as people who knew nothing about the subject and lacked standing. This attempt to delegitimize opponents was effective particularly with members of Congress. Mass mailings were sent out to seed companies and journalists describing opponents as "rural activists" and even "rural revolutionaries." The attacks became more personal in threats to sue journals publishing my articles and in telephoned threats of physical violence against Pat Mooney and his family. (By this time Mooney was devoting complete attention to seed patenting and related issues for the Saskatchewan Council for International Cooperation and later the International Coalition for Development Action.) While much of the industry had now been acquired by large transnationals, it seems evident that the unsophisticated response of the industry was engineered by those still running their seed company subsidiaries — holdovers from previous managements, people who were unaccustomed to a public arena and public scrutiny. These actors engaged in political debate as newcomers with incomplete understanding of the process.

The seed industry attempted to downplay the importance of the bill. In an interview with the *New York Times*, Harold Loden of the American Seed Trade Association pleaded, "It's the most insignificant little piece of legislation. It allows you to protect six little vegetables, when you've already got 222 other food crops covered. So what?"[17]

Loden's statement was more a plea for the controversy to end, for surely the bill was not really insignificant. The importance of the bill was tacitly acknowledged in the "Final Impact Statement," part of the routine review process undertaken by the USDA on all new proposed legislation. In this case the review was made by the USDA's Director for Economics, Policy Analysis and Budget, Howard Hjort. Signed in January, 1979, the Statement made clear that "the proposed changes would make U.S. requirements compatible with the requirements of the International Union for the Protection of New Varieties of Plants (UPOV). This would allow the U.S. to join UPOV and thus facilitate international trade."[18] Hjort further noted that "the inclusion of the six vegetables under the Act are [sic] no longer resisted by the large soup companies." He claimed that "the proposed amendments have no bearing on health, safety, civil rights or other human concerns." Hjort concluded, therefore, that public comment was "not applicable."[19]

Since 1970, the joining of UPOV and the related facilitating of international trade had become the most important reasons for extending coverage to the excluded vegetables.[20] For the seed industry the issue was no longer protection of domestic markets. The global markets in which the large seed companies now operated was a very different context.

Given the pace of seed company takeovers[21] (a list of the known significant takeovers in the United States at the time of this controversy is given in table 6) and the rapidly expanding international scope of seed company operations, membership in UPOV was not "insignificant." Without UPOV membership, the U.S. would be hard pressed to safeguard reliably its seed "patents" in foreign markets. During the 1960s and 1970s some 17 countries including most of the big markets for U.S. corporate seed exports (except Canada) had joined UPOV and pledged to observe each others' grants of protection. Seed exports were increasing in importance precisely to that sector of the seed industry affected by PVPA and specifically to producers of seed of the six excluded vegetables. As expansion of the PVPA was being considered, exports of corn seed were still a relatively small percentage of overall sales. But half the vegetable seed produced in the United States was destined for the export market even without the protection of PVPA. In volume, U.S. seed exports grew 12 percent a year between the mid 1970s and the early 1980s.[22] The granting of reciprocal rights for U.S.-protected varieties would help solidify market position and surely increase sales.

Furthermore, pharmaceutical[23] and chemical companies which were now the dominant force in the U.S. seed industry were predisposed to regarding patent protection as being important. A survey of one hundred companies (excluding small ones) in twelve industries indicated that more than any other industry, companies involved in pharmaceuticals and chemicals felt that patents were crucial to the development and introduction of their products. In fact, of all industries surveyed, only pharmaceuticals respondents stated that over half their products would not have been developed or introduced without patents.[24] Given all of these factors, one can assume that extension of PVPA was more than "minor housekeeping" to certain corporations. Defeat of the bill would send a very discouraging message to other countries considering PVPA legislation, especially to Canada, a major potential market for proprietary American seeds. Canada had no intellectual property protection for plants at all. Attempts to introduce the legislation there had been met with stiff resistance from farm groups stirred up with Mooney's help. A defeat in Washington would kill the bill in Ottawa and slow the pace of internationalization, the restructuring of the seed industry,[25] and "protected" seed exports.

As the fight over the amendment to the PVPA received increasing exposure, more people became interested in it, bringing with them yet more "issues" and preventing by their very interest a change of arenas for the seed industry. The arena was Congress surrounded by the media and constituent onlookers. The attempt to portray the legislation as a minor, housekeeping measure had failed.

In Europe, a Common Catalog system had been instituted.[26] The Common Catalog had an indirect link to European seed regulations. Governments there ostensibly created a list of plant variety synonyms — different names being used for the same variety. They then declared that as of a certain date, companies would no longer be allowed to sell varieties using those names. The bill however included not just synonyms, but distinct varieties, gardener and farmer-bred varieties. For example, in the United Kingdom the government listed the "Bedfordshire Champion" onion and the "Up-to-Date" onion as synonyms for the same variety, when government publications had previously described "Up-to-Date" as having the most resistance to downy mildew and "Bedfordshire Champion" as being very susceptible to the same disease.[27] Eleven synonyms for "Ormskirk" cabbage and seven synonyms for "Alexander no. 1" cabbage were identified. Remarkably, a variety called "Late Market" was claimed to be a synonym for both. In fact, fewer than half the varieties deleted were actually synonyms. The Common Catalog was not intended simply to eliminate the confusion over names. In effect, the Common Catalog would make illegal the sale of varieties that were important to small seed companies without large breeding programs. There were indications from Europe that the Common Catalog was also an attempt to "clear the decks" for seed patenting and make enforcement easier, a slightly less credible explanation. The industry itself explained that the Common Catalog was a consumer protection device. Government bureaucrats were simply rescuing farmers from inferior varieties by outlawing them and eliminating confusing synonyms at the same time. The mention of "illegal vegetables" was enough to capture the attention of the press and many American gardeners. The seed trade angrily denied that it had intentions of establishing such a system. While opponents never really accused the amendment of establishing such a system, proponents scored points by charging me and others with misrepresentation of the facts.[28] This flurry of charges and countercharges served to distract attention away from more pertinent issues.

It is doubtful that the other issues being raised by opponents could have sustained a long debate, even if they served to bring in new constituencies, which they did. On the other hand, the seed industry's arguments found no natural constituency among the public. The industry was reduced to arguing about incentives to research and the "rights" of the plant breeder. In the end, it appeared that the public (to the extent that people were aware of the controversy) was simply afraid of the spectre of transnationals in the garden. And they had an uncomfortable feeling about the propriety of patenting forms of life. This found expression in statements from religious leaders from the national offices of the American Baptist Church, the Presbyterian Church, and from Catholic bishops in

**Table 6.** Known Seed Company Acquisitions, 1980[30]

| New Owner | Acquired Companies |
| --- | --- |
| Anderson Clayton (ACCO) | Paymaster Farms, Tomco-Genetic Giant |
| Cargill | Dorman Seeds, Kroeker Seeds PAG |
| Celanese | Capril Inc., Joseph Harris Seed Co., Moran Seeds |
| Central Soya | O's Gold Seed Co. |
| Ciba-Geigy | Funk Seeds, Louisiana Seed Co., Stewart Seeds |
| DeKalb | Ramsey Seed |
| FMC Corp. | Seed Research Assoc. |
| Garden Products | Gurney Seeds |
| Grassland Resources | Taylor-Evans |
| Hilleshoeg/Cardo | Inernational Forest Seeds Co. |
| International Multifoods | Baird Inc., Lynk Brothers |
| ITT | Burpee, O. M. Scott |
| Kent Food Co. | L. Teweles Seed Co. |
| Kleinwanzieberer Swtzucht AG | Coker's Pedigreed Seed |
| NAPB (Olin & Royal Dutch Shell) | Agripro Inc., Tekseed Hybrid |
| Occidental Petroleum | Ring Around Products |
| Pioneer Hi-Bred | Lankhart, Lockett, Peterson, Arnold Thomas Seed Co. |
| Pfizer | Clemens Seed Farms, Jordan Wholesale Co., Trojan Seed Co., Warwick Seeds |
| Purex | Advanced Seeds, Hulting Hybrids |
| Rorer-Amchem | Jacques Seed Co. |
| Sandoz | National—NK, Northrup-King, Rogers Brothers |
| Southwide Inc. | Delta and Pine Land, Greenfield Seed |
| Tate and Lyle | Berger and Plate |
| Tejon Ranch Co. | Waterman-Loomis Co. |
| Union Carbide | Ferry-Morse, Keystone Seed Co. |
| Upjoin | Asgrow Seeds, Associated Seeds |

twelve midwestern states. After an exhaustive series of some 400 meetings on land and agricultural issues these bishops, representing 43 dioceses issued the following statement:

> stewardship of land and life itself are both symbolically and naturally joined in the life-generating capacity of the seed. We must preserve for ourselves and for future generations the genetic variety of plants necessary to protect humanity from the hazards of inbreeding. We note with concern that inbreeding has become a major practice in our present agricultural system as greater yields and profits have been pursued. We also are disturbed by the acquisition of seed companies and patents by multinational corporations. The control of seeds, because it implies also the control of food production and indeed of life itself, should not be appropriated to itself by any company or nation. We therefore urge a careful review of present and pending seed patent legislation.[29]

Kenneth Dahlberg, a social scientist at Western Michigan University, raised a similar and prophetic concern: where should the credit go for new plant varieties? Dahlberg commented that 90 percent of all plant breeding has been done by nature itself and 9.9 percent by subsistence farmers and our Neolithic ancestors. Should modern plant breeders doing 0.1 percent of the work reap all the credit and all the rewards, he asked?[31]

The first congressional hearings were opened under Representative Kika de la Garza in the Agriculture Subcommittee on Department Investigations, Oversight, and Research on July 19, 1979. De la Garza had also presided over the 1970 hearings on the PVPA. He represented a southern Texas district which is a major pepper and carrot producer — a district dominated by large commercial farms. As a cosponsor of the bill in question, de la Garza was in the enviable position of being able to preside over hearings on his own bill. The congressman was not in a good mood. According to aides, he had been told by the industry and the USDA that there would be no controversy. He had agreed to cosponsor the bill, as had many others, simply as a favor. Nine people testified. Six from industry and the USDA testified in favor, three were against. Due to the controversy, the scheduled vote clearing the bill out of the subcommittee never took place. Instead, de la Garza hinted that more hearings would be necessary to clarify the inaccurate information raised around the bill. Another hearing was eventually scheduled for April 22, 1980.

Cooperation between the USDA and industry was  evident. (In form this was reminiscent of 1970 when the House Committee used Allenby White's testimony to form the basis of its own report.) Again, USDA and industry statements on certain issues concerning amendments to the PVPA were strikingly similar. See table 7 (on next page) for an example:

**Table 7.** USDA and Seed Industry Statements Similar[32]

| USDA Statement on Consolidation in the Seed Industry | ASTA Statement on Consolidation in the Seed Industry |
|---|---|
| "If a seed company has been successful in its research and has protected varieties which are acepted by the consumer, then they are more attractive, not only for takeovers, but for their owners." | "Plant patent laws may make seed companies attractive for takeover by large corporations. So what! ... If a seed company has been successful in its research and has protected varieties which are accepted by the consumer, then they are more attractive for not only takeovers but for their owners . . ." |

Following the second set of hearings in the House, hearings were scheduled for June 17 and 18 in the Senate Agriculture Subcommittee on Agricultural Research and General Legislation chaired by Senator Donald Stewart of Alabama.

Stewart's opening remarks signaled that the hearing would be different than that conducted by de la Garza. "I am concerned about the germplasm preservation effort by the Department of Agriculture, and that is an understatement," Stewart said. "I intend to hold hearings on this important subject later in the summer, and would perhaps hold this bill until we can get some kind of amendatory language into the legislation that would strengthen our efforts as a department . . ."[33]

Exchanges between Stewart and USDA officials were pointed from the beginning. Two connected examples will suffice:

> *Barbara Schlei (USDA):* A patent provides the opportunity for a farmer to recoup the venture capital which goes into that research. Plant breeding requires unusually painstaking research . . . To develop one variety, breeders make hundreds of crosses and raise thousands of seedlings for evaluation, a process that usually requires 7 or more years to produce a marketable result.

> *Senator Stewart:* Well, then, Barbara, are we really talking about a little old farmer out there making those kinds of investments? Does that actually occur?

> *Barbara Schlei:* Yes, sir, it does occur, and it occurs in very large numbers.

> *Senator Stewart:* Could you give me some idea of what those numbers — the reason I ask that question, I was in Montgomery for about 8 years, and there was a fellow who always used to stand up on the floor and

say that, "I am here representing those little old pulp wooders down in my part of the State." I would always go along with him. I would vote for whatever proposal he had because I had a concern for the little pulp wooders in his part of the State and my part of the State. And I found out that the little old pulp wooders he was representing were International Paper Co., Scott Paper Co., and I got a little concerned after that . . . It may not seem to be a very important problem for some, but it is a hell of a problem to me, and I am not going to let this alone. If I thought for a minute that our patenting process was being utilized by large-size concerns to control the seed-producing industry, your bill would never get out of my committee.

*Barbara Schlei:* . . . if we believe that that is too much concentration, then we have a set of antitrust laws available to us to deal with that problem . . .

*Senator Stewart:* Hogwash. Those things have not been used since they were put on the books, not effectively, not successfully; have not been used since they were put on the books. That is just hogwash. I am sorry, but if the antitrust laws are relied on to weed out concentration in the economy of the agricultural sector of our economy, or anything else, you could not depend on those if your life depended on it. They just do not work.

*Barbara Schlei:* Sir, I think that if our antitrust laws are inadequate at this time, then what we properly should be addressing is an amendment to that set of laws.

*Senator Stewart:* No, ma'am. You are Wrong about that. Government policy, in many, many areas, makes concentration possible; tax policy, research policies . . .

*Barbara Schlei:* Mr. Chairman, I stand corrected, and I agree with your point that we must scrutinize all legislation to ensure that it does not have —

*Senator Stewart:* Can we do it?[34]

Stewart's promise later in the hearings that he was going to be "the germplasm and the seed area expert in the U.S. Senate" must have sent a chill through the seed industry as it contemplated its chances of getting the PVPA amendments out of his committee.

ASTA officials decided to contact Senator Herman Talmadge, chairman of the Senate Agriculture Committee, in an effort to get him to remove the bill from Stewart's jurisdiction. This is a rare move and one senators find very offensive. Talmadge was reluctant but not completely unwilling. Back in Alabama, however, Stewart was up for reelection and he was in trouble. He faced tough opposition in the Democratic primary and even more problems from a probe by muckraking journalist, Jack

Anderson. Anderson was questioning how Stewart could have real estate mortgage debts of over a half million dollars and a campaign debt of over two hundred thousand dollars on a Senate salary of slightly more than sixty thousand dollars a year. Questionable campaign financing was Anderson's answer.[35]

On the House side, ASTA officials were trying to persuade de la Garza to have the bill considered under a suspension of the House rules which would have restricted debate and eliminated the possibility of introducing amendments. De la Garza might have done almost anything to get rid of the bill at that point, but why go to extraordinary lengths to get the bill through the House if Stewart was going to block it in the Senate? Talmadge and de la Garza sat back to watch the Alabama election results.

When the votes were tallied, Stewart had lost. After Congress returned for its post-election "lame-duck" session, de la Garza had the House rules suspended and pushed through the bill on a voice vote. And in the Senate, Talmadge took control of the bill from Stewart and his subcommittee and the bill was passed without debate, without ever having actually been approved by the subcommittee which held hearings on it. For the third time in 50 years a plant patenting bill was on the way to the president's desk without ever having experienced a recorded vote.

Still the battle was not quite over. As in 1970, there were dissenting voices within the Administration urging a veto. Carter's Department of Agriculture had brought in some progressives. Specifically two associates from the old Agribusiness Accountability Project were now in powerful positions with the very office at the USDA that had prepared the "Final Impact Statement" endorsing the bill on behalf of the department. One, Susan Sechler, was now Deputy Director. She and her associate, Susan DeMarco, were political and personal friends of mine and we had a number of other friends in common who were urging them to take some action. One such friend was Lynn Randels, who was working with the president's Commission on World Hunger. In the 1970s, Randels had taken it upon herself to visit the National Seed Storage Laboratory, the nation's biggest gene bank. She was appalled at what she saw. Her brief, unpublished, but scathing report was circulated among a few "activists" and for some years was the only outside account of the problems at the facility. The commission adopted a statement of "concern" over the patenting issue. Randels, whose Washington home was a "home away from home" for both DeMarco and me on our trips to Washington, pushed for aggressive action from DeMarco and Sechler. This was ultimately successful. Their office reversed its position and recommended a veto. The president's Council on Environmental Quality also recommended a veto, and further calls for a veto came from the Resources Agency of the State of California, National Farmers Union, National Sharecroppers Fund, American Baptist Church, Environmental Defense Fund, Environmental Policy Center, Center for Rural Affairs, National Family Farm Coalition, International Federation of Agricultural Producers, National Center for Appropriate Technology, Seed Savers Exchange, Peoples' Business Commission, Sierra Club, Ozark Institute, National Coalition for Development Action, Consumers Federation of America, Rural America Inc., Agribusiness Accountability Publications, Public Citizen Congress Watch, Interreligious Taskforce on U.S. Food Policy, and a number of academics from Harvard, MIT, and other universities.

Despite the last minute pleas for a veto, President Carter signed the amendment to the PVPA in December, 1980. With Carter's signature, the seed industry had protection for breeders of new varieties — through patents in the case of the Plant Patent Act of 1930 and through the *sui generis* Plant Variety Protection Act of 1970 as amended in 1980. Viewed biologically, both laws provided protection for varieties, that is, for certain combinations of genes. The genes themselves were not made patentable. Breeders were left free to use patented varieties (with unpatented genes) to produce new combinations of genes and new patentable varieties. Furthermore, even in 1980, the industry was not able to challenge the farmer's "right" to save his/her patented seed for replanting (or for resale, if the farmer was not principally in the business of reselling protected varieties).

The PVPA must be seen essentially as a marketing tool, not as a civil rights issue or as a means to encourage research as claimed by the industry. Research expenditures as a percentage of sales had been increasing long before the 1970 act and in fact the rate of increase actually slowed afterwards.[36] The importance of the act lay in its control over varieties and variety names in the marketplace. As new varieties were being bred by companies large enough to employ breeders, the PVPA was most useful to larger companies. Table 8 (on next page) indicates PVPA-patent control by crop. This table indicates strong concentration, which over time would tend to translate into considerable marketplace power. The targets of litigation under PVPA, not surprisingly, have been smaller seed companies and bold, enterprising farmers who have tested the limits of the law or the patience of the big companies.

The amendments also helped American law conform to international standards represented by UPOV, thus facilitating participation in UPOV and the granting of reciprocal protection, important for marketing American seed varieties in Europe.

**Table 8.** Concentration of Ownership, PVPA Certificates, by Crop, 1980[37]

| Crop | Number of Dominant Corporate "Patent" Holders | Percentage of "Patents" Held by Those Companies |
|---|---|---|
| Beans | 3 | 80% |
| Cotton | 4 | 45% |
| Lettuce | 4 | 60% |
| Peas | 4 | 62% |
| Soybeans | 4 | 48% |
| Wheat | 4 | 36% |
| Barley | 4 | 69% |
| Cauliflower | 2 | 100% |
| China Aster | 1 | 100% |
| Eggplant | 1 | 100% |
| Sweet Peas | 2 | 100% |
| Tobacco | 3 | 100% |

## THE U.S. COURTS AND BIOTECHNOLOGY LAW

Scientific development did not cease, nor did the interplay between science, economics and the law come to a halt with the hybridization of corn or the establishment of intellectual property rights for plants. Quite the contrary, important work was taking place which would further reveal the structure and mechanisms of heredity.

Frederick Griffith, in the late 1920s, conducted bacterial experiments which indicated the presence and operation of a "transforming principle." Though DNA (deoxyribonucleic acid) had been discovered by a Swiss physiologist, Friedrich Miescher, in 1869, its function was not known. Not until a team of Rockefeller Institute researchers — Oswald T. Avery, Colin MacLeod and Maclyn McCarty — published the results of their work in 1944 was that transforming principle identified. Profoundly and simply, they stated: "The evidence presented supports the belief that a nucleic acid of the deoxribose type is the fundamental unit of the transforming principle of Pneumococcus Type III." They had solved the riddle left by Griffith in his experiments with Pneumococcus and mice.

Experimental pathologist and bio-ethicist Marc Lappé tells us:

While all the members of the team undoubtedly knew they had discovered a way in which the properties of organisms change from one generation to the next, Avery was transfixed by the notion that they had in fact discovered a way to *control* that change.

Writing to his brother Roy in 1944, the year of the initial discovery, Avery pointed out that their finding was "something which has long been the dream of geneticists. Up until now, the mutations (have been) . . . unpredictable and random and chance changes." Now, Avery believed, scientists had the ability to direct that change.[38]

As Nicolai Vavilov, the Soviet scientist who formulated the concept of "Centers of Origin"[39] in cultivated crops was dying of starvation in a Saratov prison for his adherence to genetics (in opposition to Lysenko, the politically powerful proponent of the inheritance of acquired characteristics, and to Lysenko's patron, Stalin), several scientists were on their way to breaking the genetic code. Erwin Chargaff elucidated base-pairing, and Linus Pauling had discovered the helical structure in proteins. James Watson and Francis Crick, working in a British laboratory, studied Pauling's 1939 book on chemical bonding and began to tinker with plausible models of a helix structure for DNA. Crick learned that bases in DNA always paired the same way. And Watson confirmed the helical structure of DNA.

Chargaff had no training in X-ray crystallography which would eventually allow one to visualize the binding of bases in a complete molecule. And Pauling's own theoretical models of a DNA structure were flawed by a mistake or oversight in chemistry by this Nobel Prize-winning chemist. Watson and Crick's model of a double helix with paired bases seemed the logical and simple structure. On a visit to Cambridge, Pauling agreed. Without ever actually having seen what they had discovered, the two published a 900-word article in *Nature*.[40] The "Age of Biology" was blossoming.

As we have seen so often before, scientific discoveries do not automatically translate into commercial techniques or applications. An appropriate social context is required. Watson and Crick's "discovery" was no exception. That it was major and historic was beyond question. But how was it going to be used?[41]

In 1952, Joshua Lederberg discovered that bacteria exchange genetic material through plasmids. Soon it was learned that plasmids consist of small bits of DNA. And it was learned that sequences of DNA in the chromosome constitute a gene, which in turn can be viewed as a set of instructions to produce a certain protein. Werner Arbor, studying phages (viruses that can infect bacteria) observed that some bacteria defended themselves by producing enzymes which split the phage DNA. Arber found that the split ends of the DNA were "sticky," that is, that genes split by these enzymes at the same location will recombine there in the absence of the enzyme, thus recombinant DNA.

A single gene was first isolated in 1969. Four years later, Stanley Cohen and Herbert Boyer, using restriction enzymes with plasmids and single isolated genes ushered in genetic engineering. Again, the concept is relatively simple. Enzymes are used to cut a piece of DNA out of the plasmid. New DNA from another source is then placed in the plasmid. The plasmid transfers the DNA to a bacterium where it becomes a part of the genetic make-up of that bacterium and of future generations of that bacterium. Shortly, fruit fly and frog genes were being transferred into *E. coli*. The patent on this process clearly anticipates the importance of the discovery:

> The ability of genes derived from totally different biological classes to replicate and be expressed in a particular microorganism permits the attainment of interspecies genetic recombination. Thus, it becomes practical to introduce into a particular microorganism . . . functions which are indigenous to other classes of organisms.[42]

In 1976, Boyer and Robert Swanson each put up $500 of their own money and launched Genentech. On October 14, 1980, they took the company public. They offered about 16 percent of the company (1.1 million shares) at $35 a share. Within twenty minutes the price had risen to $89 a share. The company's value was over $500 million.[43] There was no doubt that biotechnology was hot.

Genentech's success in raising capital added to the quickening pace of discovery and spawned dozens of new "biotech" companies, a number specializing in agriculture. It should be noted that the real breakthroughs initially came from scientists in the public sector at Berkeley, Stanford, the University of Wisconsin, and other universities. In short order, these university researchers either jumped ship with offers of big salaries and equity positions in new companies or they signed contracts which turned their publicly-funded research into private hands the moment it became patentable, if not before.[44]

Genentech's incorporation was risky not just because the technology was new and commercially untested, but also because it came four years before the Cohen-Boyer patent mentioned above (or any other biotechnology-related patent) was issued. The technology was racing ahead of the legal or regulatory systems' ability to handle it. Patent attorneys could not have been unaware of the seed industry's difficulty in winning patent and patent-like protection for plants and most recently for varieties of six "little old vegetables." Did they also notice that seed industry officials had reassured Congress by saying that they would never return asking for gene or animal patents?

Despite the promise of the technology, forging a patent system for biotechnology through the Congress would have been nearly impossible in the 1970s or early 1980s. Was it ever seriously considered? Probably not. At the time the industry did not even have a trade association of its own. In any event it is doubtful that it would have wanted to be locked in to a specific law fashioned when fears and concerns about the technology's potential were first surfacing.

Since 1974, two cases had been bouncing between the Patent Office and various courts. One was filed by General Electric the other by Upjohn. The Upjohn case involved a patent application for a biologically pure strain of an antibiotic-producing bacteria. The GE application (filed under the name Chakrabarty, for the GE scientist involved in the work) was for a cell fusion-created bacteria which ate oil. GE's bug, however, could not withstand the rigors of the real world. Unlike Upjohn's, it could have no commercial value in itself. But Upjohn's was a "derived" bacteria, and thus Upjohn could not make as strong an argument that its bug was not simply a "product of nature." Significantly, both patent applications were being filed not to protect the companies, their inventors or their inventions, but to try to establish a legal precedent. Late in 1979, Upjohn dropped its application in an attempt to force the courts to deal with the clearer and stronger GE claim.[45] Let it be observed here that while Upjohn had had some experience with PVPA through its seed company subsidiaries, both it and GE had had far more experience with utility patents and with securing patent coverage through legal as opposed to political means. The legal approach not only made sense pragmatically, but it also fit with the *modus operandi* of the two companies.

The U.S. government, through the Patent Office, opposed both Upjohn's and GE's claims, arguing that had Congress intended bacteria to be patentable it would have specifically provided for such in a law like the Plant Patent Act of 1930 or the Plant Variety Protection Act of 1970.

When the GE case reached the Supreme Court (in Diamond v. Chakrabarty), the Peoples' Business Commission, an activist group headed by Jeremy Rifkin, filed an *amicus* brief in support of the government's position. In this brief, the commission attempted to expand the issue before the court. Using material Pat Mooney and I had written, it cited the deleterious effects of patent laws covering plant varieties and called attention to the loss of genetic diversity.[46]

The court sidestepped these issues, however, with a ruling that was nevertheless sweeping and revolutionary. With a slim five to four majority, the court held that GE's (Chakrabarty's) discovery was patentable because the bacteria was "not nature's handiwork, but his own." The ruling came down just three months before Genentech's stock hit Wall Street.

With blessings from the Supreme Court, the Patent Office was obliged to look upon other biotechnology-related patents with favor.[47] Almost immediately, such patent claims began to flood the office. In 1982, 3116 were received. Through the 1980s, the Patent Office experienced a 20 percent rate of increase in biotechnology patents each year,[48] a rate double that of other technologies compared to 1974–80,[49] Applications for utility patents for plant varieties were accepted in the United States in 1985. Two years later the government announced that higher animals were patentable subject matter.

The GE-Chakrabarty case was a major tactical victory for the industry.[50] Not only did it secure the protection it had long sought, but it did so through a new arena, the court system. The courts were neither fast nor cheap, but they were faster and cheaper than the political process. They were also foreign territory to most advocacy groups. Note that the Peoples' Business Commission was the *only* advocacy group to intervene in the GE case — even those involved in the PVPA fight were conspicuously silent. In any case, few nongovernment organizations familiar with the issues had the experience, funding, or legal standing to pursue opposition to "life-form" patenting in the courts. Furthermore, most NGOs active in the PVPA fight were committed politically and strategically to an "organizing" and political approach rather than a legal approach. This left the legal arena virtually uncontested.

The courts gave the industry what Congress and the administration certainly would not have and they did so in a less public, less painful manner. The decision, made outside the public forum of Congress had another profound benefit to industry — it shifted the debate from "should we patent life?" to "how do we *regulate* biotechnology?" The questions that had been raised for decades over protection of plants were suddenly irrelevant for perhaps all living things. One only had to wait for future interpretations of the GE ruling from the courts and the Patent Office.

As those rulings and interpretations have been made, it has become clear that a wide spectrum of biological material is patentable. This spectrum includes microorganisms, genes, plants, and animals (and characteristics). Plant varieties previously protectable under the PPA or PVPA are now patentable under utility patent statutes. In other words, breeders may choose between legal forms of protection. They can opt for PPA/ PVPA or utility patents (the same laws that protect inventors of new mousetraps and light bulbs). Legal protection at the gene and microorganism levels was precisely what many in the new biotechnology industry desperately desired. Without this, much of the industry would have been without patents. PPA and PVPA held little relevance, particularly for those firms engaged in medical research. Even for agricultural firms, there was the fear that expensive biotechnology research embodied in a novel gene in a plant variety protected as a variety under PPA or PVPA would mean giving that research away via the research and farmers' exemptions.

Utility patents impose more stringent requirements, including the revealing of an "inventive step," but they offer much stronger protection. Under UPOV no "inventive step" is required. One can simply say that the new variety was produced "by crossing," for example.

With utility patents, no research or farmers' exemption exists. A company acquiring a utility patent for a plant variety could theoretically

**Table 9.** Comparison between UPOV (PVPA-Type) and Traditional Patent Systems

| Elements | UPOV | Utility Patent Systems |
|---|---|---|
| Scope of Protection | Product (e.g., variety) | Product<br>Process<br>Use |
| Requirements | Distinct<br>Uniform<br>Stable | New<br>Useful<br>Inventive<br>Sufficiently Described |
| Farmers' Exemption | Yes | No |
| Research Exemption (for experimental use) | Yes | Yes |
| Research Exemption (for commercial use in breeding a new variety) | Yes | No |
| Discoveries patentable? | Yes | No |

Note: Many of the terms used in this table are subject to interpretation and may differ from country to country. Several, including the patentability of discoveries and the scope of research and farmers' exemptions, are in a process of debate and revision in several countries. These are also affected by the recent UPOV Convention revision (see below). This table is intended as a general reference only.

prohibit the farmer or backyard gardener from saving seed from that variety and replanting it. (In fact, proposals to amend the PVPA to strengthen it in just this way are now being floated by the American Seed Trade Association. Instead of a farmer's right to save seed, they refer to the farmer's privilege — a privilege they now wish to withdraw.) A utility patent for a gene or characteristic would prevent other breeders from utilizing, without permission, that gene or characteristic in forming a new variety. It would give tremendous economic power in the marketplace to the holder of a patent for a gene conferring a significant characteristic.[51] In fact, the danger exists that a company could potentially come across very valuable genes and essentially gain control over an entire species through utility patents. Of course, no one would be forced to pay for or use the patented gene. Other companies or farmers could exercise their "freedom" and choose not to acquire or use the new (let us say, disease resistance or higher yield) gene, but exercising that freedom might mean sacrificing competitiveness and going out of business.

The option of strong, formal patent coverage adopted in some countries in the wake of biotechnology has put pressure on UPOV to strengthen its convention lest it become, in the words of critic Pat Mooney, "the Neanderthal of intellectual property systems." A March, 1991, meeting in Geneva formulated a new convention which sanctions double (patent and UPOV-style) protection systems and extends UPOV to all plant genera and species. (Previously, UPOV specified that member states could offer only one form of protection. The revision ratifies the reality — that many states are beginning to offer legal choices for patent and patent-like protection.)

The UPOV revision takes the extraordinary step of extending the rights of holders of protected varieties beyond the reproductive material to the harvested material and products obtained through illegal use of propagating material. This means that the rights' holder legally controls not just the seed but potentially the product of the seed as well. Such proposals must be viewed as attempts to redefine relationships and alter power. This redefinition affects not just relationships between companies and farmers, but also among the companies themselves.

The UPOV revisions also extend coverage to include varieties that are "essentially derived" from protected varieties. Companies complain that other companies take their protected varieties, engage in "cosmetic breeding" (changing one or two easy and unimportant characteristics) and then apply for protection for a "new" variety. The UPOV revision would have the effect of reducing the number of protected varieties, assuming this practice of cosmetic breeding is really a problem. But if it does that, it will damage the industry's argument that PVPA is responsible for increases in the number of varieties and lend credence to critics' claims that the new varieties are new in name only. Furthermore, the criteria that new varieties be "distinct" will surely be tested in coming years. As breeding programs proceed in a common direction toward common goals, the degree of difference between varieties declines, thus forcing redefinitions of what is "distinct." In effect, "distinct" becomes less and less distinct. Eventually most varieties may appear to be derivatively bred. New definitions will continually be needed if the law is to keep pace with changes in plant breeding practices. These new definitions will employ scientific criteria for determining "distance" between two varieties, but the definitions themselves will be rooted in a political and commercial context.

Finally, as mentioned above, the new UPOV treaty mounts a serious attack on the farmer's "right" (or is it a "privilege"?) to save protected seed and replant it. Again, UPOV would extend its rights to harvested material. The revisions would give members the *option* of taking action to allow farmers to save seed for their own use.[52] Without positive action by member states on behalf of the farmers, the right would be lost. Thus, the norm established is that farmers no longer have the right to save seeds (without violating the law or paying royalties). Exceptions can be made, but it is the exception and not the rule that farmers retain control over their harvested seed.

The UPOV revision will require significant legislative changes in national laws for adhering countries[53] — within a certain time period adhering states will be required to adopt the revised treaty — and thus it signals what will surely become a fight in a number of member states, particularly over the issue of whether farmers can legally save the seed of a protected variety for replanting. Farmers refer to this as a "right," as did Allenby White in his testimony for ASTA during hearings on the 1970 PVPA. Recently, however, seed company and ASTA officials have insisted on calling it a "farmer's privilege."[54] The use of language reveals the underlying notion of what type of relationship farmers should have to seeds and the companies that supply them. As a recent ASTA position paper on intellectual property rights clearly states, "Farmers should have restrictions on their ability to save and plant saved seed of varieties protected by PVP and varieties which contain patented genetic components."[55] This is a vision of extremely limited power for farmers, one in which the farmers are limited to one right, the "right" to return to the market each season to purchase seed.

## FURTHER DEVELOPMENT AND REFORMS IN "BIOLOGICAL MATERIALS" LAWS

Plant variety protection laws were themselves a significant departure from traditional patenting systems where inventions have to be new, useful, inventive, and described sufficiently to enable someone skilled in the art to reproduce the invention. In the 1960s and 1970s, it was not thought that plants could meet such strict criteria and they were not required to do so in *sui generis* laws. Thus, the trade which society makes with the inventor, namely the grant of monopoly rights in exchange for the contribution of the knowledge (the inventive step), was compromised.

Biotechnology poses additional problems. Are the "inventions" of biotechnology new and inventive in the legal sense? Or are they products of nature? Can they be described adequately? If not, traditional patent systems offer no protection and new systems, new laws are needed. In the United States, a series of court and Patent Office decisions have ameliorated some of these problems. In contrast, in Europe, the European Patent Convention in Section 53b expressly prohibits the patenting of plants and animals — a formidable obstacle.

Constructing new patent laws to accommodate biotechnology might be the most logical thing to do, but political opposition to this would be far too great in most countries. Instead, there have been and continue to be a multitude of efforts to modify existing patent laws through regulatory, administrative, and judicial decisions. Space does not allow me to do more than generalize. In various countries, these accommodations are taking a number of forms: New microorganisms are being redefined so that they are no longer considered products of nature (and thus excludable from many patent laws), but rather products of human inventiveness. Invention is being redefined to include discovery. Discovery is not treated differently from invention explicitly in U.S. patent statutes, but in Europe discoveries are not generally patentable. This is changing. A new organism, for example, is not one that has never existed before, but one not in a public culture collection or obtainable with more than minimum effort.

The scope of coverage is broadening to include genes and characteristics (and plants and animals). Descriptive requirements are being loosened. And the burden of proof is being reversed. Both the World Intellectual Property Organization and the European Commission, for example, are proposing that defendants prove their innocence by proving that they have not used a plaintiff's patented microorganism.[56] The result of these developments is to maintain the effectiveness of the legal mode of control and give more power and more control to the patent holder.

These moves on the international front have been supplemented by initiatives within the United States. Since the 1980 Chakrabarty case, Congress has passed some 14 laws to strengthen intellectual property protection. According to Representative Robert Kastenmeier, chair of the House Judiciary subcommittee which deals with intellectual property rights, "we're pressured to create new property rights all the time now."[57] Many of these do not deal cleanly and clearly with "the patenting of life" which might engender controversy. But some are just as crucial.

In this chapter, the importance of judicial interpretations of existing law was demonstrated. But how the law is applied and who applies it are also important factors for actors seeking legal protections. Prior to 1982, patent appeals cases were heard in all twelve U.S. Courts of Appeal. In 1982, Congress created the U.S. Court of Appeals for the Federal Circuit based in Washington as a court to hear all patent appeal cases. That court is now upholding patents in 80 percent of the cases, versus 30 percent under the old system."[58] In addition, the Reagan Justice Department relaxed its policy of using antitrust laws against companies that aggressively defended their patents, refused to license their technologies, or charged higher fees to some users than others. Injunctive relief is now possible to force an alleged infringer out of the business before the case is decided. And penalties can be assessed on lost sales, not just lost royalties. Willful infringement can result in a tripling of damages.[59] The result of these policy changes, legal reforms, and judicial rearrangements has been a dramatic increase not only in the rate of patents upheld as cited above, but also in the absolute number of cases filed — up 60 percent since 1980.[60]

In addition, the seed industry is seeking a strengthening of the Plant Variety Protection Act through tightening of the farmer exemption. According to the industry, too many farmers are using this exemption to grow and resell seeds of protected varieties for the purpose of planting. The industry claims that this is forcing them out of certain smaller markets by making breeding for these niche markets uneconomical. Privately, however, executives state that they would like to see farmers prohibited from reusing the seed of protected varieties on their own farms. As already noted, industry publications have begun referring to the farmers' right to do this (which is provided for explicitly in the PVPA) as "farmers' *privilege.*" Those exercising this "privilege," however, are characterized as "pirates." Once again there is an effort to separate farmer from seed and further commercialize and commodify seed through the patent system.

The United States has also acted to impose its own bilateral sanctions on countries deemed to have unfair trade barriers, including inadequate intellectual property laws. Since 1984, the United States has held bilateral talks with more than 30 nations, tying provision of adequate intellectual property rights to participation in the general system of preferences, which allows countries to export to the United States without restrictive tariffs.[61] Reductions in preferences have been placed into effect against Argentina, Brazil and Mexico. A trade law passed in 1988 virtually mandates sanctions against countries perceived to be engaging in unfair trade practices against the United States. Trade Representative Carla Hills (the U.S. negotiator in the General Agreement on Tariffs and Trade — GATT) has reported that 36 countries are engaging in such practices — nearly all reports include a section on intellectual property. Punitive tariffs of $39 million were in fact imposed on Brazil in June, 1988, concerning Brazil's not honoring U.S. drug patents, an act which the president of Brazil's congress termed a "gratuitous act of aggression."[62]

To summarize: the explosion of biotechnology in the 1970s and 1980s created new opportunities for the seed industry and biotechnology companies. But realizing these opportunities depended on devising a successful strategy for adapting the legal system to take advantage of the possibilities raised by the new technologies. Past experiences with legislative fights over extensions of the scope of patent law were enough to give anyone doubts about the success of obtaining gene patenting, for example, from the U.S. Congress in the 1970s. Patent rights were secured through the court system beginning in 1980, marking a major change in tactics and arenas for proponents of biological patents. Since then the court system itself has been manipulated to be even more amenable to patent holders. Furthermore, UPOV has recently strengthened its convention. In the next chapter, we shall examine the strengths and limitations of these strategies and why they have helped push the biotechnology patent debate into still new, and potentially more risky arenas, with new and very different actors.

## DISCUSSION

The account of the successful effort to expand coverage of the  original 1970 Plant Variety Protection Act to include the six vegetables excluded from it and to make other changes[63] to facilitate U.S. entry into the International Union for the Protection of New Varieties of Plants (UPOV), further exemplifies earlier themes regarding the legislative process within a larger context of rationalization, commercialization and introduction of technologies.

However, this chapter is also about the emergence of new actors, new relationships among actors, new issues, interest group behavior, and the role of bureaucracy in this particular legislative process. When the American Seed Trade Association organized to secure passage of the amendment, new actors such as various public interest groups mobilized their constituencies to oppose the amendment. The choice and creativity they displayed was limited by the legislative history of the PVPA, the commercial context, and the congressional arena. While the public arena enabled advocacy groups to make a "public" issue out of the amendment, that arena eventually constrained those very actors — by circumscribing the issues that could be effectively raised and the manner in which they were raised. (Strictly speaking, the issue to be decided was the amendment dealing with the six vegetables — not genetic erosion, seed industry concentration, or other concerns) Congress also provided a less-than-friendly atmosphere for challenges to property rights which already had precedence in the law and which were supported by large corporations.

As Weber and Collins have noted, rational capitalism is predictable and routine.[64] Laws are often sought to increase that predictability. According to Collins, mass production is impossible without predictability, which implies institutional factors and appropriate systems of law, property and finance.[65] By 1980 the seed industry had become big business. Seeds were being produced on a large scale by multinational corporations such as Shell Oil and Monsanto. The PVPA (together with participation in UPOV) were seen by industry groups as protecting their research investment and as providing a predictable, ordered business environment. This was what the effort to pass the 1980 amendment was all about. However, seed industry efforts to achieve consistency and increase rationality caused tension and led to conflict and change.[66] They drew opposition from advocacy groups, farmer organizations, and church groups, which raised new issues and created a new and more controversial context.

The entrance of these new actors in 1980 was an unexpected development from the standpoint of the bill's sponsors, and it expanded the issue well beyond property rights. Now the discussion concerned industry concentration, loss of genetic diversity, the breeding strategies of pesticide companies in the seed business, the ethics of patenting forms of life, seed prices, government plant breeding, research policies, and America's relationship with international organizations such as UPOV. Part of the reason that the range of issues expanded was that the new actors were not bound by the norms of the seed industry. Its rules did not apply to them and they were not accountable through social ties or employment to the industry. In fact, as Dietz notes, 1960s activists were "pre-adapted" to be skeptical of the exercise of corporate and government power.[67]

In this chapter we are still dealing with some of the effects of major changes in the science and technology of plant breeding. By themselves, these changes did not produce pressure to change or reinterpret laws. All technology exists in a social context: the technology influencing the 1980 legislation was embedded in commercial structures. The development of technology (in a commercial context) was linked with rule system changes.[68] Each affected the other and contributed to changing the other.

Without the proposed amendments to allow patent-like protection for the six vegetables omitted from the 1970 act, breeders of the six were unable to prevent other companies from acquiring their new varieties, producing seeds with them, and selling them to the public — all legally. Without control over the varieties, the original breeders failed to realize the profit potential of their varieties. The amendment would also allow the United States to join UPOV, which would facilitate international recognition of property rights assigned in the United States. Actors such as seed companies worked to overcome the mismatches, incompatibilities or problems that occurred when changes in technology and commerce did not coincide with existing legal arrangements. They worked to create laws such as the PVPA which would allow them to benefit more from the opportunities raised by the new technologies and related changes to commercial and market structures. Such laws can help institutionalize power, resource control, and action capabilities, allowing some actors to dominate or benefit on a systematic basis. We can begin to discern this in changing relationships between large and small companies and between breeding and nonbreeding companies. It is further revealed and confirmed in data on the concentration of PVPA certificates held by specific corporations.

Laws embody choice — purpose, plans, policies and desires.[69] But the choices are structured, limited.[70] Some theories which begin with a methodological individualism have trouble dealing with the context of the legal process, with how certain choices come to be present and with the feedback mechanisms from structure to actors.[71] In this chapter the importance of context and agency is stressed. As actors struggled, they learned and changed and they gained or lost power.[72] Power is the ability to affect others' choice.[73]

Actors act with incomplete knowledge, different levels of skill, experience and resources, and varying degrees of access to politicians and bureaucrats — all are illustrated in the history of the 1980 amendment. Conflict was heightened when actors who possessed more traditional forms of power, but who were unaccustomed to confrontational and media politics, struggled with those who were more comfortable and experienced with this style.

Laws are created by actors within a certain context; they do not spring forth from social consensus.[74] The notion that "people deserve to receive the fruits of their labors" was not enough to insure coverage or ownership under the law. Despite the fact that the 1980 law simply expanded the 1970 law, it did not become law because of the extension of legal logic, but because of the initiatives of actors, who struggled to extend (or limit) that logic. In other words, the existence of gaps in the 1970 law does not fully explain the passage of the 1980 law — the gaps could have been allowed to remain. Similarly, laws are not passed simply because a powerful group "needs" them, whatever this may seem to mean. It still takes effort, creativity, and mobilizing of resources. Law is not the inevitable result of "need." The amendment was not secured just because "the industry needed it." Were that the case, the six vegetables would never have been excluded from the 1970 act. Surely industry "needed" it then as much as it needed protection for many of the other species. By 1980 we have witnessed three legislative contests (over the PPA, the PVPA and now the expansion of the PVPA). Clearly, none of the resulting laws can be explained by simply identifying "needs." Each must be understood in the richness of a particular context. Each must be understood as having been created by actors through the exercise of agency. As I have tried to show, these are not automatons, blindly fulfilling a role or function, but creative agents engaged in purposeful activity which "makes a difference."

Laws also do not simply institutionalize custom. Burns states that general notions of property rights represent deeply ingrained norms. It would appear, however, that *intellectual* property rights concerning *biological* materials are not so deeply ingrained and there are widely differing views about what rights of ownership should be provided under law.[75]

The laws which actors secure may or may not reflect existing norms; indeed this may be the source of friction and conflict. Actors may be able to explain the new property rights they desire in traditional language, obscuring their radical content. (Is this self-deception, design, or the "veil of ignorance?") Thus property rights over plant varieties were asserted as though there were essentially no difference between light bulbs and plants, or the "inventive" process behind the two. However, in a new situation different existing norms may conflict.[76] Once expanded to include plant breeders, the granting of rights to inventors conflicted with the common ownership of plant species and varieties and the view (previously enshrined in law) that "products of nature" were not patentable. I conclude that in this particular field, redefinitions of property rights are difficult to assert in democratic fora, particularly in the presence of organized oppositional interests. In such fora, appeals can be made to conflicting norms and opposing interests may be organized. (This point will be further illustrated in the following chapter.) In fact, in 1980, amendment opponents challenged the very assumptions that seed industry actors thought had become accepted — namely their "right" to property rights over plants. The emerging opposition was one reason why some companies apparently preferred to seek additional property rights through the courts, where such assumptions were scarcely questioned.[77]

The unintended consequences of the introduction and commercialization of new technologies are not usually as quickly known as the benefits. In this case, the PVPA was effectively passed in two stages (1970 and 1980). All sexually reproduced plants except six were made eligible for patent-like protection in 1970. The six were added in 1980. By the time the amendment was debated in 1980, the 1970 Act had a ten-year history. Consequences of the act became the subject of investigation and debate in 1980. Indeed, the effects of the new sociotechnical system (including the PVPA) on genetic diversity in agricultural crops was scrutinized. (See also appendix 1.) Advocacy groups such as the National Sharecroppers Fund broadened the scope of the debate by bringing in the unintended consequences of the replacement of traditional crop varieties by modern, scientifically bred commercial varieties (which they claimed was furthered by PVPA). They asserted that this "genetic erosion" entailed great risks and undermined the very foundations of agriculture, including most directly plant breeding itself. Thus, in the political debate over amendments to the PVPA, such concerns became linked with intellectual property rights claims as part of the political context in which the law was enacted.

In 1980 the amendment was developed and introduced into Congress almost in a routine way, without fanfare. Seed industry representatives and members of Congress expected it to be dealt with quietly and quickly. (As Harold Loden of ASTA remarked to the chief congressional sponsor of the bill, "When I told you it was noncontroversial that was the biggest lie I ever told!")[78] This was an understandable miscalculation. New issues can attract attention (and the participation of new actors) and upset plans and strategies.

Often "bureaucratic politics" is more important than party politics in the modern state,[79] especially when a matter is not likely to be a public or media issue. In this case, it was not simply bureaucratic politics, but the way in which the policy system operates that was important. Support and opposition to the amendment in 1980 was not divided along party lines in Congress. As in 1970, bureaucrats within the U.S. Department of Agriculture supported the bill and actively "politicked" for it. They and other actors sought to create policy and chose to do so in ways outside any formal system of public input.

As an arena, Congress has certain rules and norms which guide how it operates. Congressional and industry representatives use these rules to thwart opponents. Individual representatives are powerful by virtue of their membership. Thus, when a senator serving as a subcommittee chairman obstructed the bill, it appeared that the bill might not move out of his committee. But when he lost his bid for reelection in Alabama, "rules" of courtesy and procedure no longer applied and the bill was removed from his jurisdiction.

After passage of the 1980 amendment, Congress appeared to key industry actors to have been exhausted as an effective arena. They needed to take concerns to new arenas — the courts and GATT (see the following chapter), for four reasons. First, the PVPA itself had now been "completed." A further broadening of property rights would probably entail not an amendment to the PVPA but an entirely new law.  Second, given the difficulties in passing the simple amendments in 1980, it was unlikely that proponents would see Congress as a fertile arena for further expansions of property rights in the early 1980s.[80] The expansion of rights now considered by certain business interests was much more conceptually and politically challenging and therefore risky, in that additional actors might be drawn into the fray and a bigger battle created. Third, PVPA opponents also wanted a more favorable arena and sought an expansion of issues, which was not easily addressed by Congress. And fourth, some industry organizations and particular corporations desired broadened, uniform, *international* patent law coverage, which was beyond the capabilities of the U.S. Congress to provide.

We have seen that new technologies are often mismatched with existing sociotechnical systems. The rapid development of the "new biotechnologies" in the 1970s presented scientists and companies involved in this field with remarkable technical capabilities and commercial opportunities. Yet, the U.S. Congress did not and probably would not have sanctioned the patenting of new genetically engineered organisms which scientists were increasingly able to "create." Budding new biotechnology companies were stymied in protecting their research investment, owning and controlling their inventions, and securing their position in the marketplace, because many of their inventions had the ability to reproduce and could do so in commercial facilities almost anywhere. The new technology permitted what existing laws did not yet facilitate or encourage — the development and commercialization of new biotechnological products.

In terms of securing property rights which would make the new technologies more useful, actors faced alternative arenas in which to pursue their goals. Indeed, these goals could be pursued in one arena or simultaneously in more than one. Different actors with complementary interests could be involved in different arenas. This last possibility is more likely with well-organized, highly motivated and well-financed interests dealing with issues of broad applicability.

The existence of a law does not tell us how it is interpreted, used or enforced. Not all changes occur by passing new laws. Actors can attempt to change the way in which laws are routinely interpreted and enforced. They can even attempt to change who does the interpreting and enforcing, as we see with the Reagan Administration's reorganization of the courts dealing with patents.

As certain actors pursued an amendment to the PVPA in the late 1970s and in 1980, several corporations pursued increased patent protection by asking the courts to reinterpret existing patent law in order to expand the applicability of those and other laws. These corporations were knowledgeable about utility patent law and the appeals process for patent applications. While Congress posed problems, the court system was familiar.

Arenas are action settings. As previously noted, they have certain rules (formal, informal or both). These rules prescribe which issues can be addressed, in what manner (and with what potential result), through what procedures, by which actors, as well as where and when this may take place. Such rules influence the ways in which issues can be framed and the resources that can be used, and require new resources and different skills. One may lobby Congress, for example, but not the courts. The peculiar characteristics of an arena therefore affect relations among actors, influence the recruitment and involvement of allies, and give some actors advantages and power while placing others at a disadvantage. Certain arenas favor some actors over others. The favored actors may have better "standing," more experience, more resources, and more power in those arenas than others. Their goals may be more tailored for or appropriate to the arena than those of other actors. Thus, actors seek to use arenas most comfortable, appropriate, and useful to the pursuit of their interests.

In the 1970s, two corporations cooperated to fashion a powerful test case which was brought through a series of courts all the way to the Supreme Court. This case was not aimed at securing a patent for a particular microorganism, for it was acknowledged that the organism concerned had no commercial value. Instead the case was filed for the purpose of obtaining a ruling to expand the scope of the existing law to cover forthcoming inventions. The corporations in question had legal standing in the court, and a compelling "case" strengthened by the financial and technical expertise to present it. Potential adversaries were disadvantaged by lack of experience, knowledge and finances in this arena. Furthermore, NGOs which fought the expansion of rights in Congress saw their role as organizers and advocates, not as litigants.[81] The case was won by General Electric, which argued that its creation was not a product of nature but of human manufacture. However, the rights won in the U.S. courts are geographically bound, and the private sector was not willing to settle for such constraints.

## NOTES

1. Quoted in Cleaver, Harry, "Contradiction of the Green Revolution." *Monthly Review*. June, 1972.
2. Anonymous, *Changes in Farm Production and Efficiency*, 1978. Washington: U.S. Department of Agriculture. January, 1980: p. 18.
3. Quoted by Douglas Learmond, *Journal of Commerce*, November 24, 1971.
4. *Congressional Record*, November, 1973, p. 268.
5. *Wall Street Journal*, August 10, 1961, p. 1.
6. Emergency Committee for American Trade, "The Role of the Multinational Corporation in the United States World Economies," Sections A-1 and A-2 in Subcommittee on International Trade of the Senate Finance Committee, Multinational Corporations, 93, 1, p. 837–848. The obvious exception to the trends noted above was in plantation agriculture. At this time, Henry Frundt tells us, "The growth rate of U.S. transnational corporations in plantation agriculture was the lowest of all growth rates among the various sectors of U.S. corporate investment abroad." (Frundt, Henry, *American Agribusiness and U.S. Foreign Agricultural Policy*. Ph.D. dissertation, Rutgers University. 1975: p. 168.)
7. Vaupel, James W., and Joan P. Curhan, *The World's Multinational Enterprizes: A Sourcebook of Tables*. Boston: Harvard Business School. 1973: p. 344.
8. Anonymous, *Business Week*. November 21, 1970: p. 30.
9. See, for example, McMullen, Neil. *Seeds and World Agricultural Progress*. Washington: National Planning Association. 1987.
10. Quoted in Doyle, Jack, *Altered Harvest: Agriculture, Genetics, and the Fate of the World's Food Supply*. New York: Viking. 1985: p. 104.
11. Harlan, Jack, "Genetics of Disaster." *Journal of Environmental Quality*. Vol. 1, No. 3. 1972: p. 213, 215.
12. His childhood home was decorated with maps in virtually every room. His only sibling, a brother, has also pursued international work through a career with the Canadian foreign service.
13. I also wrote a pamphlet entitled "Seeds of Life or Destruction?" for the Agricultural Marketing  Project of the Vanderbilt University Medical School. The pamphlet was distributed by farmers at open-air markets in Tennessee and Alabama in 1977.
14. Fowler, Cary, Open letter dated July 4, 1979.
15. Telephone interview with Harold Loden (former seed company official and president and top staff officer of the American Seed Trade Association), Athens, Ga., July 9, 1992.

16. Brown, George Jr., Letter to Representative Kika de la Garza dated November 8, 1979.
17. Crittenden, Ann, "Plan to Widen Plant Patents Stirs Conflict." *New York Times*. June 6, 1980: p. 1.
18. Hjort, Howard, "Final Impact Statement." USDA. January 9, 1979: p. 1.
19. Ibid., p. 2, 3.
20. Also important was the fulfillment of the informal agreement ASTA had made with members adversely affected by the dropping of the six vegetables in 1970 that it would attempt to secure the inclusion of the vegetables at the earliest possible time.
21. McMullen (1987: p. 92) cites a survey of 100 corporate takeovers in the seed industry. Only two occurred prior to passage of the PVPA in 1970. Sixty-one occurred between 1970 and 1979. Nineteen occurred in the 1980s and the dates of the rest are unknown. Neil McMullen, *Seeds and World Agricultural Progress*. Washington: National Planning Association. 1987: p. 92.
22. McMullen, op. cit., p. 131.
23. Drug companies had rather recently become involved in animal and plant health products, including pesticides. The link between this activity and plant breeding was and is an obvious factor in their interest in the seed business.
24. Mansfield, Edwin, "Intellectual Property, Technology and Economic Growth." in *Intellectual Property Rights in Science, Technology, and Economic Performance: International Comparisons*, Francis W. Rushing and Carole Ganz Brown (eds.). Boulder, Colo.: Westview Press. 1990: p. 224–225.
25. In a government-sponsored survey, two-thirds of the public sector plant breeders and four-fifths of the private sector plant breeders "felt PVPA has increased the acquisition of seed companies by non-seed companies." In *The Impacts of Patent Protection on the U.S. Seed Industry and Public Plant Breeding* by L. J. Butler and B. W. Marion. Research Division, College of Agricultural and Life Sciences, University of Wisconsin-Madison. September, 1985: p. 51.
26. Note reference to related matters in the previous chapter. American companies took a different position on this than did their European counterparts. In the United States in the early 1960s, companies feared that plant breeders' rights might be a Trojan horse for "germplasm control" with the government deciding which varieties could or could not be sold.
27. Jabs, Carolyn. *The Heirloom Gardener*. San Francisco: Sierra Club Books. 1984: p. 79–80.
28. This was encouraged by a poorly written Associated Press wire article which clearly stated that the bill might outlaw certain vegetable varieties. The industry charged opponents with feeding false information to the journalist, but opponents themselves denied ever having had contact with the journalist. See "Farm Bill Could Make Growing of Some Vegetable Varieties Illegal," *The Farmers Forum*, Fargo-Moorhead, September 7, 1979: p. 9.
29. Fowler, Cary, quoted in "Testimony before the Senate Agriculture Subcommittee on Agricultural Research and General Legislation on S. 23, An Amendment to the Plant Variety Protection Act. Washington. June 17, 1980: p. 13.
30. Ibid., p. 7ff. These were acquisitions known of by opponents to the legislation. A more complete listing could probably have been made by those associated with the seed industry, but none was made public.
31. Dahlberg, Kenneth, "Testimony before House Subcommittee on Department Investigations, Oversight, and Research on H.R. 999." Washington. April 22, 1980: p. 140 (of Hearings).
32. Fowler, Cary, "A Brief Guide to the Issues Involved in Plant Patenting and Amendments to the Plant Variety Protection Act (H.R. 999, and S. 23) Which Would Expand Coverage of Our Plant Patenting Law." (Unpublished) National Sharecroppers Fund: 1980. Statements are taken from the official record of the hearings.
33. Stewart, Senator Donald, "Statement." Hearings before the Subcommittee on Agricultural Research and General Legislation of the Committee on Agriculture, Nutrition, and Forestry, United States Senate, on S. 23, S. 1580 and S. 2820. June 17, 1980: p. 2.

34. Hearings before the Subcommittee on Agricultural Research and General Legislation of the Committee on Agriculture, Nutrition, and Forestry, United States Senate on S. 23, S. 1580, and S. 2820. June 17, 1980. p. 12 ff.
35. Anderson, Jack, "Stewart Is Yet To Answer Questions About Ethics," Syndicated newspaper column. October, 1980.
36. Fowler, Cary, "Testimony," p. 2. (Data derived from seed industry sources.)
37. Data compiled from the *Journal of the Plant Variety Protection Office* and from various sources regarding ownership and takeovers in the seed industry. This table gives a sample of the most patented crops (the first six) with some of the least patented crops (the final six in the table).
38. Lappé, Marc, *Broken Code: The Exploitation of DNA*. San Francisco: Sierra Club Books. 1984: p. 15.
39. Vavilov's Centers of Origin are more commonly referred to as Centers of Diversity today, in large part because the latter places emphasis on the utility of the insight. If one can determine the Center of Diversity of a particular crop, it can help guide collecting efforts when new genetic material is needed for crop breeding programs. While Vavilov based his Centers of Origin on where he found the greatest diversity, he never actually used the term, "Centers of Diversity."
40. Watson, J. D. and F. H. C. Crick, "Molecular Structure of Nucleic Acids: A Structure for Deoxyribose Nucleic Acid." *Nature*. Vol. 171. 1953: p. 737–738.
41. When interviewed recently, James Watson was asked if in 1953 he had any idea that his research would spawn an industry. Watson replied "None whatever . . . " Watson then proceeded to explain the importance of others' work and claim that Boyer and Cohen, not Watson and Crick, were the "parents" of biotechnology. See "From the Double Helix to the Human Genome," in *Biotech 90: Into the Next Decade*, by G. Steven Burrill with the Ernst & Young High Technology Group. New York: Mary Ann Liebert, Inc. 1989: p. 171ff.
42. United States Patent Office, "Patent 4,237,224 :  Process of Producing Biologically Functional Molecular Chimeras." Washington: U.S. Patent Office. 1980: p. 1.
43. McAuliffe, Sharon, and Kathleen McAuliffe, *Life for Sale*. New York: Coward, McCann & Geoghegan. 1981: p. 27–28.
44. Kenney, Martin, *Biotechnology: The University-Industrial Complex*. New Haven: Yale University Press. 1986.
45. McAuliffe and McAuliffe, op. cit. p. 199.
46. Peoples' Business Commission, Parker v. Chakrabarty,  Brief in the Supreme Court of the United States, October Term, 1979, No. 79–136. p. 6ff.
47. In 1985, the Patent Office´s Board of Patent Appeals and Interfaces ruled that a corn plant containing an increased level of a certain amino acid could be patented. This ruling, *Ex parte Hibberd,* firmly established that the government would allow  utility patents for plants under 35 U.S.C. 101. Two years later in *Ex Parte Allen* the board ruled that multicellular animals were patentable. A year after that, the first animal patent was issued to Harvard University for its genetically engineered mouse.
48. International Biotechnology Association, "Backlog in Biotechnology Patent Applications," *IBA Reports*. July-August, 1988: p. 9.
49. Lacy, William and Lawrence Busch, "The Changing Division of Labor Between the University and Industry: The Case of Agricultural Biotechnology," in Molnar, Joseph, and Henry Kinnucan (eds.), *Biotechnology and the New Agricultural Revolution*. Boulder, Colo.: Westview Press for the American Association for the Advancement of Science. AAAS Selected Symposium 108. 1989: p. 34–35.
50. It also affected research expenditures according to Buttel and Barker. They say that the PVPA and the Chakrabarty case stimulated "a trememdous amount of private investment in agricultural biotechnology in general and plant-related biotechnology in particular." Frederick Buttel and Randolph Barker, "Emerging Agricultural Technologies, Public Policy, and the Implications for Third World Agriculture: The Case of Biotechnology," *American Journal of Agricultural Economics*. Vol. 66, no. 2. December, 1985: p. 1172.

51. See, for example, the case of Hilleshøg and sugar beets described in Berg, Trygve, Åsmund Bjørnstad, Cary Fowler, and Tore Skrøppa, *Technology Options and the Gene Struggle*. NORAGRIC Occasional Papers Series C. Ås: Norwegian Centre for International Agricultural Development. Agricultural University of Norway. March, 1991: p. 124.

52. UPOV, Diplomatic Conference for the Revision of the International Convention for the Protection of New Varieties of Plants. "Final Draft, International Convention for the Protection of New Varieties of Plants." Geneva: UPOV. March 19, 1991.

53. Elgin, J. H. "Briefing Paper — Impact of the 1991 Revised UPOV Convention." Unpublished USDA internal document. April 5, 1991.

54. Studebaker, John, "PVP: Where Are We Going From Here?" *Seed World*. July, 1991: p. 18.

55. American Seed Trade Association, "ASTA Position Statement on Intellectual Property Rights for the Seed Industry." Approved by the ASTA Board of Directors, June 29, 1990. Washington: ASTA. 1990: p. 2.

56. Newman, Peter, "A Modest Proposal for European Patents," *Bio/Technology*. Vol. 7, January 1989: p. 26.

57. Dwyer, Paula, "The Battle Raging Over Intellectual Property," *Business Week*, May 22, 1989: p. 78.

58. Ibid., p. 79.

59. Anonymous, "Pay Attention to Patents, Says Management Expert," *Research & Development*. December, 1988: p. 16.

60. Dwyer, op. cit., p. 78.

61. Gadbaw, R. M. and T. J. Richards, (eds.), *Intellectual Property Rights; Global Consensus, Global Conflict?* Boulder, Colo.: Westview Press. 1988: p. 7.

62. Dwyer, op. cit., p. 87. ("Super-301," as the relevant section of this Act was called, expired in 1990. The main target, according to an economic advisor to GATT's director-general, was Japan. "India and Brazil were thrown in, mainly because they had irked America's trade negotiators at the Uruguay round by objecting strenuously to American positions on services and intellectual property." The effectiveness of Super-301 is debatable. See Bhagwati, Jagdish, "It's the Process, Stupid," *The Economist*, Vol. 326, no. 7804, March 27, 1993: p. 83.)

63. Such as lengthening the effective period of the PVPA certificate from 17 to 18 years to conform with the UPOV standard. This change — largely irrelevant and not needed by the industry — further demonstrates the link between the 1980 amendment and the desire of its promoters to have the United States join UPOV.

64. Collins, Randall, *Max Weber: A Skeleton Key*. Beverly Hills: Sage Publications. 1986: p. 32.

65. Ibid., p. 86.

66. Ibid., p. 74.

67. Dietz, Tom, personal communication, November 23, 1992.

68. Burns, Tom, and Helena Flam, *The Shaping of Social Organization: Social Rule System Theory with Applications*. London: Sage Publications. 1987: p. 293, 13.

69. Chambliss, William, and Robert Seidman. *Law, Order, and Power*. Second Edition. Reading, Mass.: Addison-Wesley. 1982: p. 10.

70. Burns, Tom, Thomas Baumgartner, and Philippe Deville, *Man, Decisions, Society: The Theory of Actor-System Dynamics for Social Scientists*. New York: Gordon and Breach Science Publishers. 1985: p. 8.

71. Van Den Broeck, Julien. *Public Choice*. Dordrecht, The Netherlands: Kluwer Academic Publishers. 1988: p. 46ff.

72. This will be quite evident with both nongovernment organizations (NGOs) and the seed industry from this point onward.

73. Chambliss and Seidman, op. cit., p. 89.

74. Ibid., p. 34.

75. Witness the diversity of opponents — religious, farm, consumer, environmental, scientists (academia).
76. This is one reason that religious organizations are drawn into the controversy. Some feel that it is not right to patent "life" or otherwise claim responsibility for having invented something like a plant or animal.
77. It is also one reason behind the move of NGOs to the FAO. At FAO, such basic assumptions can be challenged and presented in their political and economic context.
78. Interview with Harold Loden.
79. Rourke, Francis, *Bureaucracy, Politics, and Public Policy.* Second Edition. Boston: Little, Brown and Company. 1976: p. 184.
80. Adding coverage of six vegetables to the existing PVPA was controversial enough without considering the difficulties of securing patentability for microorganisms, animals, genes, etc.
81. Several environmental groups such as the Environmental Defense Fund and the Natural Resources Defense Council do have experience in litigation. However, they were late in expressing concern over biotechnology. Furthermore, their involvement in agriculturally oriented biodiversity issues has been slight, thus they have not had significant, ongoing relationships with those NGOs most active in this area.

# PART III: DEFINING PROPERTY RIGHTS IN INTERNATIONAL ARENAS

*New Issues and Actors, Unsettled Conflicts*

CHAPTER **6**

# New International Initiatives:
# GATT, FAO and Keystone

Biotechnology is actually a collection of technologies which open up new possibilities for the directed manipulation of genetic materials, and in so doing create a situation in which genetic diversity potentially becomes quite valuable. These developments in technology also represent changes in relationships among actors, and form the framework for conflict and the redefinition of rights and relationships.

By their very nature, many of the products of biotechnologies can be produced almost anywhere. Often the laboratory or fermentation vat is the environment.[1] The fact that bacteria and plant varieties can reproduce and light bulbs cannot means that methods of control (including questions of access) are qualitatively different with biotechnology than with most previous technologies. To profit fully from this technology and to protect against its misappropriation, a system of control which is international in scope is necessary. Without such a system, even strong domestic patent laws would only provide a consolation prize to American companies.

The scientific and commercial development of biotechnology raced ahead of the legal protections in the 1980s. While Congress was debating patent protection for plant varieties, the industry was anticipating the immediate need for gene patenting, characteristic patenting, and microorganism and animal patenting. It is probably safe to say that neither the public nor the Congress had had enough time to become comfortable with the new technology. The prospect of legislating patent protection for new forms of life engineered in the laboratory must have been daunting indeed to corporate strategists. Instead, as we have seen, some companies chose a legal arena. But as with congressional action, a limitation of this approach was that it only applied to the United States. Another change of arenas developed — one designed to bring patent laws for biotechnology by fiat to virtually all countries, but without the necessity of going through a time-consuming and unpredictable debate country by country. As with the legal route, this new arena — the General Agreement on Tariffs and Trade (GATT) also puts opponents at a disadvantage.

The U.S. courts and GATT were (and are) unlikely arenas, of course, for the expansion of rights and benefits sought by nongovernment organ-

171

izations (NGOs — advocacy groups such as the Rural Advancement Fund International and the International Coalition for Development Action) and certain Third World governments for the biological materials found in the fields and forests of Asia, Africa and Latin America. By the early 1980s, these actors had succeeded in securing a new and more sympathetic forum for their concerns — the UN Food and Agriculture Organization in Rome.

In the final part of this chapter, we look at a novel effort to "settle" some of the issues which had flared up in the sometimes raucous and unpredictable forum of the FAO. I examine a new effort designed to negotiate the terms of access away from the political pressures of the more public, more ideological FAO. This is also an effort on the part of some actors to defuse an otherwise unpredictable situation at FAO, and on the part of others to realize some gains from past battles. This avenue seems to lead toward major concessions to the Third World. But ultimately the benefits may be greater for others. The structure of the new arena allows for and seems to encourage actors' loosening their traditional positions. In negotiations, adversaries can share at least one common goal — a successful resolution of the conflict. In the Keystone Dialogue, this appears to shape behavior.

The entrance of the Keystone Center as a new actor and facilitator of the negotiations holds the possibility of introducing significant, unpredictable change. The Keystone "rules" are different than those that have governed past interactions. They push strongly towards compromise and away from confrontation. And through breaking down personal barriers between individuals and organizations, the process holds the possibility of bringing order to the debate — if only for a moment!

## INTELLECTUAL PROPERTY RIGHTS AT GATT

The legal breakthroughs of 1980, both with PVPA and Chakrabarty, were important in expanding the scope of patent protection in the United States, but they did little to protect American business outside the country in the case of biotechnology. Five years later, patent authorities were still able to say that "the field of biotechnological inventions is the most prominent example of the existence of a considerable gap between the state of the art and the state of the law."[2]

Biotechnology, perhaps more than any other technology this century, came about as an international technology. From the beginning a web of investments, contracts, joint ventures, and research projects linked together different companies and research institutes around the world.

Additionally, this is the first major industry to emerge within a context of global telecommunications and computer databases, and in a milieu of international business as a norm in the corporate world. Concretely, foreign sales by biotechnology companies are expected to more than double in the next decade as a percentage of all sales.[3]

The biotechnology industry is unusually committed to research. As the Organization for Economic Cooperation and Development (OECD) put it, biotechnology is a "science push" rather than a "market pull" development such as semiconductors.[4] Agricultural biotechnology companies currently devote 146 percent of product sales to research and development costs. R & D expenses as a percentage of sales for biotech therapeutic drug firms are 125 percent.[5] Few industries could match such expenditures and the biotechnology industry will not be able to do so very long itself. At current rates of R & D expenditures over sales, only a fifth of all biotechnology companies can survive more than 36 months. Nearly 40 percent cannot survive a year.[6]

With so many companies facing collapse, the importance of patents becomes immense. According to a study by Linda Miller, a vice president at PaineWebber, biotechnology companies cite obtaining patents as the second most significant risk to their business.[7]

Few products can be developed, tested, approved by regulatory agencies, and on the markets in time to generate enough cash to save most biotechnology companies. For many companies, the patent becomes the product — the product that can be dangled before the investment community for more funds, or the product that can literally be sold to other companies.

With no more than a handful of biotechnology products actually on the market, there are more than 8000 biotechnology patents pending before the U.S. Patent Office. Increasingly, patents are the force guiding research decisions. One example published in *Business Week* will suffice. In late 1987, Genetics Institute (a Cambridge, Massachusetts company) had to decide which of four potential products to pursue. It did not have the funding to work on all four. A meeting was called at the company headquarters. The scientists argued for the one that had done the best in research. The attorneys argued for another. It had not performed as well, but it could garner the most powerful patent. The attorneys' view prevailed. According to the company's patent attorney, Bruce Eisen, "researchers used to be up in arms if such crass decisions were made." But now, "the strength of the potential patent position is a leading factor in what research to pursue."[8] Indeed, at least one company was created in the United States whose "main business," according to the *Wall Street Jour-*

*nal*, "is buying up patents and then suing other companies for alleged infringements . . ."[9]

Not only do companies expect researchers to produce patents, they expect them to produce broad patents, patents which anticipate future developments in the science and try to cover these developments within the scope of the patent. The famous patent issued for a transgenic mouse in the United States was, in fact, for much more than a mouse. The claim was for "a transgenic non-human mammal all of whose germ cells and somatic cells contain a recombinant activated oncogene sequence introduced into said mammal, at the embryonic stage."[10]

While an enormous amount of capital and research is involved in biotechnology, the actual commercial application of the technology can be rather simple. A genetically engineered microorganism, the result of an intensive research effort, may as happily produce its product in a competitor's fermentation vat as in the inventor's. Traits given a plant through genetic engineering may simply be reproduced in the seed and as simply transferred to another variety through conventional breeding techniques. Unlike light bulbs or spark plugs, many products of biotechnology will be capable of reproducing themselves. The difference between the better mousetrap which is patented and the better mouse, patented or not, is enormous.

National legal systems have been unable to keep pace with the rapid development of the biotechnologies. The European Patent Convention and the UPOV Convention were instituted "when the biological sciences were just at the verge of comprehending the natural movement of genes from one bacterium into another and of identifying plasmids and phages as vehicles (vectors) for carrying genes into bacteria . . . this development in natural sciences, with industry closely following suit, has yet found few parallels in the legal sphere."[11]

With biotechnology potentially affecting so many of the items in world commerce (up to 40 percent of all world trade according to some estimates), and with patent coverage seriously outdated, a major problem exists for the new industry. To protect its research, to protect its market which is increasingly international, and to guard against easy piracy due to the biological nature of its products, the industry desires patents. And it wants these patents to apply not just in the United States, but around the globe. To complicate matters, many countries, particularly in the Third World, are openly hostile to the patent systems of the industrialized world. Nineteen fields of economic activity are excluded from coverage by various of the 97 members of the Paris Convention. Twelve of these fields are related to biotechnology.[12] Coverage of chemicals under patent laws is a relatively recent phenomenon. Twenty-two countries still do not allow for patents on chemicals. In the mid-1980s, Norway and forty-four other countries still did not honor pharmaceutical patents. Forty-two countries do not recognize patents for biological processes for producing plant or animal varieties. And seven do not even allow patents for substances obtained by microbiological processes. Pushing life-patenting statutes through every government in the world would be daunting indeed. A rewriting of the Paris Convention was long overdue and theoretically such a rewriting could engineer international agreement on reforms to accommodate biotechnology. But the Third World has had its sights trained on the Paris Convention and been more in the mood for a rolling back of coverage than an expansion.[13]

Business interests in the United States were also frustrated with progress on patent reform in the World Intellectual Property Organization. In a radical departure from past practice, the U.S. Chamber of Commerce and others urged the administration to pursue patent reform in the current Uruguay round of negotiations at the General Agreement on Tariffs and Trade (GATT) in Geneva.[14]

A series of laws passed in the United States in the mid-1980s indicated the growing concern of the government over protecting "American" intellectual property rights abroad. These laws, beginning with the Trade and Tariff Act of 1984, also set the tone and the objectives for American negotiators. The International Trade and Investment Act required the U.S. Trade Representative to prepare a report on trade barriers affecting intellectual property rights (IPR) and stated that its goal was to remove such barriers. At about the same time Congress criminalized trafficking in goods and services with a counterfeit trademark.[15]

Congress significantly escalated the battle for intellectual property rights (IPR) with the passage of the Generalized System of Preferences Renewal Act of 1984. This act:

> added intellectual property protection . . . barriers to the eligibility criteria for developing countries to receive duty-free treatment for exports of certain products to the United States. The law explicitly directed the President, in reviewing a beneficiary country's eligibility, to "give great weight to . . . the extent to which such country provides adequate and effective means under its law for foreign nationals to secure, to exercise, and to enforce exclusive rights in intellectual property, including patent, trademark, and copyright rights."[16]

Corporate concern over foreign protection of IPR which might be presumed in the passage of the above-mentioned laws found organizational form in the founding of several corporate coalitions to push these interests. The Multilateral Trade Negotiations Coalition (chaired by William Brock, a former U.S. Trade Representative, U.S. senator and food industry executive) brought together a number of large financial institutions, manufacturing concerns, agribusiness corporations (including Cargill and others with seed businesses) and trade organizations.[17] Among these were the Intellectual Property Committee, a coalition of thirteen big companies including a number of drug and chemical companies with seed and biotech concerns.[18]

The interest of companies in pursuing intellectual property rights issues at GATT is well illustrated by a Conference Board survey to which 164 companies responded. (Respondents included a number of companies not likely to be active in the patenting field, thus the results may be "conservative.") Over half said they were working to influence intellectual property laws. Next, sixty-six said they were working to affect GATT. Fifty-three were working on the Paris Convention. Significantly, nearly all companies were working to increase levels of protection, except that almost half of those working on the Paris Convention admitted to simply trying to maintain current levels of protection. The number of companies thinking success was likely or possible with GATT was second only to those thinking it was likely or possible with home country laws. Only four companies out of 59 lobbying GATT thought success was unlikely.[19] With 40 percent of the companies in a survey that failed to cover even half of the "Fortune 500" saying that they were working to promote expansion of IPR through GATT and expected some success, it is not difficult to imagine the government being under some pressure to use GATT as an arena. As an arena, it offered a voting procedure weighted to favor industrialized countries, and a general focus on issues that provided these countries with great bargaining strength.[20]

At the beginning of the current Uruguay Round, agreement was reached on the scope of negotiation. In the "General Principles Governing Negotiations (paragraph v of section B) industrialized countries formally agreed that they did not expect developing countries "to make contributions which are inconsistent with their individual development, financial and trade needs. Developed contracting parties shall therefore not seek, neither shall less-developed contracting parties be required to make, concessions that are inconsistent with the latter's development, financial or trade needs."

There had been no long history of IPR negotiations within GATT. Discussions had almost entirely been limited to trade in counterfeited trademarked items. IPR was not on the list of subjects to consider for a

GATT work program following completion of the Tokyo Round in 1979.[21] The terms of reference for the new GATT round, referred to above — reached after long, arduous negotiation — seemed to limit the scope of what GATT would do in the field of IPR.

Despite this limitation and the conventional wisdom that agricultural subsidies were the target of the new GATT round, others saw things differently. According to William Brock of the Multilateral Trade Negotiations Coalition, "agriculture is not the issue . . . rather it is the linchpin to agreement on issues of greater magnitude, issues that really matter, like intellectual property protection . . . ."[22] The risk that IPR might be lost, traded off in the rough and tumble of tough negotiations at GATT, was thought minimal by former U.S. Attorney General Nicholas Katzenbach (who for seventeen years was senior vice president and general counsel of IBM, one of the most aggressive corporate promoters of international recognition of IPR[23]). Katzenbach observed that "while theoretically such risk exists, there seems to be no reason to be concerned: The critical importance of meaningful protection of intellectual property to developed countries offers the best guarantee."[24]  In this context the challenge was made. The United States put forth a novel and stunning position: the absence of intellectual property rights protection (at a minimum level similar to that offered by the United States) constitutes an unfair trade barrier and should be subject to trade sanctions under GATT.

The United States was asking for no small concession. The U.S. International Trade Commission estimated that the country lost $61 billion to foreign competitors from theft of intellectual property in 1986, the year the Uruguay Round began,[25] a figure in the neighborhood of Third World debt payments. Moreover, the United States asserted that patent protection must extend to everything regardless of subject matter — to all classes of biological materials from genes upward. This point must be emphasized: rather than going through the traditional channels to affect patent law changes (such as WIPO and the Paris Convention) the United States has chosen to link trade negotiations and intellectual property negotiations in a forum for trade negotiations. Strategically, the threat of trade restrictions is being offered to coax countries into adopting foreign levels of patent protection through the only forum in which such a tactic might work across the board. Such a framework clearly serves certain interests. In addition, the structure of negotiations themselves reinforced the already overwhelming strength of industrialized countries at the table. Carlos Correa, director of the Center for Advanced Studies at the University of Buenos Aires asserts:

The actual drafting process was confined, in practice, to a few countries. U.S.A., E. C., Japan and Canada were those that provided the basic texts on which further discussions took place in a so-called "five-plus-five" drafting group, composed of five developed and five developing countries. The agreements reached in this group were later on transferred to a broadened "ten-plus-ten" group. With the exception of the members of these groups, the remainder countries have hardly had any real opportunity to influence the output of the drafting groups. In addition, unlike the negotiations on the existing intellectual property conventions, no record of discussions was made for TRIPs [trade related intellectual property]. Proposals have no recognized source and only direct participants know who and why certain provisions were adopted or not. The TRIPs negotiations have been, hence, the most non-transparent negotiations ever conducted on IPRs [intellectual property rights]. Since GATT staff is prevented from revealing such an information, in addition, contracting parties will lack any background material to interpret the proposed rules and, particularly, to better understand the premises and intent of the adopted texts.[26]

Correa points out that working group composition was determined by the chairmen and was not the result of consensus or an effort to have balanced representation. Thus, he claims, "African countries were almost systematically excluded from participation in the key drafting groups."[27]

The ability to leverage trade sanctions against intellectual property rights concessions is not the only advantage GATT offered. The way in which negotiations are organized and structured gives a substantial advantage to industrialized countries which they would not receive in all fora.

As outlined by Michael Gadbaw (an attorney formerly with the Office of the U.S. Trade Representative) and Timothy Richards, the American strategy is fourfold:

1. Attempt to persuade Third World countries of the value of intellectual property rights;

2. Threaten loss of access to U.S. markets;

3. Offer increased or decreased research and development funding through the private sector, and;

4. Pursue agreements on minimum patent standards through GATT.[28]

If approved, a GATT agreement would authorize trade sanctions against countries not having acceptable intellectual property laws or not enforcing those laws. "The primary thrust of the Uruguay Round efforts," according to Gadbaw and Gwynn, "is to draw the developing countries into a new set of rights and obligations."[29]

As *The Economist* bluntly put it:

Countries that are poor, indebted or ex-communist — often all three — must be able to sell farm produce, textiles and other basic goods abroad; rich countries must be able to export patents, copyrights and skills in the services that are coming to be their area of advantage; and the rules of trade must be strengthened to cope with modern forms of protectionism. All these are promised by the Uruguay round.[30]

Interestingly, if GATT succeeds in setting minimum global standards for IPR including standards outlined by the revised UPOV treaty, Third World countries will find that the door opened to agricultural exports by one provision in GATT (reduction of barriers) will be closed by another (control over the products of patented varieties). Under UPOV, it would be illegal to export products produced by varieties protected by breeders' rights in one country but not in the producing country. In other words, if a Third World country wanted to use a modern protected variety and then export the product, it would have to adopt plant breeders' rights legislation. The possibility of using protected varieties for breeding purposes would also be curtailed. However, it is not clear how effective GATT-imposed IPR would be. Few Third World countries have the administrative infrastructure to enforce IPR. It remains to be seen whether and how GATT could effectively force the creation of such an infrastructure or what the consequences would be to countries unable or unwilling to provide it.

American initiatives at GATT must be placed in the larger context of the growing importance of patents to transnational corporations. A number of indications of this are provided above. Patent coverage of biotechnological innovations is just one aspect of this context. No claim is made that the U.S. strategy of pursuing IPR extension through GATT is because of the desire or need for this type of patent coverage. While many of the corporations lobbying for increased coverage through GATT have commercial interests in biotechnology and seeds, it is unclear to what extent this piece of their business prompted their pushing the U.S. government to use GATT as a forum. Nor is it clear to what extent American representatives at GATT are aware of the importance of that forum to biotechnology interests.[31] The sheer complexity of the issues prevents individuals from comprehending the full picture and provides an opening for special interest groups to supply that expertise. (As the Italian foreign minister remarked during a 1988 debate, "I sit there talking about soybeans, and I don't even know what the miserable things look like."[32]) Despite this, the issue of ownership of biological materials could be profoundly affected by developments at GATT.

## THE UNITED NATIONS FOOD AND AGRICULTURE ORGANIZATION

The extension of intellectual property rights through the legislative and judicial process (without improvement in efforts to conserve genetic diversity) was a sign to nongovernment organizations that a new arena was needed. In order to continue there also needed to be a redefining and repackaging of the arguments and the goals. It was no longer sufficient simply to be against plant patenting laws. The interests of the NGOs had always been wider than patenting. The challenge, nevertheless, was to develop a new strategy and set it to work in a new but potentially friendlier arena. This section explores that process and looks at the way in which the strategy was developed to protect the "property rights" of the Third World through challenging industrialized countries' access to genetic diversity. It shows how new arenas can help radically alter power relationships, encouraging various responses from the disadvantaged — including a search for yet new arenas. The development of new technologies adds fuel to the political fire by adding potential value to the botanical materials found in the Third World.

The political battles over intellectual property laws in North America helped give training and experience to a number of activists opposed to such laws. Of these, Pat Roy Mooney, a Canadian, has been most influential. His 1979 book, *Seeds of the Earth* was followed in 1983 by "The Law of the Seed," a book-length issue of the journal *Development Dialogue*, published and distributed by the Dag Hammarskjöld Foundation in Uppsala, Sweden.[33] In it, Mooney focused on the battles over intellectual property rights for plants. But he linked this issue to broader ones including the question of national sovereignty over genetic resources and questions about access to and ownership of material already collected and stored in northern gene banks.

"The Law of the Seed" was widely circulated in Europe and the Third World. It gave fuel to rising concerns in diplomatic quarters over the propriety of proprietary rights for materials which largely originated in the Third World. And it gave ammunition to the national groups which had sprung up to oppose plant patenting laws. By the mid-1980s, groups were active in Australia, New Zealand, Norway, Germany, Holland, France, Italy, and Canada, and rumblings were being heard in the United Kingdom, Ireland, and Austria. Mooney, a polished public speaker and skillful debater, virtually lived on airplanes, sometimes making well over a dozen trips a year to Europe and the Third World during the 1980s. On these trips, he met with nongovernment organizations, scientists and government officials, blending organizing, research, and lobbying.[34] In doing so the breadth of his exposure to the different actors in the different camps, as well as his access to various sources of information was probably greater than anyone else's.

The issue became international and political in 1981 at the biennial conference of the United Nations Food and Agriculture Organization (FAO).[35] Both Mooney and I had attended an earlier technical conference on plant genetic resources and had been moved and energized by the urgency with which the world's most prominent plant geneticists and germplasm curators spoke of the problem of loss of genetic diversity. Mooney had also been involved with various youth activities at the FAO years earlier and with the World Food Conference. Significantly and uniquely among the people of NGOs, he was both familiar with and not intimidated by the FAO as a forum.

Prior to the 1981 FAO conference, Mooney and I were given consulting work (through Dr. Art Domike of American University, whom I had met while working on *Food First* and later while consulting with the UN Centre on Transnational Corporations) to outline the issues and options in the area of genetic resources for the president of Mexico.[36] We were told that the president had a personal interest in this subject and that our report would receive his close attention.

The Mexican ambassador to the FAO came to the 1981 conference armed with a briefcase full of proposals concerning genetic resources including one for the establishment of an international gene bank under the auspices of the FAO and another which called for an international legal convention governing the exchange of plant genetic resources. These proposals capped growing unrest in the Third World over the handling of genetic resources — unrest which was not limited to Mexico. In 1977, Ethiopia ceased allowing collection or export of coffee germplasm. Ethiopia was not alone. India was embargoing some genetic material. In East Asia, scientists were calling for more national control over these resources.

The 1981 conference thus marked the beginning of a shift toward new arenas and new actors and toward an initiative from certain Third World governments to gain more control over plant genetic resources. To a certain extent this shift in arenas marked the first time NGOs, or opponents of plant patenting, had taken the initiative with their own proposals. Moving the debate to FAO allowed for this to happen because it shifted the power base from American to Third World interests. Furthermore, it extended the debate beyond patenting in the narrow sense, and thus moved the debate onto territory NGOs are most comfortable with — the connections between patenting and genetic conservation, and the between these and development issues. This happened also to be more appealing to the politically oriented Third World delegates and to the press. While this shift to the FAO might seem logical enough ten years later, it did not seem so automatic in 1981. Few NGOs had been to Rome. Few FAO delegates knew what "genetic resources" meant. The pivotal role of Pat Mooney must be underlined here. After submitting the consulting report to American University, Mooney contacted Mexican officials in Mexico and Rome. The proposals of the Mexican delegation did not come out of thin air or even a consulting report. They were worked out in close cooperation with Mooney. This in turn began a ten-year period of cooperation and planning between Mexican officials in Rome and NGOs on this issue, which grew particularly close when José Ramon Lopez-Portillo, son of the former Mexican president, arrived in Rome to be Mexico's ambassador to the FAO.

The beginnings of this initiative in the FAO took place, of course, in the larger framework of the establishment of intellectual property laws for plant varieties based on genetic material from the Third World. But before looking at the controversy that erupted at the FAO, it might be helpful to pick up the botanical garden thread left dangling in an earlier section. The flows of germplasm from the Third World to the industrialized countries were a powerful part of the context which led to the 1981 resolutions and they continue to be at the center of the debate even today.

In 1974, the Consultative Group on International Agricultural Research (CGIAR) founded the International Board for Plant Genetic Resources (IBPGR). The IBPGR, a self-described "purely scientific and technical body" was to serve as a "catalyst" for plant genetic resource conservation activities.

CGIAR is the parent body of a network of international agricultural research centers (IARCs) including the International Maize and Wheat Improvement Center (CIMMYT) in Mexico and the International Rice Research Institute (IRRI) in the Philippines (see Table 10 next page). These centers have been major collectors and storage sites for germplasm and have played a key role in the breeding of new varieties for the Third World. Consequently they have also played a major role in genetic erosion and in the commercialization of Third World agriculture. The regional origin of staff and trustees of these centers reflects the influence of industrialized countries. Slightly over half of the staff and just under half of the trustees of CGIAR institutes (ten of thirteen of which are located in the Third World, excluding the Washington headquarters of the CGIAR itself) come from Europe, North America and Australia/New Zealand. Industrialized country trustees hold half or more of the positions on seven of the boards.[37]

Table 10. CGIAR Centers[38]

| CGIAR Cener | Major Crop(s)/Objectives | Location of Center |
|---|---|---|
| CIAT | Cassava, Field Bean, Pastures, Rice | Colombia |
| CIMMYT | Barley, Maize, Triticale, Wheat | Mexico |
| CIP | Potato, Sweet Potato | Peru |
| IBPGR | Plant Genetic Resources | Italy |
| ICARDA | Barley, Chickpea, Faba Bean, Lentil, Wheat | Syria |
| ICRISAT | Chickpea, Millet, Peanut, Pigeonpea, Sorghum | India |
| IFPRI | Food Policy | United States |
| IITA | Cassava, Cowpea, Maize, Rice, Soybean, Sweet Potato, Yam, Plantain | Nigeria |
| ILCA | Pastures, Livestock | Ethiopia |
| ILRAD | Theileriosis, Trypanosomiasis (animal diseases) | Kenya |
| IRRI | Rice | Philippines |
| ISNAR | National Research Systems | Netherlands |
| WARDA | Rice | Cote d'Ivoire |

CGIAR itself is governed loosely by a board which represents the "donors," in this case meaning donors of funds. It is headquarted at the World Bank. The CGIAR was formed on the initiative of the Ford and Rockefeller Foundations to unite once privately funded centers like CIMMYT into a coordinated network. The hope was to escape the bureaucracy and control of the UN system while still appearing to be part of the system.

Central to the founding of the IBPGR — the center that concentrates on genetic resources — were M. S. Swaminathan, who brought the Green Revolution to India and was later to be the director of the International Rice Research Institute; Otto Frankel, a cranky Australia-based scientist; and Richard Demuth, a Washington lawyer for the State Department, who had long had ties with the Agency for International Development. Upon its founding, Demuth retired from the State Department and became the first to chair this "purely" technical and scientific body.

IBPGR is headquartered at the UN's Food and Agriculture Organization in Rome.[39] Indeed, IBPGR's founding virtually eliminated FAO's active program in genetic resource conservation. FAO staff and programs simply became IBPGR staff and programs. FAO continued to pay their salaries, but IBPGR exercised supervisory and programatic control. The structure was what IBPGR itself called an "historical anomaly."

Since the founding, the board has had a distinctly northern flavor. On the surface the ratio of industrialized to Third World members does not seem unreasonable — a few more from the "North" than the "South," though by 1988 the North held nine of fifteen seats. But the tenure of those from the North is nearly twice as long as those from the South, indicating in this case that power is being accumulated. And an analysis of the grants made by IBPGR shows that 57 percent have gone to scientists and institutions in industrialized countries, 10 percent to fellow CGIAR institutes, and less than a third to Third World countries — this to protect a resource which is overwhelmingly found in the Third World. Indeed, some industrialized countries have actually received more in aid from IBPGR than they have contributed.

This data would be nothing more than titillating were it not reflective of the manner in which IBPGR has handled the genetic resources themselves. Only 15 percent of the samples collected have been designated for storage in Third World collections. Fully 85 percent has been stored in industrialized countries and IARC gene banks. This data must be given in the context of the system of "world" and "regional" collections established by IBPGR.

IBPGR's rather meager budget ($5 million a year during much of the 1980s) belies its historical importance. With relatively small grants to developing and developed countries alike, IBPGR was able to exercise great influence over the direction of conservation activities. Its panels of experts decided not only which crops were most endangered, but where they were threatened and which should be collected in what priority. Equally important, IBPGR assumed the authority to designate certain gene banks to hold world base and regional collections, thus determining who would have ready, convenient, and guaranteed access to the materials and information about the collections.

This channeling of genetic resources also affected the ownership of the resources. Technically, these "world collections" were not owned by "the world." They were, in fact, the property of the facility in which they were stored. This might be a government gene bank, for instance, making the seeds the property of that government in the strict sense.

In 1987, 67 of the world base crop collections were in western industrialized countries. Another 26 were in CGIAR institutes and four were in eastern Europe. Just 22 were held by Third World countries, one fewer than assigned to the United States.

IBPGR has been particularly generous to the United States when it has come to designating sites for global and regional storage responsibility. Over 200 crops are produced in or imported into the United States. The top 15 account for over three-quarters of the economic value of the total. These are the 15 crops most important to the United States. Of these, the country has been given global storage responsibilities for five and regional responsibilities for three. Three are mandated to others, two are for crops which are only imported into the United States and for two others the IBPGR has established no storage responsibilities at all. Of the top 15 crops, the United States ranks among the top four germplasm holders in the world in 11.[40]

One might expect a rational, technical reason for the situating of so many of the world's important germplasm collections in the United States. The country, presumably, would have better facilities than those in the Third World. Ironically, this may not be the case, particularly considering the newness of many of the Third World gene banks. A steady stream of reports from the 1970s onward, prepared by both U.S. government and various scientific bodies, has been very critical of the American germplasm conservation system. In 1981, the General Accounting Office found that "indications are that germplasm protection and preservation mechanisms are inadequate, and comprehensive plans have not been made to cope with present and future problems."[41] The GAO charged that the government even failed to "adequately perform the housekeeping chores of collection, maintenance, and evaluation of germplasm stock."[42]

Criticism of IBPGR's policies has also been heard within the larger CGIAR system. David Wood of the International Institute for Tropical Agriculture (CIAT) wrote an open letter to gene bank directors in the system claiming that "There is a relation between the amount a country donates *to* IBPGR, and the number of collections designated to that country *by* IBPGR" [his emphasis].[43]

In determining storage responsibilities, IBPGR has considered not only technical capabilities as noted above, but also questions of control and access. Stored in the United States, genetic resources were accessible to scientists and breeders much as material in botanical gardens was accessible to colonial powers. The benefits of having the world collection of wheat based in the United States rather than in a gene bank in the Center of Diversity should be obvious. Were situations to warrant it, the United States could then exercise control over the material, denying access if need be. In 1977, T. W. Edminster, head of the Agricultural Research Service of the USDA, wrote to the chairperson of the IBPGR outlining the terms under which the United States would accept storage responsibilities and acknowledging exactly that point: "They (the collections) would become the property of the U.S. Government . . . As you know it has been our policy for many years to freely exchange germplasm with most countries of the world. Political considerations have at times dictated exclusion of a few countries."[44]

Trevor Williams, executive secretary of IBPGR, was aware of and sympathetic to the American position. As he stated in a letter to George White, USDA plant introduction officer, "As far as the IBPGR is concerned, all genetic resources samples entering the USA enter the US germplasm system."[45] Furthermore, the designation of so many base collections in the United States by IBPGR took place even though Williams apparently knew of periodic American embargoes. A telegram from the U.S. Embassy in Rome to the U.S. Secretary'of State in 1984 described a meeting with Williams:

> Williams also commented that while he understands U.S. has never formally denied request for germplasm, there have been instances when the word went out that "for diplomatic reasons" answers to germplasm requests should be slowed down, not acted on, or answered through intermediaries . . . [46]

As genetic resources began to be raised as a political issue in the early 1980s in the FAO, delegates had mixed feelings about this history. Some viewed IBPGR as a source of grants and had no knowledge about the larger flows of germplasm. Some delegates (including several from Latin America) had been involved in national germplasm programs and had had personal and sometimes negative experiences with IBPGR. Virtually all were agitated over the American policy concerning ownership of materials donated by the Third World. Mostly, delegates approached the issue desirous of establishing more Third World influence over the direction of conservation activities. Data concerning historic flows of germplasm and funding tended to cast the debate in a North/South context which is familiar territory to most diplomats, even if in this case the reality is much more complex.

Thus, as Mexico tabled its resolutions at the 1981 FAO Conference, Third World delegates were becoming aware of:

1. The loss of genetic diversity in agricultural crops;

2. The disparity of designated storage facilities between North and South and the related issues of access and control;

3. The advances in biotechnology which were drawing more attention to and giving more value to genetic diversity at the gene level;

4. The efforts by many industrialized countries to establish patenting systems for varieties, genes, characteristics, etc.

5. The absence of international governmental political control over IBPGR.

Each of these points was to become even better known among ambassadors to FAO during the course of the 1980s. Mexico in 1981 simply began the process. The resolutions finally adopted called for the director-general of FAO to draft the elements of a legal convention and report back to the next conference in 1983 on the feasibility of establishing an international gene bank. The resolutions were hotly opposed by industrialized countries, particularly the United States, England and Australia, but they won unanimous acceptance from Third World countries. Mexico lobbied skillfully among Latin American countries and cultivated its ties with Spain. African and Asian diplomats were less active, but were lobbied by representatives of nongovernment organizations such as the International Coalition for Development Action (ICDA) for whom Pat Mooney worked, and others, who attended using press credentials granted by sympathetic newspapers and journals.[47] The NGOs arrived more knowledgeable about the issues than most of the delegates and the delegates rather quickly came to view the NGOs as a resource to whom they could turn for information and analysis.[48] Perhaps it was one of the few times that the press was answering more questions than it was asking. NGOs also played a crucial role in bridging the communication gap between Latin American delegates and those from Asia and Africa.

The outcome of the 1981 conference precipitated furious behind-the-scenes activity. At the FAO headquarters there was division. IBPGR employees saw the international gene bank proposal as a threat to their own delicately crafted system. Would such a bank draw attention to the restrictions to access employed by IBPGR's designated sites? More importantly, would Third World nations begin to specify that collections go to this new bank which would be under FAO as opposed to IBPGR or national control?

The seed industry saw the proposed legal convention as the bigger threat. How would a legal convention dealing with exchange of genetic resources affect their own efforts to privatize and "commoditize" these resources?

The March, 1983, meeting of FAO's Committee on Agriculture (COAG) saw a number of these issues discussed rather openly. But the debate, in which Sweden (typically sympathetic to Third World concerns) took a hard stand in favor of IBPGR (chaired at the time by a Swede) and against the convention and international gene bank, served only to solidify the emerging North-South division on the issue.

An FAO survey of gene banks and assorted research institutes attempted to gauge the degree to which germplasm was being restricted. A low return rate of the questionnaire flawed the results, but what emerged was the clear picture that industrialized countries did not want to consider elite breeding lines or patented varieties as material that could or should be freely exchanged. Material that was highly variable and material that was to be found in the Third World (the so-called primitive cultivars or landraces) constituted the "common heritage of mankind." Patented varieties were private property.

Scientifically, the dividing line between these categories is blurry. What may be a primitive cultivar to one breeding program might be a breeding line to another. With the United Kingdom's attempt in 1982 to redefine the terms of its Plant Varieties Bill, the distinction became even more confusing. It was proposed that the definitions for "plant" and "variety" be deleted as no precise definitions could be agreed upon. Critics quickly exclaimed that if there was no plant and no variety, there should be no bill. But the exercise was indicative of a deeper problem, namely that germplasm categories and definitions are political and legal — not scientific — constructs.

After 1981, the U.S. government became increasingly alarmed at events in Rome. Given both the plans and capabilities of their "adversaries," the USDA fears were exaggerated. Misperceptions of the threat apparently began to fuel an increasingly hostile and reactionary response to events. A "briefing paper" penned by two senior USDA staffers prior to the 1983 FAO conference listed three implications of proposals before the upcoming conference:

1. They "would politicize germplasm policies."

2. They "would probably drive primary donor countries out of system, e.g., U.S. would never grant FAO control to National Seed Storage Laboratory."

3. "International centers, i.e., IRRI and CYMMT [sic], would be subject to FAO control."[49]

The 1983 FAO conference provided ample fireworks. Third World positions had become more refined. Instead of an international gene bank, Third World delegations, again led by Mexico, called for the establishment of an international system of gene banks. The demand for a legal convention was softened to a legal "undertaking," a mild and voluntary agreement. The appropriate legal drafts for such an "International undertaking on plant genetic resources" had been prepared by FAO before the conference.[50] And, significantly, a new demand emerged — for the creation of a commission on plant genetic resources, as a body where governments as governments could meet to discuss matters concerning genetic resources and monitor the Undertaking.

The debate at the three-week long conference was emotional from the beginning. The undertaking specified that all categories of germplasm should be freely available and proceeded to list those categories, which predictably included patented varieties and breeding lines — a direct threat to plant variety protection. Interestingly, Third World delegates and NGOs were still promoting the principle of "free availability" of germplasm — a reactionary position against efforts to privatize the resource through patenting. Neither had made the leap to advocating Third World sovereignty over the material. That would come later in response to the intransigence of the North in the debates.

The proposal for a commission, however, struck some as an attack against IBPGR, an attempt to set up a parallel body with the political power and legitimacy of the UN. The details of this Conference as important as they might be, will not be explored here. Suffice it to say that the major proposals for an undertaking, a network of gene banks, and a commission were approved with unanimous Third World support and almost unanimous (but for Spain) opposition from Europe and North America.

The first meeting of the Commission on Plant Genetic Resources opened in March, 1985. Delegates from 93 nations dashed in from a steady week-long rain to participate in an agenda devoted solely to genetic resources. In a memo circulated to allies, the U.S. had urged a boycott of the meeting. That suggestion however failed totally and in the end the U.S. delegates appeared and found seats at the back of the hall with NGOs in a section reserved for "observers."

At this time, the position of the American Seed Trade Association was virtually "determining" the official United States position, according to a high-ranking official of the USDA who was a senior member of the U.S. delegation at the FAO meetings.[51] Indeed, these delegations to FAO routinely included a representative of the seed trade who was not a government employee (the only delegation containing such an industry representative). ASTA's attitude was quite hostile. In a 1984 position paper, ASTA charged that the undertaking:

strikes at the heart of free enterprise and intellectual property rights . . .
The definition includes unimproved and obsolete varieties, land races, wild
and weedy species, all of which the seed industry believes appropriate to be
preserved and freely exchanged. However, it also includes improved elite
varieties and breeding lines within the definition of plant genetic resources
. . . This puts the Undertaking in direct conflict with the rights of holders of
private property . . . .The anti-private business bias of the Undertaking is
clear. To stand mute to an international Undertaking, albeit voluntary and
without force of law, would imply approval and provide moral justification
to other governments to appropriate private property.[52]

ASTA bluntly staked out a position which claimed property rights for
seed companies, but no property rights for farmers or others over the
landraces, or raw materials used by seed companies. ASTA concluded its
paper with a list of five recommendations. First, that the United States
reject the undertaking. Second, that the United States lobby other governments to reject it. Third, that the United States attempt to strengthen the
IBPGR. Fourth, that it consider helping IBPGR move outside of FAO.
And fifth, that it "condition future financial support to, and participation
in, FAO on whether the Undertaking in its present form is effected."[53]

U.S. government position papers, one dated just three weeks after
ASTA's and the other prepared for the first meeting of the FAO commission in March, 1985, reflect the seed industry's view. "The Undertaking's
principles are inconsistent with U.S. law and practice," stated the position
paper prepared by the Department of State. It went on to voice support for
IBPGR and speak of the duplication inherent with the establishment of the
commission.[54]

Officials inside the U.S. government were beginning to sense not just a
threat to proprietary rights over plant varieties but also to the related
traditional rules of exchange which made "Third World" genetic resources both free and freely available.[55] In a draft position paper on the FAO
undertaking, Quentin Jones, then head of the U.S. genetic resources
program, (referring to major U.S. crops) discussed the importance of
continued access and confided:

> . . . clearly, we are dependent on other countries for our crop germplasm.
> If we were denied access to these sources, we could be in very serious
> trouble because we still have a long way to go toward having the genetic
> diversity of these crops represented in our genebanks. Corn may be a near
> exception.[56]

J. T. Williams of IBPGR was no less concerned. In June of 1984, he
wrote a letter marked "CONFIDENTIAL" to Quentin Jones in which he
discussed IBPGR-FAO relations. "I am sure you can see," Williams

stated, "that all too easily control will come little by little."[57,58] Some six weeks later in a draft paper for the IBPGR executive committee meeting in Leuven, Belgium, Jones laid out the problem expressing concerns over germplasm availability and control quite clearly:

> Cause for Concern: "Seeds of the Earth" and "Law of the Seed" by Pat Roy Mooney and colleagues [sic] is [sic] having a divisive affect [sic] between developing and developed nations, and among nations of each category, that is being expressed in erosion of cooperation, goodwill, and trust in the free exchange of plant germplasm. The situation is being taken advantage of by FAO to achieve its own objectives.

> The signals are clear: Protestations to the contrary, FAO is seeking to bring world leadership for biological conservation (not just plant genetic diversity) directly under its unilateral control. There are probably some attendant political objectives as well . . . It is no time for the Board to assume a position of "All is well; business as usual . . . "

> The Board must conceptualize and implement actions that will minimize the impact of Mooney and Company through stimulating mutual confidence and goodwill between "North" and "South."[59]

ASTA's similar analysis of the dangers of the "voluntary" undertaking misjudged the direction of the threat. ASTA feared that the undertaking might be upgraded to a binding legal convention that would destroy years of effort they had put into establishing intellectual property rights for plants. This option has certainly occurred to Third World ambassadors and their NGO allies, but it has largely been dismissed as too ambitious. Such a legal convention would only garner the signatures of Third World states and thus would not mean much.

The undertaking was seen in the Third World camp as a different sort of tool. Compliance was indeed voluntary. This meant that the Third World had a tool — now agreed to by over 100 nations — that set out guidelines for the exchange of genetic resources. Industrialized countries could, within the spirit of the undertaking, exclude certain categories of genetic resources from exchange. By the same token, Third World countries could exclude certain categories. As patented varieties designed for northern agricultural systems were of limited use in the Third World and as elite breeding lines were of even less utility, the Third World was sure that industrialized countries would be hurt more in such a swap. The goal, of course, was not to hurt industrialized countries. Third World ambassadors interpreted the undertaking to mean that they were obligated to exchange all their resources only with others who had signed the undertaking without restrictions. Countries not cooperating fully with the Third World could not expect the Third World to cooperate fully with them.

Third World delegates argued that if industrialized countries demanded recognition of "plant breeders' rights" (the term most often used in Europe for plant variety protection), then they should be prepared to recognize "farmers' rights."

As a political idea, "farmers' rights" dated back to Mooney's work and my own in the early and mid-1980s. But in fact the notion was really older. Kenneth Dahlberg, a social scientist who testified against seed patenting in the United States, had called attention to the inequities of rewarding only modern plant breeders for the minuscule amount of improvement they made to varieties compared to our Neolithic ancestors. Jack Harlan before him had spoken of the "amateurs" who had really created the genetic diversity we now wrangle over. "Farmers' Rights" as used in the FAO debates beginning in 1987 became shorthand for the view that farmers both past and present are plant breeders, and that they have made valuable but unrewarded contributions.

Third World delegates to FAO claim that their part of the globe has a more informal, less visible, less recognized, and totally unrewarded system of innovation. The argument is a political argument which will be decided politically. But the political position rests on the assertion that farmers have in fact contributed to diversity — that this diversity is not simply, as modern patent laws might put it, "a product of nature." To the extent that Third World farmers are and have been plant breeders, the argument for a parallel system of compensation to plant patenting is strengthened politically. Let us examine, quite briefly, what sorts of things are known about the steps of the plant breeding process at the farm level in the Third World.

In the Andes, Dr. Steve Brush has described sophisticated taxonomy systems for potatoes among that region's farmers. Similar studies have shown up to five levels of classification for rice among farmers in Asia.[60]

Farmers may be able to describe and classify their plants, but do they know about heredity? The Pima and Tepehuan people in Mexico have ways of describing introgression of wild and weedy genes into cultivated crops and "a sophisticated sense of the relationship between domesticated and spontaneous species," according to Dr. Gary Nabhan, an ethnobotanist.[61]

Can they use such knowledge of heredity? In the 1960s Dr. Garrison Wilkes observed harvests of hybrids of Indian maize with teosinte. Farmers would bring maize seed in to be grown around and exposed to teosinte. According to them the result was flintier kernels and greater yield.[62]

In the most far-reaching study of its kind to date, Dr. Paul Richards found that farmers in Sierra Leone can distinguish among 70 different rices. These are differentiated according to length to maturity, ease of husking, proportion of husk size to grain size and weight, susceptibility to bird and insect attack, appropriateness in different soils and with different levels of moisture, color of plant parts, cooking time and qualities, and taste, among other characteristics.

When harvesting, these farmers stay clear of the boundaries between different "varieties." They harvest panicle by panicle, saving the interesting material for future experiments. They also rogue off-types when they desire to keep a variety "pure." They have trial plots. They record data. They test germination rates. They try to match their rice to the local ecological niches. (Do the traits uncovered in this process constitute discovery or invention in the legal sense? Does it matter?) They multiply promising new varieties and they conduct field tests.[63]

In summary, Third World farmers have been found to employ taxonomic systems, encourage introgression, use selection, make efforts to see that varieties are adapted, multiply seeds, field test, record data, and even name their varieties. In short, they do what many northern plant breeders do, except that they do not apply for patents — the one step in the process that requires skills (and money) which they do not have. These practices should come as little surprise to the reader, given the activities of U.S. farmers in the 1800s and early 1900s, as described in chapters 1 and 2. But the question arises as to whether the work of Third World farmers deserves any less recognition or reward than that of the 14-year-old American boy who, as described in chapter 3, discovered the world's first thornless rose, and the company which eventually got the patent for this "innovation"?[64]

If the actions of Third World farmers can so closely resemble the steps taken in more formal plant breeding programs, and if the product of their labors is valuable, then the argument can be made that the genetic diversity of the Third World cannot simply be considered a "raw material." At least it is not a raw material in the way that copper or iron ore might be, for the genetic resources of the Third World are improved resources — resources to which value has been added by human creativity and labor. This point was first explicitly articulated in a meeting with Norwegian parliamentary leaders at the end of the 1980s. If the Third World could construct a philosophical argument to complement its physical possession of genetic diversity, some sort of accommodation would be more difficult to deny. The apparently "logical" basis of existing rules regarding ownership of this material would have been challenged. This alone would not be enough to change those rules, but it would help in political organizing.

The actions of Third World farmers may meet the requirements of patent or plant breeders' rights laws, but the plants themselves do not. These plants may be new, distinct, and useful. (Indeed, they may be "priceless," though without a system to assign an appropriate value, they have very little market value.) But they are rarely uniform. This alone can keep them from being patentable under existing statutes. The obvious question is, why should they be uniform? Uniformity is a quality promoted in industrialized agricultural systems and always required by patent laws, but its agronomic appropriateness in the Third World is highly suspect. In any case, the Third World farmer's field is at once a seed bank, a test plot and a production site. How could it be uniform? How can the Third World farmer be asked to be innovative and to produce uniformity simultaneously in one small plot? The difficulty, it seemed, was that this form of innovation could not be accommodated by existing statutes. The rules simply did not fit the new situation in which the inventiveness of Third World farmers was being realized. Dr. Melaku Worede, director of Ethiopia's renowned gene bank, provides a useful example. He tells the story of an American scientist who collected a high-lysine sorghum there some years ago. After testing in the laboratory this scientist announced his discovery — a high-lysine sorghum. The locals had a name for this variety, which the scientist had not bothered to learn. It was called "Why Bother With Wheat?" They already knew the sorghum's qualities. Who made the discovery?[65]

It is readily acknowledged that collected seeds in gene banks are poorly documented. Often there is little "passport" information such as where the material was collected. There is almost no information on local uses, names, etc. In such a situation, attributes bred by "folk science" can become anonymous attributes, a gift from nature, disconnected from the labor and creativity of real people — the common heritage of mankind. In the extreme, this material can even become patentable. In this regard one conclusion of an exclusive meeting cosponsored by the American Society of Agronomy, the Crop Science Society of America, the American Agricultural Economics Association, and the American Society of Horticultural Science is particularly interesting: "It is important to support better characterization of material in gene banks so that characterization is known and in the public domain, available, and therefore not subject to intellectual property rights."[66] This statement serves to highlight how patents may come to be used in relation to Third World genetic resources. Are these organizations not suggesting that material (potentially the "Why Bother With Wheat?" sorghum) might be patented if efforts are not soon made to catalog what is contained in gene banks?

Whatever the scientific or ethical merit of the case for farmers' rights, the urgency remained to find a way to make it operational. Proponents were not interested in devising a scheme to reward individual farmers or communities. It would be nearly impossible to assign credit for a particular variety or gene to an individual. For this reason the model of the western industrial patent system was clearly inappropriate. For similar reasons it would be almost as difficult to try to allocate compensation based on national contributions. An added problem is that the value of Third World farmer innovation may not be immediately evident. Plant breeding literature is full of stories of what ASTA calls "obsolete" farmer-bred varieties being collected and only years later being discovered to have value, much as in the "Why Bother With Wheat?" example given above. Finally, any compensation scheme had to function in such a way as to maintain Third World solidarity, for that would be necessary if the scheme were to survive the expected political opposition of northern governments.

As a solution, FAO (again, after much debate and the now-common North/South division) established an International Fund for Plant Genetic Resources. This fund was defined by the conference as being designed for genetic conservation and utilization work. It is administered by the FAO Commission on Plant Genetic Resources. Politically, this fund met most of the above criteria. Compensation for farmers' rights (the philosophical equivalent of royalties to a patent holder) would go to the fund. This fund would then finance projects concerned with conservation and utilization (plant breeding, for example). Financing of utilization was important, the Third World delegates and NGO allies argued, because it would benefit and reward the innovators, the farmers. A purely conservation-oriented fund would mainly benefit industrialized countries. Administration by the FAO Commission on Plant Genetic Resources would accomplish the desire for governmental control in contrast to the IBPGR structure. If the North demanded recognition of plant breeders' rights, then the South would tie that to recognition of farmers' rights. The establishment of the fund and the linkage to plant breeders rights finally gave teeth to the voluntary Undertaking without actually turning it into a legally binding convention. Once again, much of the strategy behind these maneuvers was Mooney's.

The fund was approved by the FAO conference and by 1989 was legally established. But this alone was not enough. FAO resolutions stated that countries could donate money to the fund in recognition of farmers' rights. Mexico and others argued that the fund had to have a mandatory funding mechanism. Royalty payments to patent holders are not voluntary, it was argued. Why should we speak of donations to the fund and not of compensatory payments? A voluntary fund would be a fund without money and would be effectively negate any rights Third World governments might claim over genetic resources.

Purely as a tactical maneuver, NGOs proposed a $150 million-a-year fund. No one seriously thought approval would be forthcoming, but it gave Third World ambassadors room to negotiate, perhaps for $50 million. But there was no agreement at FAO and no overt signs of impending negotiations.

Over the course of a decade, Third World governments at FAO had constructed a structure to challenge the exclusive ownership rights to biological materials granted by patent laws to corporations in the industrialized countries. Through a series of step-by-step moves at biennial conferences, Third World delegates had established mechanisms to begin squeezing industrialized countries into concessions. Industrialized countries could not fully adhere to the undertaking, so the Third World was justified in not adhering. If industrialized countries did not wish to adhere to or recognize farmers' rights, then the Third World might begin to deny access to its genetic diversity to foreign collectors, and furthermore would not honor foreign plant patents. In such a stand-off, the Third World would not lose anything it already had. Industrialized countries, however, would lose access to much needed genetic diversity, the raw material for plant breeding, the fuel for the new biotechnologies. The trade-off was not a good one. As U.S. Secretary of Agriculture Richard Lyng put it, the United States is "completely at the mercy" of the Third World for germplasm.

Events at the FAO were causing the American government to reevaluate its view of what constituted "control" of genetic diversity. The philosophical framework of "common heritage," which underpinned a system of free access and exchange, was beginning to appear vulnerable. How could private property rights be maintained and enforced for the "inventions" of the seed trade, while assuring that this industry would continue to have access to the necessary raw materials as free goods? This was the question that confronted various northern governments at the end of the 1980s.

## THE KEYSTONE DIALOGUE

Throughout much of the 1980s the battle lines in the fight over control of genetic resources were rather clearly drawn. They remained clearly drawn even as the battles moved from the U.S. Congress to the FAO and to the

GATT. Neither side offered compromises. And personal animosities were frequently present. The escalation of tensions had its risks. The United States feared loss of access to germplasm and an increasingly tense battle over intellectual property and genetic resources with an uncertain outcome. Third World leaders and NGOs feared a Pyrrhic victory in the UN and the break-up of their fragile coalition. Significantly, both sides were alarmed by continuing erosion of genetic diversity in the field and in inadequately staffed and maintained gene banks.

The first signs of a thaw were seen around 1987. Ciba-Geigy, the Swiss pharmaceutical giant with over $150 million annual seed sales,[67] began inviting adversaries in for tea and discussions. The talks were informal, respectful, even cordial. Ciba-Geigy's stated purpose was to explore the possibility that there might be common ground in the dispute. At approximately the same time, overtures began to be made by the new head of the U.S. Plant Germplasm System to the NGO community. Dr. Henry Shands, a friendly, self-effacing scientist from DeKalb-Pfizer had replaced the abrasive Quentin Jones. Shands seemed eager to form his own opinions about the controversies and, because he was new, was less inclined to defend programs and positions which he had not created.

The National Academy of Sciences (NAS) and the Office of Technology Assessment both undertook major studies on genetic resources and in the process encountered all of the main actors in the debate. Drs. Michael Strauss and John Pino of the NAS both served as intermediaries assuring each side of the other's best intentions and willingness to communicate.

At this time, William Brown, former president and CEO of Pioneer Hi-Bred, chair of the U.S. National Board for Plant Genetic Resources, and easily the most important and influential figure in the seed industry, contacted Pino at the National Academy. Brown's concern was that events at the FAO had gone too far and were threatening to "get out of hand."[68] Brown suggested that a way be found to defuse the situation.

This led to a request to the Keystone Center in Colorado, U.S.A., to hold a dialogue on plant genetic resources.[69] The Keystone Center was established in 1975, to provide a neutral, safe, off-the-record site for discussions among key participants in contentious debates when the time seems appropriate for compromise or resolution of the problem. Keystone's board is liberally constituted with representatives of big, mostly American corporations: First Boston Company, Cetus, Warner Brothers, ABC, SmithKline Beecham, Monsanto, Exxon. There are also representatives of various conservation groups, including the National Wildlife Federation and National Audubon Society. Keystone employs a rather small staff skilled in meeting facilitation and conflict resolution. After a series of small planning sessions, Keystone convened its first plenary meeting in Keystone, Colorado, August 15–18, 1988.

The sources of funding for that first meeting are indicative of the desire of the corporate world for negotiation, or at least resolution of the controversy in the late 1980s. The funders included Ciba-Geigy, Pioneer Hi-Bred, and the Wallace Genetic Foundation (established by the founders of Pioneer and still closely linked with the company), DeKalb-Pfizer Genetics (Shands' former employer), the USDA's Agricultural Research Service (Shands' present employer), the Ford Foundation (a member of the CGIAR board and major funder of the International Rice Research Institute, whose immediate past director would be named chair of the Keystone dialogue), the German Marshall Fund, and the W. Alton Jones Foundation (with prior interests in tropical forest conservation issues).

Forty people participated in the meeting. They included the heads of the government genetic resource programs for the United States, the U.S.S.R., China, Brazil, Peru, the Netherlands, Ethiopia, and the Nordic countries. Both IBPGR and the FAO Commission on Plant Genetic Resources were represented, as were the World Bank and the CGIAR system. From the corporate side, the president of Cetus, the vice president for research as well as the president of the microbial genetics division for Pioneer, the director for public affairs/seeds for Ciba-Geigy, and the executive vice president of DeKalb-Pfizer Genetics were present. The U.S. National Academy of Sciences and the U.S. Agency for International Development also were represented. And the Republican staff director of the U.S. House Agriculture Committee was present. NGO participation centered around the Rural Advancement Fund International (with invitations to both Pat Mooney[70] and myself) and Third World NGOs that had participated in FAO lobbying activities. The Mexican ambassador to FAO (and son of a former Mexican president) who had led the fights in Rome during much of the 1980s was also present. Rounding out the forty were several well-known academics with a long history of involvement in genetic resources or patenting, such as the former director of the Cambridge Plant Breeding Institute and a Stanford law professor. At least one invited group, the Environmental Policy Institute, declined to participate saying that it feared the effort was one meant to co-opt dissent.

The chair of the dialogue was Dr. M. S. Swaminathan. He had recently retired as Director of the International Rice Research Institute (perhaps the CGIAR system's most respected research center) and he was now president of the International Union for the Conservation of Nature and Natural Resources. He was the independent chair of the FAO and he had important ties with the Ford and Rockefeller Foundations. In short, he

commanded respect from the "establishment." His sympathetic performance as chair during some of the acrimonious debates at FAO had mostly
neutralized what might have been some harsh feelings from the NGO and
Third World side.

I have gone to some length in describing the participants in the Keystone International Dialogue on Plant Genetic Resources, because their
positions gave weight and legitimacy to the proceedings of the meeting. It
is not an exaggeration to say that many people were looking on to see if
anything constructive might come from the talks.

The format of discussions at Keystone is also important to mention.
Keystone dialogues operate on the basis of certain specific rules. Participants are asked to speak as individuals, not as representatives of their
organizations — this to encourage discussion and discourage the need to
"go back and get clearance." All discussions are held off the record.
People may not be quoted outside of the meeting. And finally, any report
coming out of the meeting must be adopted by consensus. That is, each
person must be able to live with every word of the report, or it is not
printed. While this gives each person the power of an individual veto, in
practice there is great social pressure not to be a lone objector. In most
cases, individuals who are bothered by something tend not to object if
others with whom they are allied decide not to object.

The meeting produced a 33-page report, remarkable if only for its
length. Much of the report contained observations and recommendations
that were hardly controversial ("There needs to be improvement in, and
distribution of training aids . . ."). But important ground was broken in
two areas — in defining the notion of genetic resources as "common
heritage" and in the emerging concept of "farmers' rights."

Participants agreed that funding for genetic conservation should include provisions to encourage "utilization of appropriate genetic varieties
. . . .The value of a resource to a country depends on the country's present
and future ability to utilize them. It follows that support for genetic
resources conservation should be supplemented by support for plant
breeding activities." Furthermore, the report stated: "There is a need for
effective public and farmer operated breeding programs as well as private
breeding programs to provide options."[71]

The meeting tiptoed around patenting, simply saying that farmers
should have choices, that different systems might be needed in different
countries, and that the system should "promote the continuing development of new varieties." It is not difficult to see how corporate executives
might agree to such conclusions. But from the corporate side, there was no
strategy of how to use, develop or extend such statements. On the other

hand, the agreements on farmers rights — "that landraces have *value* as a result of the *labors* of many farmers" — contain powerful implications of unfinished business. An agreement that landraces are valuable as a result of labor makes landraces hardly distinguishable from patented varieties, which also draw their value from labor, except for the fact that no compensation mechanisms exist for the landraces. The meeting ended without further elaboration or development of this point. Participants, however, did outline a long list of contributions that farm families could make to genetic resources work thus serving to legitimize grass-roots participation in genetic conservation and breeding work.

The results of the meeting were well received by the outside world. But perhaps more importantly, the meeting had begun to change adversaries' views of each other making further negotiation possible — the Keystone strategy, it seemed, was working. Corporate executives emerged saying that NGOs could be "constructive." NGOs emerged with respect for the candidness and honesty as well as the concern for genetic diversity shown by corporate executives. Don Duvick of Pioneer Hi-Bred was particularly important to the process. Duvick is from "the old school." He grew up on a midwestern U.S. farm without electricity, where values of honesty and hard work obviously made their mark. He is quiet, and can be viewed at first as almost humorless, but few would doubt his personal commitment to farmers or genetic conservation. As vice president of the world's largest seed company (annual sales approximately $900 million), it was interesting to see that this family background still very obviously played a role in the formulation of his opinions even when it conflicted with certain corporate interests.[72] Shands of the USDA struck people as being similar in honesty and openness. Mooney, for his part, appeared not to have horns and disarmed some former opponents with his humor and broad grasp of the subject. In short, the lines of communication had been pried open. The key players were in place. A new arena had been established. A second meeting was planned for 1990, in Madras, India.

Communication continued and even improved between meetings. NGOs organized an informal "Keystone alumni" dinner at the 1989 FAO Conference, for example. And a number of participants were in frequent contact with each other regarding plans for the next meeting. Specifically, NGO and corporate representatives both urged that "tougher" corporate people attend the next meeting.

As participants climbed aboard the bus for the hour-long trip from the Madras airport to an isolated, walled hotel in the countryside, expectations were decidedly modest. Despite the fact that adversaries could now tentatively refer to each other as "friends," the second session's agenda would be centered on farmers' rights and compensation. No one expected agreement, much less consensus. Mooney quietly predicted that no report at all would come from the meeting and speculated that the meeting might end in a walk-out of one side or the other. These predictions proved to be far off base.

Most of the participants from the first session returned for the second. A few people were dropped from the list and a few others, most notably the president of the Rockefeller Foundation, the past president of ASSINSEL (International Association of Plant Breeders for the Protection of Plant Varieties), the minister of the environment of Indonesia, and executives from Ciba-Geigy and Kleinwanzlebener Saatzucht (KWS), were added.

The resulting report was equally long, but much more detailed. It credited intellectual property laws with both encouraging development of new varieties and encouraging genetic erosion and uniformity. It criticized the effort to insert intellectual property rights for plants into the GATT negotiations and urged countries to "assess the potential impact of the negotiations on the preservation and exchange of plant genetic resources."

The conclusions on "farmers' rights" and an international fund, likewise, were surprising:

> Farmers' Rights recognizes that farmers and rural communities have greatly contributed to the creation, conservation, exchange and knowledge of genetic and species utilization of genetic diversity, that this contribution is ongoing and not simply something of the past, and that this diversity is extremely valuable. Yet, neither the marketplace nor current intellectual property systems have any way of assigning a value to this material. A concrete way of recognizing Farmers' Rights would be a fund, such as the fund currently existing at FAO, which supports genetic conservation and utilization programs particularly, but not exclusively, in the Third World. The fund would not be designed to reward or compensate individual farmers, farm communities, Third World Countries, or governments nor to compensate anyone or anything based strictly on their contributions of germplasm.[73]

At first glance it might appear that this could not possibly be a consensus statement. But there was virtually no debate over the need for or advisability of establishing such a fund. People from industry insisted on a few points: first, that the fund be mainly but not exclusively for the Third World; and second and more importantly, that the fund not be described as "compensating" any individual or government. The fund would recognize farmers' rights, not compensate them. This distinction would have been unacceptable to Third World representatives and NGOs were it not for industry's surprising concession that contributions to the

fund not be voluntary, but mandatory. This agreement was also conditioned on the explicit understanding that NGOs would not push for the
funds to come from taxes on the seed industry. Interestingly, corporate
opposition to a tax was simply pragmatic. The industry will not support
this agreement if there is a tax and we need the industry's support if the
governments are to agree, was what was said. The proposal by NGOs at
FAO three years earlier for a $150 million a year fund had been scoffed at
as a wild fantasy. The Keystone dialogue endorsed a $500 million annual
fund. The meeting reaffirmed its support for an "agreed interpretation" of
the categories of germplasm included in the FAO undertaking. This
interpretation, suggested by the first Keystone meeting, worked out in
specifics in a small group of Keystone participants in Washington, and
formally accepted by FAO, essentially retracted the demand for free
exchange of breeding lines and patented varieties. The eagerness for a
resolution to the fights of the 1980s was evident to everyone.

The report from the Madras meeting was greeted with shock by members of the genetic resources community. In scope and number, agreements had far exceeded expectations. But few were second-guessing the
conclusions. Instead there seemed to be relief that a resolution might be in
sight. Other, slightly less visible developments followed the Madras
meeting: Mooney was asked to join the board of Keystone (he declined)
and I was appointed to serve as the first "outsider" on the U.S. National
Plant Genetic Resources Board, a group which advises the secretary of
agriculture on policy.

Following several working group sessions in 1990 and 1991, the final
plenary of the Keystone dialogue was held outside of Oslo, Norway, May
31–June 4, 1991. Participants warned that Third World governments
should not be pressed into adopting inappropriate IPR through the GATT
process. The group further agreed that while IPR may "stimulate innovation in certain market conditions . . . it could have a negative impact on the
farmer-breeders who still actively maintain important genetic diversity as
a part of their traditional activities."[74] Third World countries adopting IPR
were cautioned to allow farmers to plant back seed from protected
varieties.

Much of the time and energy at the last session was consumed in
designing a structure, work plan, and budget for a "Global Plant Genetic
Resources Initiative." The Initiative was an attempt to solve the continuing genetic erosion crisis and to give substance to the concept of farmers'
rights by financing local conservation and utilization (plant improvement)
projects. While the initiative would not guarantee an end to NGO or Third
World opposition to IPR for plants, it would defuse the political charge

that only Third World innovation is unrewarded and only Third World resources are "free." At the same time, the initiative would provide a tangible victory to activists and Third World interests. The wording of the final Keystone report reflected the origins of the process. Though William Brown died just weeks before the final plenary, he would have been pleased with the report's conclusion: The new Global PGR Initiative is designed to create "the basis for a general cooperative venture based on mutual benefit. The Global PGR Initiative, taken as a whole, will inevitably create a new environment of trust and exchange."[75]

Since the conclusion of the Keystone dialogue, participants have actively lobbied for government, corporate, and NGO support for the initiative. Representing a consensus of disparate views, the report may be a convenient blueprint for politicians looking for "direction." Writing shortly after the conclusion of the Keystone plenary, it is not possible to judge its impact. But like any "invention" or idea, the challenge will be to put it into practice. This will call for organization and political skills, and the exercise of power — questionable attributes of the *group* constituted temporarily as the "Keystone Dialogue." The ability of actors to maintain consensus, coordinate resources, and implement the initiative will profoundly influence the future course of struggles over intellectual property rights for biological materials. Short of concrete implementation, however, the consensus achieved at Keystone may well shape public opinion and provide the basis for a new vision of what is acceptable and desirable. If so, it could become an important part of the ideological context for future developments.

Were the "Keystone process" to stop now, the chief beneficiaries might not be the Third World governments or NGOs. In a private letter to Keystone staff prior to the final plenary, Pat Mooney outlined what he thought each side had gained and lost. Mooney concluded that through or as a result of the Keystone dialogue, "progressives" had:

1.  . . . implicitly acknowledged the right of breeders to seek protection and the right of countries to grant protection;

2.  redefined categories covered under the FAO Undertaking in order to exclude breeders' lines and patented varieties from automatic exchange;

3.  worked behind the scenes to facilitate the U.S. and Canada joining the FAO Commission;

4.  presented their strategy for a Code of Conduct on PGR Introduction, a sequal [sic] to the Code of Conduct on Germplasm Collecting introduced at FAO in 1989;

**5.** significantly defused the tense and confrontational atmosphere around the IPR/genetic resources debate.

While the agreements reached at Keystone were remarkable and even progressive, they were only agreements. They were not yet real. As Mooney described it: "Nice words on GATT, but it won't stop GATT. Nice words on farmers' rights — but no rights for farmers. Nice words on community approaches — but no facility or funds to back them up."[76] Again, it is too early to judge the importance or impact of the dialogue from anyone's perspective.

These efforts, which may in some years' time provide some answers to the question of compensation (or recognition) for Third World genetic resources and innovation, still leave open the debate over the extension of patent laws to cover the new developments in biotechnology. The United States is still pushing for extensions through GATT, an effort which may totally derail the agreements reached at Keystone. NGOs are raising issues in the UN Conference on Trade and Development (UNCTAD). Revisions of the UPOV convention have been made and await only individual member adoption. Patent law reform is under way in Europe and is still being defined in North America. And the UN is seeking to make more concrete and implement a broader biodiversity convention signed in Brazil in 1992 by most of the nations of the world, excluding the United States.

## DISCUSSION

In this chapter we examine efforts of actors to solve problems in three very different arenas. In the first, the U.S. government attempts to link intellectual property rights protection with trade issues at the General Agreement on Tariffs and Trade (GATT) in Geneva. It does so hoping to force others to adopt certain patent standards if they wish to avoid trade sanctions under GATT. In the second, developing countries and NGOs seek to put pressure on developed countries and carve out concessions through the vehicle of establishing farmers' rights. In the third, a diversity of important figures in the genetic resources debate gather for private negotiations under the auspices of the Keystone Center.

In terms of theory, this chapter specifically concerns new arenas and the negotiation process. But again, actors, agency, and context are central to the development of the chapter. The influence of new technologies and the desire by some actors to fashion new rules in response to this is also evident.

Earlier we saw some actors facing problems in pursuing new property rights through the U.S. Congress. Patent law, as van den Belt and Rip point out, "is a social accomplishment that creates new solutions for new situations."[77] "Solving" one situation, however, created a new situation and a new strand for the fabric. Equilibrium proved elusive.

After gaining new rights through the court system, actors still faced certain obstacles to full international commercialization — how to protect the intellectual property of expanding biologically based export businesses. The problem was particularly acute with biotechnology since the "export" often carried with it the ability to reproduce itself. To address such a problem, actors could attempt to change rules on a country by country basis or seek arenas where international agreements might be possible. Perhaps because the position of industrialized countries is powerful in GATT (the voting formula is skewed in their favor and trade sanctions can be painful to less developed countries), a number of actors focused on GATT as a possible arena for securing new agreements on property rights.

The theoretical assumptions regarding new arenas are similar here to those offered for the last chapter. New arenas offer new possibilities and outcomes. They may involve new actors and call for different skills and resources. Actors have choices about how to pursue their goals. These choices are not without constraints, of course. One choice may involve arenas when more than one arena is technically possible.

Additionally, we see here that new arenas allow for different kinds or qualities of discourse. Privacy is conducive to policy deliberations in a negotiation forum.[78] Actors can explore options shielded to some degree from the public accountability present in other fora. Compromise can be more easily agreed to in private, where responsibility for decisions is obscured.[79] This may particularly be the case when a wide range of issues is being negotiated, a multiplicity of interests involved, and a number of actors present. In such a situation, a broader range of problems and solutions can be discussed and trade-offs made on seemingly unrelated matters as part of larger "solution packages." At Keystone, tacit acceptance of the right of commercial plant breeders to benefit from their inventions was part of the price paid by NGOs for the support by other actors of a global initiative on the conservation and use of plant genetic resources. No one actor need take responsibility for the compromise. The process offers participants the protection of "plausible deniability" to grease the machinery.

In different arenas, actors endeavor to "frame" the issues in a manner that benefits them. For example, we have a trade issue at GATT; a fight for intellectual property rights in Congress; a narrow yet sweeping patent application in the courts; and a fight over genetic resources and farmers' rights at FAO. Different arenas can facilitate the framing and linking of issues. The United States could not easily link intellectual property rights issues with trade sanctions at FAO. It could and does at GATT. Thus the choice of arenas (which can be experienced by others as the imposition of arenas) can virtually determine who will be able to frame or define the issue and how — a very useful position for an actor.

Events in one arena can affect events in another. Arenas are connected by actors, issues, resources, and rules — and by the obvious fact that they affect one another. Changes or developments in one arena help redefine norms of opposition and discourse, and the opportunities in other arenas. They change relationships between actors and the power, opportunities, and liabilities they have. These changes can even facilitate the incorporation of critics into the discussion and decision-making processes of some of the institutions they had previously opposed.[80] The Keystone dialogue encouraged participants to step out of traditional roles as representatives of interests. This, of course, is not completely possible, but the atmosphere Keystone created reduced tension among actors and probably contributed to a lessening of controversy at FAO.[81] At Keystone, actors agreed that the FAO undertaking which calls for the full exchange of all categories of genetic resources really should not apply to breeding lines and patented varieties. This "agreed interpretation" (adopted by FAO) helped facilitate U.S. entry into the Commission on Plant Genetic Resources.

At the UN Food and Agriculture Organization, NGOs found an arena more favorable to their interests. This arena provides more power to the numerically superior forces of Third World governments. As a political forum, it makes possible the insertion of additional issues and the framing of debate in ways quite different than in the U.S. Congress or judicial system. Resolutions are based on statements by governments and the content of the debate which can be quite far-reaching. In addition, the range of political viewpoints is far broader in the FAO.

With a different configuration of power, such as that found at FAO, actors could question old assumptions and challenge existing relationships. New issues were created and the possibility of unintended consequences rose. At FAO we see that actors can change strategies, in this case from simply opposing a bill in Congress to proposing new and different notions of property (farmers' rights, national sovereignty vs. common heritage), and relationships. This was an attempt to create a rule system to mobilize resources for a collective end.[82] Other actors were hampered by lack of experience with the workings of this arena and by an incomplete and flawed understanding of the motivations, plans and capabilities of opposing actors, particularly in the context of a new arena and a newly framed set of issues. Certainly the seed industry exhibited misunderstanding of NGOs and fueled the conflict.

If the desired outcome requires negotiation, or some consent on the part of opposing actors, then actors disadvantaged by a change of arenas must be enticed into the new arena. There are a number of factors which might entice them there (or if already present, encourage them to participate), including the risks of leaving the issue uncontested in an arena with certain decision-making capabilities. Such was the case with the involvement of the United States in the FAO debates. Over a period of years, the United States pursued a clearly defensive strategy, never mounting a new initiative of its own in this hostile arena. The importance of arenas and even their legitimacy as arenas can be affected by the recognition which key actors (including nonparticipants) afford to the arena.

The legal and scientific complexity of the issues would seem to argue against bold new initiatives or meaningful intervention in any arena by people with little formal expertise in these subjects. But, on the contrary, actors not bound by the constraints of specialization can become very important assuming they have competence and carry out their strategies wisely. Such actors here reshaped analyses, made new and provocative connections between various issues previously thought to be distinct, and in the process they drew new people and institutions into the debate. Rules changed. The lobbyist — virtually an unknown animal at FAO — had become a fixture at biennial FAO conferences by the end of the 1980s. Those portrayed as having "no standing" had gained standing through the acquisition and exercise of political power.

Arenas differ in terms of the access and influence they afford to political pressures — interest groups, the media, "public opinion." Different outcomes are possible on similar issues from arena to arena. Different decision-making arenas give different degrees of importance to the same criteria in making decisions. Some even stress entirely different criteria. Interests which are politically unpopular in one arena may avoid the negative consequences of that by shifting to another arena which is less concerned about or even largely disinterested in the unpopular position. Of course, a position which is unpopular in one arena may be quite popular in another. Contrast the decisions reached by the U.S. courts with those of the FAO, for one example.

Property rights accrue to those with the power to formulate, legislate, and enforce. Just because farmers are innovative does not mean that their creativity will be legally recognized. Prior to the meetings at the FAO, there had been no clear attempt to secure rights for farmers related to their plant breeding and conservation activities. The assertion of new rights was really a call to redress old problems and establish new relationships.

Physical ownership does not necessarily guarantee the right or ability to control what is owned or to benefit from its exploitation (in the case of biological materials). One may own but not control. One can, for example, own an object without owning the formula for that object or any of the object's component parts. Unlike seed companies, Third World farmers have no intellectual property rights over the diverse and variable landraces they "own." They own seeds, not varieties or formulas. Without this intellectual property right, they are not able to sell their seeds without at the same time legally handing over the right to reproduce "their" variety or "expropriate" any valuable genes or characteristics found therein.

The fact that some actors can exploit resources that others own yet cannot exploit means that the owners do not fully control their resources or fully benefit from their ownership. At the FAO, Third World government representatives may be aware at some level that while they own resources, they are not in a position to control their full development. Without this ability, they are stuck with a lot of "primitive" seeds instead of breeding materials and valuable genes. The difference is not in the seeds themselves, but in how they can be exploited and by whom. This situation is an important piece of the context of the debate at FAO.

While legal protection is secured for the products of the new technologies, it is opposed by certain actors for the products of the old, farmer-utilized technologies. Some actors promote the notion of "common heritage" to justify their access to and nonbeholden benefit from a whole class of biological materials — those "possessed" by Third World farmers. These actors defend this informal, customary approach to these resources even as they endeavor to construct very formal and rigid legal systems of recognition for biological materials developed under their care. The attempt to expand property rights over biological materials through the law effectively means an encroachment on the informal rights of others. It shifts the effective locus of control. While Third World farmers may *possess* valuable germplasm they do not *own* it in a way that allows them to exploit it fully. Possession itself is only partial (quite apart from the issue of "ability to use"). Farmers' development of the material through breeding is unattached to intellectual property rights which would allow them to claim benefit from it as a corporate plant breeder might. Peasant farmers can eat their seeds, perhaps sell them to others who will eat them, or replant. To the corporate plant breeder, however, this very same genetic material is a resource which can be fashioned into something that can be legally owned and protected. This protection can and does specify certain enforceable rights and relationships which in scope and power far exceed those of the farmer who may initially have been responsible for the unique and useful characteristic in the material. As for farmers' materials, one is reminded of Rudyard Kipling's question, "It's pretty, but is it Art?"[83] In the eyes of the law, it is not.

Some new technologies are so complicated and their commercialization so far into the future that patents themselves become a product. Companies' fortunes rise and fall based not on the performance of products in the marketplace, but the procurement of patents. Thus, the complexity of technology and the related difficulty of commercializing it can combine to create new and different values for both products and patents. This situation becomes part of the context in which actors struggle to redefine property rights and relationships.

Property rights indicate relationships. The use of language both reveals and promotes actors' interests. Seed industry representatives spoke of "farmers' rights" during the campaign for the PVPA as a way of acknowledging the limits of the law and perhaps reassuring skeptics. Fewer than twenty years later, such actors now repudiated those rights, preferring to speak instead of the farmers' *privilege* to save seeds. It may be difficult to attack what one recognizes as a right. A privilege, however, is fair game. This one came under attack as the seed industry attempted to redefine its relationship with farmers.

The concept of common heritage or common ownership, which indicates open access to genetic resources, also conflicts with assumptions of national sovereignty over resources. Whereas Third World governments began the 1980s advancing "common heritage" at the UN, many ended the decade having signed the FAO undertaking with "reservations." These reservations were made to allow for the exercise of national sovereignty and the protection and control of certain resources which they view as being *their* property and not common property.

In fact, the principle of common heritage/common ownership, which was supposed to govern the handling of genetic resources, never really did completely. It was a way of describing behavior which effectively disguised the real social relationships — relationships which experienced stress, challenge and redefinition in the 1980s. When collections are made in a Third World country, for example, ownership is not transferred from that country to the "world community." In fact, material from a Third World country normally is taken to a gene bank which is under another nation's or organization's control, where it becomes the property not of the world community but of whoever collected or received it.

Some rule systems (they do not have to be laws, but can be "principles" or norms such as "common heritage") facilitate some actors benefiting, dominating, and/or controlling on a systematic, ongoing basis. This is the case with the intellectual property rights secured through the courts and is, in fact, what actors sought at FAO with the proposal of an international gene fund.

In the context of struggles over property relationships, previously held "principles" or norms can be used or interpreted in unforeseen ways. As noted above, the principle of "common heritage" was cited as a justification for free collecting of resources in the Third World. But Third World delegations at FAO used the same principle of common heritage to make claims on patented varieties and breeding lines in developed countries.

New rules can be created by actors for very different reasons. New rules which benefit one industry, for example, may be an "unintended consequence" of the efforts of other actors in their quest for new rules for themselves. Not all actors pushing for reforms through GATT are seed companies interested in intellectual property rights for biological materials. Some are computer software companies. Others are drug companies or book publishers. Seed companies may be a small part of the overall effort. Yet, if GATT establishes minimum patent standards enforced through trade sanctions, seed companies will be among the beneficiaries. Other actors may be totally unaware of or unaffected by the concerns of seed companies.

Actors learn, become conscious of common interests, and change, and this alters power balances among actors. Their actions are influenced by expectations about the future.[84] Policy positions of actors need to be viewed in the context of long-term as well as immediate goals. GE was interested in more than the patent on a single microorganism. Certain actors at FAO were interested in establishing a commission on plant genetic resources, but not just for the sake of creating another commission. They saw the advantages of creating a new arena as an ongoing forum likely to be sympathetic to their interests. In such a situation, the success of actors in creating this new arena was viewed as a threat by those whose control was enhanced in other arenas. In this case, a more public, "democratic" decision-making forum threatened private control — especially when the shift to that forum was made to take advantage of this characteristic.

Linear history does not stress the blind alleys or the paths not taken. Keystone may someday be seen as a blind alley in *some* respects.[85] These blind alleys may be failures in terms of contemporary expectations. The action of actors escapes them when it enters the social world and they cannot fully know or anticipate what the effects will be. We may think of efforts like Keystone (or GATT?) as blind alleys because they fail to produce the main results actors strive for in those arenas. Still, these efforts become part of a larger context and may play an important enabling or constraining role in other action. The fight at GATT will certainly affect future trade negotiations. The Keystone dialogue has changed relationships among actors and their perceptions of problems. Even if the agreements at Keystone are not implemented, actors will have gained knowledge about each other through the process of negotiation.

Keystone is what Burns and Flam term a "negotiative-contractual form," where procedures are essential to the legitimacy of the outcome.[86] The rules of the dialogue were stressed by the organizers, and it would appear generally upheld by participants. Legitimacy was a crucial element in the Keystone exercise, but it may not be enough to guarantee success.

Attempts at dealing with large issues, contentious issues and/or financial issues by "subgovernments"[87] are problematic. To some extent, Keystone was an effort to solve problems by "insiders," — something fairly similar to a subgovernment. To be successful, negotiations must include the actors who have the power to enforce agreements. At Keystone, some actors could "deliver," others could not.

Bureaucrats have more power over policy and programs than over budgets and funding. Keystone participants coming from governments appeared to have the power to negotiate successfully certain policy problems (U.S. entry into the FAO commission). But U.S. government officials in attendance had neither the authority nor the influence to speak for their government in committing any substantial funding. Negotiated decisions involving both policy and money are vulnerable if made only by those who do not exercise power over budgets. Inequality of power in hierarchies means that views of those on top are important simply because of their status, not because of their intrinsic worth. Thus there can be a disjunction of power and knowledge.[88] The highest ranking bureaucrat actually working on a particular subject may have more knowledge about the field than anyone else, but may not have enough power to make substantial funding or policy decisions.

Due to the differing abilities of actors to enforce agreements, the outcome of negotiations such as Keystone is particularly uncertain. This uncertainty is compounded by the fact that agreement from this arena must be transferred to other arenas with different actors, rules and power configurations, if they are to be implemented fully.

## NOTES

1. Plant varieties are not as adaptable to production/distribution in all climates as are certain products of biotechnology. With plant varieties companies are careful to control breeding material. Release of breeding material may help competition within the geographic range of the particular crop variety. However, national laws can sometimes provide protection within this range. With many genetically engineered organisms, however, the "range" of the organism is practically unlimited. If the organism is obtained by competitors it can be used practically anywhere — easily in countries which do not provide reciprocal patent rights.

2. Beier, F. K., and J. Straus, "Patents in a Time of Rapid Scientific and Technological Change: Inventions in Biotechnology. In Beier, F. K., R. S. Crespi, and J. Straus, *Biotechnology and Patent Protection*. Paris: Organization for Economic Cooperation and Development. 1985: p. 15.

3. Burrill, G. Steven, with the Ernst & Young High Technology Group, *Biotech 90: Into the Next Decade: Fourth Annual Survey of Business and Financial Issues in America's Most Promising Industry*. New York: Mary Ann Liebert, Inc. 1989: p. 30.

4. Beier and Straus, op.cit., p. 16

5. Burrill, op.cit., p. 69.

6. Burrill, op.cit., p. 46.

7. Yoo, John, "Biotech Patents Become Snarled in Bureaucracy," *Wall Street Journal*. July 6, 1989: p. B2.

8. Dwyer, Paula, "The Battle Raging Over Intellectual Property" *Business Week*. May 22, 1989: p. 78.

9. Lambert, Wade and Arthur S. Hayes, "Investing in Patents to File Suits Is Curbed." *Wall Street Journal*. May 30, 1990: p. B8.

10. In Cook, Arthur G., "Patents as Non-Tariff Trade Barriers." *TIBTECH*. October, 1989: p. 262.

11. Beier and Straus, op. cit., p. 29.

12. Straus, Joseph, "Biotechnology and its International Legal and Economic Implications." Undated draft. p. 22.

13. Were the Paris Convention to be renegotiated, the United States would not enjoy the advantage of being able to leverage trade sanctions against Third World concessions on IPR. For this and other reasons (including Third World experience with the Paris Convention and relative inexperience in GATT), industrialized countries have more of an advantage (in relation to the Third World) in GATT than in negotiations on the Paris Convention. Dietz, Rycroft and Stern have noted the importance of defining issues and related this to the determination of arenas. They argue that "we also need better information on how issue frames influence policy outcomes." This would seem to be a clear case of where a policy outcome will probably be influenced and as such might be a candidate for the further research suggested. Dietz, Thomas, Robert W. Rycroft, and Paul C. Stern, "Framing and Power in Policy Systems: The Case of Environmental Risk." Unpublished draft, October 23, 1992, p. 21.

14. The developments at GATT have their own exceedingly complex context, which for various reasons I have not been able to present here. This context includes both past and present efforts to open up markets for trade and investment in many fields. I do not mean to suggest here that United States efforts at GATT are driven exclusively or even mainly from the desire to obtain intellectual property rights for biotechnology.

15. Bradley, A. Jane, "Intellectual Property Rights, Investment, and Trade in Services in the Uruguay Round: Laying the Foundations," in *Stanford Journal of International Law*. No. 23. 1987: p. 74.

16. Ibid., p. 74.

17. Peng, Martin Khor Kok. "Transnational Corporations: The Interests Behind GATT." *The Ecologist*. Vol. 20, no. 6. November–December, 1990: p. 209.

18. Weissman, Robert, "Prelude to a New Colonialism: The Real Purpose of GATT," *The Nation*. March 18, 1991: p. 336.
19. Berenbeim, Ronald, "Safeguarding Intellectual Property." *Research Report* no. 925. New York: The Conference Board. 1989: p. 4–5.
20. GATT is also virtually "off-limits" to nongovernment organizations. Unlike at the FAO, NGOs are not permitted easy access to meetings or delegates. Additionally, some NGOs would find Geneva to be prohibitively expensive for long-term efforts.
21. Bradley, op.cit., p. 60. Interestingly, the first case brought to GATT concerning patent infringement was brought by the United States against Canada — not the typical Third World "pirate" nation — over export of auto parts the U.S. believed were protected under its patent laws.
22. Peng, op.cit., p. 209.
23. For example, "by the end of 1987 IBM had been involved in eighty court and police actions in Taiwan" alone. Despite this large number, it had earned only $650,000 in damages according to Ashoka Mody of the World Bank, "New International Environment for Intellectual Property Rights," in *Intellectual Property Rights in Science, Technology, and Economic Performance: International Comparisons* edited by Francis Rushing and Carole Ganz Brown. Boulder, Colo.: Westview Press. 1990: p. 227.
24. Katzenbach, Nicholas deB., "The International Protection of Technology: A Challenge for International Law Making." *Technology in Society*. Vol. 9. 1987: p. 137–138.
25. Dwyer, Paula, op. cit., p. 78.
26. Correa, Carlos M., "TRIPs: An Asymmetric Negotiation," Unpublished draft, June, 1993: p. 3–4.
27. Ibid., p. 4.
28. Gadbaw, R. Michael, and Timothy J. Richards, "Introduction," in Gadbaw, R.M. and T.J. Richards (eds.), *Intellectual Property Rights: Global Consensus, Global Conflict?* Boulder, Colo.: Westview Press. 1988: p. 20.
29. Gadbaw, R. Michael, and Rosemary E. Gwynn, "Intellectual Property Rights in the New GATT Round," in Gadbaw, R. M., and T. J. Richards, op. cit., p. 40.
30. Anonymous, "Uruguay and Apple Pie." *The Economist*. Vol. 309, no. 7709. June 1, 1991: p. 15.
31. However, the United States government has acknowledged that it refused to sign the Convention on Biodiversity at the UN Conference on Environment and Development due to lobbying from biotechnology interests, which perceived in the convention a threat to the U.S. negotiating position on IPR at GATT. This would seem to indicate that biotechnology interests may have significant influence in the formulation of U.S. policy at GATT.
32. Runge, C. Ford. "The Developing Countries and the Uruguay Round." Staff Paper P-91-9. St. Paul, Minn.: University of Minnesota Institute of Agriculture, Forestry and Home Economics. February, 1991: p. 8.
33. Publication of this journal was planned to coincide with an important meeting of the FAO conference in 1983.
34. Mooney and I made many of these trips together and closely coordinated our work with each other even prior to our working with the same organization.
35. The issue had been mentioned earlier. M. S. Swaminathan, the "father of the Green Revolution" in India and the independent chair of the FAO Council had made note of concerns over the topic at the 1979 FAO conference. He later told Pat Mooney that he had been inspired to do so by reading Mooney's book, *Seeds of the Earth*. In addition the Spanish delegation had proposed a strengthening of existing structures for genetic resources. Still the issue was not fully "engaged" nor framed in a political manner. See Esquinas-Alcazar, Jose T., "Plant Genetic Resources: A Base for Food Security," *Ceres*, No. 118, 1987: p. 43.
36. Goodman, Louis, with Arthur Domike and Charles Sands, *The Improved Seed Industry: Issues and Options for Mexico*. Washington: Center for International Technical Cooperation. 1982.

37. Consultative Group on International Agricultural Research, *Annual Report — CGIAR, 1988/89*. Washington: CGIAR. 1989: p. 58.
38. Ibid., p. 51. (Note: CGIAR is in the process of adding new centers to its network. This list will therefore not be complete at the time of publication.)
39. As of late 1992, IBPGR is in the process of legally separating from FAO. While still technically under FAO, it already has moved into a separate building and enjoys an increasing amount of autonomy.
40. Fowler, Cary, and Pat Mooney, *Shattering: Food, Politics and the Loss of Genetic Diversity*. Tucson: University of Arizona Press. 1990: p. 190–191.
41. General Accounting Office, "The Department of Agriculture Can Minimize the Risk of Potential Crop Failures," Report to the Congress by the Comptroller General, GAO, April 10, 1981: p. iv–v.
42. Ibid., p. iii.
43. Wood, David, Letter addressed to "Genetic Resources Units: IARC's," Annex. September 15, 1987. Emphasis in original.
44. Edminster, T. W., Letter to Richard Demuth, chairman, IBPGR, January 19, 1977.
45. Williams, J. T. Letter to George White. November 30, 1982: p. 1.
46. U.S. Embassy — Rome. Telegram to Secretary of State, U.S. Department of State. October 1, 1984: p. 1.
47. Mooney joined the Rural Advancement Foundation International (RAFI), a part of the National Sharecroppers Fund/Rural Advancement Fund during this period. At ICDA his work was ably taken over by Henk Hobbelink. ICDA ceased its seed-related activities when Genetic Resources Action International (GRAIN) was created as an independent organization with Hobbelink as its head.
48. NGOs generally arrived several days prior to the FAO conferences to participate in intensive training and educational sessions hosted by sympathetic Italian NGOs and organized by ICDA and RAFI. Often briefing papers had already been sent out, allowing participants to study the issues and discuss them with colleagues before arriving.
49. Murphy, Charles, and Quentin Jones, "Briefing Paper." Internal USDA document. October 26, 1983: p. 1.
50. The "undertaking" established voluntary guidelines for the conservation and exchange of plant genetic resources. See FAO Document C 83/II REP/4, 5. 1983.
51. Denny, Wayne, personal discussion, Washington, D.C., October 16–17, 1990. T. B. Kenney (Administrator, USDA) in a telegram to George Dietz, First Secretary at the U.S. Mission to UN-FAO also noted (April 19, 1984): "The seed trade (ASTA) is responding very negatively to both the Undertaking and the Commission. They will undoubtedly have an influence on any official U.S. reaction." In fact, ASTA, IBPGR *and* CGIAR officials participated in internal meetings at the USDA to develop USDA policies, according to a letter from Orville Bentley, assistant secretary of agriculture to Secretary of Agriculture John Block, on June 7, 1984. IBPGR-USDA cooperation is further evidenced in the fact that a letter I wrote to Trevor Williams at IBPGR in Rome in 1981 was found to be in the possession of the USDA when they released it as part of the interrogatory process during the lawsuit filed by the Foundation on Economic Trends against the USDA. An unpublished agenda of a small Rome meeting of activists working on the campaign at FAO also turned up in the USDA files.
52. American Seed Trade Association, "Position Paper of the American Seed Trade Association on FAO International Undertaking on Plant Genetic Resources." Washington: ASTA. May 5, 1984: p. 1–2.
53. Ibid., p. 6.
54. U.S. Department of State, "U.S. Position on FAO Undertaking and Commission on Plant Genetic Resources." March, 1985: p. 1–2.
55. A certain level of concern may be evidenced in the fact that five documents, all cables, were denied to lawyers representing the Foundation on Economic Trends in their lawsuit over USDA's custodianship of genetic resources. Henry Shands of the USDA in a letter to the foundation's attorneys stated that the documents had been designated as "classi-

fied" by the Department of State. Two sent in November, 1983, concerned the FAO conference of the same month and were between the American embassy in Rome and the secretary of state in Washington. An additional one was from the American embassy in Brussels to the secretary of state in November, 1983, concerning the FAO gene bank proposal. One was from the secretary of state to the American embassy in Bogata in April, 1983, concerning the FAO Committee on Agriculture. The fifth, sent in January, 1985, concerned an FAO meeting and was from the secretary of state to OECD capitals. (From Henry Shands, Letter to Foundation on Economic Trends attorneys, May 25, 1988: p. 1.) Later, in November 1992, I was informed by Dr. Shands that the material had been classified not because of sensitive references regarding genetic resources, but because classified materials concerning other countries and other matters not connected with genetic resources happened to be contained in the same document. The subject of the part of the documents of relevance to the foundation's lawsuit was given to the foundation by USDA. According to Dr. Shands, the USDA did not intend to imply that this was the only subject addressed in the document or that its classification was based on material related to genetic resources.

56. Jones, Quentin, Draft Report on FAO Undertaking. Internal USDA document. May 3, 1984: p. 2.
57. Williams, J. T., Letter to Quentin Jones. June 19, 1984: p. 1.
58. Richard Demuth, the first chairman of IBPGR, also wrote Jones and spoke of the need of "finally freeing the Board from the tenacles of FAO." Letter dated March 8, 1985: p. 1.
59. Jones, Quentin, Draft for the IBPGR Executive Committee Meeting in Leuven, Belgium on IBPGR and the FAO Undertaking. August 6, 1984: p. 1–2.
60. Conklin (personal communication), cited in Brush, Steve, "Genetic Diversity and Conservation in Traditional Farming Systems," *Journal of Ethnobiology*, Vol. 6, no. 1, Summer, 1986: p. 158.
61. Nabhan, Gary, *Enduring Seeds: Native American Agriculture and Wild Plant Conservation*. San Francisco: North Point Press. 1989: p. 33.
62. Wilkes, H. G. "Hybridization of Maize and Teosinte in Mexico and Guatemala and the Improvement of Maize." *Economic Botany*. Vol. 31. July–September, 1977: p. 271ff.
63. Richards, Paul, *Coping With Hunger: Hazard and Experiment in an African Rice-Farming System*. London: Allen & Unwin. 1986: p. 134ff.
64. Kneen, O. H. "Plant Patents Enrich Our Lives," *National Geographic*. March, 1948.
65. Personal communication with Melaku Worede on a number of occasions in the late 1980s and early 1990s.
66. Anonymous, "Quandary over Plant Patenting Brings Diverse Group of Experts Together." *Diversity*. Vol. 4, no. 2–3. 1989: p. 36.
67. Fowler, Cary, Eva Lachkovics, Pat Mooney, and Hope Shand, "The Laws of Life: Another Development and the New Biotechnologies." *Development Dialogue*. Uppsala: Dag Hammarskjöld Foundation. Nos. 1–2. 1988: p. 77.
68. Personal interview with John Pino, Sundvolden, Norway. June 5, 1991.
69. Originally, promoters of the dialogue intended to exclude "activists" such as Pat Mooney. The purpose of the meeting would then have been less to negotiate with adversaries than to develop a common strategy against them. But this original view did not prevail and a broad range of interests were represented at the first meeting.
70. Mooney joined the Rural Advancement Fund International staff in 1984.
71. Keystone Center, "Final Report of the Keystone International Dialogue on Plant Genetic Resources: Session I: *Ex Situ* Conservation of Plant Genetic Resources." Keystone, Colo.: Keystone Center. August 15–18, 1988: p. 13–15.
72. Duvick retired from this position during the course of the Keystone dialogue series. He retained his interest and influence in genetic conservation issues, serving as chair of the National Plant Genetic Resources Board.
73. Keystone Center, "Final Consensus Report of the Keystone International Dialogue Series on Plant Genetic Resources: Madras Plenary Session." Keystone, Colo.: Keystone Center. January 29 — February 2, 1990.

74. Keystone International Dialogue Series on Plant Genetic Resources, "Final Consensus Report: Global Initiative for the Security and Sustainable Use of Plant Genetic Resources." Oslo Plenary Session. Pre-publication draft. Keystone, Colo.: Keystone Center. June 21, 1991: p. 3.
75. Ibid., p. 33.
76. Mooney, Pat, Letter to Michael Lesnick and John Ehrmann (executive vice presidents of the Keystone Center), May 7, 1991: p. 1ff.
77. Van den Belt, Henk, and Arie Rip, "The Nelson-Winter-Dosi Model and Synthetic Dye Chemistry," in Bijker, Wiebe, Thomas Hughes and Trevor Pinch, *The Social Construction of Technological Systems: New Direction in the Sociology and History of Technology*. Cambridge, Mass.: MIT Press. 1987: p. 155.
78. Rourke, Francis E., *Bureaucracy, Politics, and Public Policy*. Second Edition. Boston: Little, Brown & Co. 1976: p. 137.
79. Ibid., p. 138.
80. Note, for example, my appointment by the U.S. Secretary of Agriculture to the National Plant Genetic Resources Board.
81. Through the "agreed interpretation" and the absence of major new, controversial initiatives at FAO during the late 1980s and early 1990s.
82. Burns, Tom, and Helena Flam, *The Shaping of Social Organization: Social Rule System Theory with Applications*. London: Sage Publications. 1987: p. 17.
83. Quoted in Sherwood, Morgan "The Origins and Development of the American Patent System," *American Scientist*. Vol. 71. (September–October, 1983): p. 503.
84. Burns and Flam, op. cit., p. 28.
85. Winner, Langdon, *Autonomous Technology: Technics-out-of-Control as a Theme in Political Thought*. Cambridge, Mass.: MIT Press. 1987: 63ff.
86. Burns and Flam, op. cit., p. 370.
87. Ripley, Randall B., and Grace A. Franklin, *Congress, the Bureaucracy, and Public Policy*. Homewood, Ill.: Dorsey Press. 1976: p. 6.
88. Rourke, op. cit., p. 131.

# Some Observations & Conclusions

Looking back at the 12,000 year history of agriculture, one cannot fail but be impressed by the remarkable changes that have occurred just in the last century. Behind many of these changes, it would seem, has been the powerful driving force of modern technology.

I began this study with the aim of studying intellectual property rights associated with biological materials — in simple language, plant patenting. Among other things, I might have expected to tie advances in technology — for example, the advent of scientific plant breeding following the rediscovery of Mendel's laws of heredity in 1900, or the development of biotechnology in the 1980s — with the changes in patenting law which seemed to follow closely on their heels. Indeed if one were looking for technological determinism, one might believe it could be easily found here. At first glance, the introduction of new technologies would seem to have led almost inevitably to the passage of these laws.

As I began to study the technology, the law, and the law-making process in more depth, however, I found that no simple causal connections could be drawn. In one case, the law covered products not produced by the new technology and excluded those that were. In another, both the technology and the law preceded the development of marketable products. There was no single pathway. No one pattern of rule or law-making held for each case.

What I found instead were much more complicated realities — complex social processes. Having noted the complexity, this is not to say that the subject is beyond some degree of explanation or even understanding. But how can we describe this research theoretically? Can a theoretical framework help in furthering our understanding of the subject?

The fact that there seemed to be different pathways leading to the creation of law indicated the importance of considering law and law-making in its social and economic context, and of trying to understand how that context might help account for the different pathways. As the context of various laws is never the same (problems differ, actors change, relationships differ), the laws themselves are never created in exactly the same way, by the same influences.

Laws reflect and are derived from context-dependent problem situations and problem solving. This is not to say that laws are created by or because of situations. It is *actors* who experience the problem situations (or opportunities). They experience the constraints and enabling features of that

ever-changing context — a context they are never completely free to
choose. They are also a part of that context and are experienced by others.
Actors can perceive and define problems and opportunities and formulate
goals and plans. Within limits, actors engage in problem solving and can
effectively alter their circumstances. Neither actor nor action is predetermined by the context. Both evidence creativity, change and effectiveness.
But both are in context.

In this study, certain *processes* are evident — processes of commercialization, legislation, and technological innovation. Each has certain characteristics and again, each must be considered as a product of actors acting in
a particular context. We may consider the effect and impact of these
processes upon one another mediated by actors and the material world.

Finally, we note the importance of *structures*. Here we are dealing
primarily with legal and political structures. These structures have properties and rules (and resources).[1] It is through these properties that actors
experience and deal with the legal structure, for example.

All of the major elements of complex social processes — actors, processes and structures — exist in a certain context and the interaction among
elements takes place in a larger societal and material context including the
nature and qualities of the plants themselves, as previously noted. Each
element forms part of the context of the others, and affects and is affected
by the others.

The framework, which for convenience has been termed "complex
social processes," has certain abstract characteristics that have now been
identified: actors, processes, and structures. The overall process generates
problems and provides the context for solving them. In pursuing this study
I have tried to link the elements of these complex social processes together,
having found that it is not profitable to focus on just one or to consider all
separately without linkages. In this sense my effort falls within the tradition of Giddens (structure-structuration), Burns (actor system dynamics),
and of Weber. This tradition finds actors making their own history. But the
history is made in structurally conditioned ways. The efforts and strategies
of actors, as well as the constraints, opportunities, and "freedoms" they
have, may often be actor-created, but they are also inevitably context-
dependent. As the story is told, we discern many intricate relationships and
more than one context-dependent pattern. Instead of speaking of "causality" in the traditional sense, however, we see these relationships as being
more intertwined. That which affects is also affected.

Such an interpretation discourages one from adopting a more traditionally Marxian approach. The most compelling and tempting example is
provided by Kloppenburg in *First the Seed*, an impressive, rich, and well-
written account of the "political economy of plant biotechnology." Having

provided a sophisticated and detailed context, Kloppenburg abstains from exploring the actual *process*, the turning points during which legislation is constructed. The Plant Patent Act itself is given a little more than a page. The 1980 passage of the expansion of the PVPA, the most hotly and publicly contested battle over plant-related intellectual property rights in U.S. history (or perhaps any other), receives less than a complete paragraph. One is left with the impression — intentional or not — of a monolithic and nearly omnipotent force, namely capital, which works its will.[2] The conclusion appears foregone if only because the actual struggle and process through which the laws were created receive such scant attention. The pecularities of certain actors, their interests, the context as *they* experienced and perceived it, are not fully picked up or appreciated by such an approach. The more fundamental problem is that this approach does not particularly encourage one to examine such processes. The story, as I see it, is still more complicated, still more contingent in the sense that it is not so determined.

There is no single pathway to the creation of intellectual property rights laws concerning biological materials. How biological materials can be used, developed, and commercialized changes over time. The part or aspect of the plant which companies and breeders consider valuable and desire to control (e.g., the species, variety, gene, or characteristic) changes. Such changes alter the context in which actors perceive problems and opportunities, and attempt solutions. The circumstances surrounding the passage of the 1930 Plant Patent Act are different in so many ways from those around the 1980 Chakrabarty Supreme Court decision, to cite but one example, that one should not expect to find a single pattern to fit both. To explain these outcomes we look to certain complex social processes as identified above. These processes do not manifest themselves as a single pattern. Nevertheless, they seem to have three, basic, common, abstract components. In the following pages I provide three figures representing different patterns.[3]

In the case of the Plant Patent Act of 1930, the commercialization of agriculture and the commodification of planting materials presents certain problems and opportunities to seed and nursery companies. Nursery companies in particular perceived the lack of a means to control the varieties they sold — specifically their inability to prevent others from pirating their varieties and selling them. This was an obstacle to business expansion and profit-making. Through their legislative initiatives, they were able to secure passage of a plant patenting law giving them a different type of ownership (over the variety) and more control over how others could use it. A simple pathway leading to the Plant Patent Act of 1930 might be represented as in figure 3.

Within this rather simplified pathway, we can identify more complex social processes. Commercial, legislative, and technological innovation processes, form a background or context which presents actors with certain problems as well as possibilities for fashioning responses or solutions. Commercialization largely eliminated the farmer seed saver and made farmers more dependent on the marketplace for their planting materials. It also helped place a premium on certain varieties — those which were especially productive or desirable to consumers, for instance. Certain technological innovations, including improvements in transportation and refrigeration, facilitated commercialization. These helped farmers produce for the marketplace and they helped seed and nursery companies sell to the farmers. But interestingly enough, new scientific knowledge about inheritance used by some plant breeders in planned and directed breeding programs was not widely employed by those seeking patent law in 1930. However, the growing awareness of scientific plant breeding and public appreciation for plant "inventors," such as Burbank, were part of the emerging scientific and commercial context in which actors approached Congress. The legislative process existed, obviously, as a tool which could be used.

Particular actors commercialize, innovate, make policy, legislate. They do so in creative, not predetermined ways, as I have often stressed. As circumstances change, their perceptions of those circumstances can also change and lead to new goals and strategies. As they act, their actions enter a social world and unintended consequences occur. There are feedback mechanisms from processes and actions to actors. Learning can then take place and actors can change. Furthermore, new situations may encourage new actors to participate.

To pass a patent law, however, actors must deal with a legal structure. Legal structures do not themselves pass laws. Law is not developed through the magical extension of revealed logic or through the codification of social consensus. The legal structure has certain rules and resources with which actors must contend. In 1930, actors literally had to write a new law designed for their purposes. This new law was considered necessary in part because existing patent laws were not regarded as applying to plants. Court processes and new legal interpretations would not suffice.

As we look at other efforts to gain control over biological materials, we find that the sequence of events and the pattern involved is different. Again, different contexts, actors, problems, and goals help produce different patterns even though the end result may be another law or mechanism for extending control over biological materials. In chapter 5, I discussed

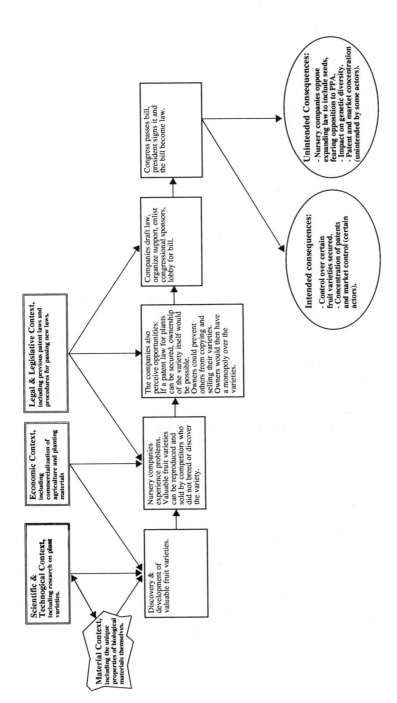

**Figure 3.** Background and Passage of Plant Patent Act of 1930 (PPA)

how actors endeavored to broaden the scope of existing law to include genetically engineered organisms. A simple pathway for this process might look like figure 4.

Here the "use" of technology *precedes* commercialization. In 1930, it largely *follows* commercialization.

While it is important to note that the pattern or pathway is different, it is also important to observe certain similarities in the two stories. The similarities are of the type that allow us to use a common framework — complex social processes — in attempting to explain and better understand the patterning of events. As in the earlier chapters, one must examine the actors, processes and structures within their given context. While these elements are the same, the specifics we find are quite different. Technological developments have altered actors' capabilities of manipulating biological material tremendously. New actors realizing this seek new, more favorable arenas which the legal structure allows to pursue their interests.[4] In doing so, they bypass the need for the cumbersome and sometimes unpredictable political and legislative efforts characteristic of previous attempts to expand ownership and control. No commercial products yet exist. In a sense, commercialization awaits the legal changes which will in turn facilitate the venture financing needed to develop products and bring them to the market.

Figure 5 presents a pattern in which actors define problems in certain ways so as to facilitate addressing those problems in particular arenas. Intellectual property rights issues concerning biological materials came to be discussed at GATT because corporations were successful in framing the problem as a trade problem and in lobbying the U.S. government to pursue the issue within the framework of trade negotiations. Meanwhile, various NGO advocacy groups combined with several Third World governments saw the problem in a different way, not surprisingly. They saw it as a "justice" issue, a "North-South" issue involving unequal transfers of resources. Framed politically, it became possible to fashion proposals to deal with this problem in a forum in which sympathetic Third World governments have considerably more power than they do at GATT.

Dietz, Stern and Rycroft assert that:

> conflicts that are defined as "economic" are those in which the use of material resources is considered more legitimate than the use of other resources, conflicts that are defined as "political" are those in which public support is considered the most legitimate of resources, and conflicts that are defined as "scientific" or "technical" are those in which expertise is considered the most legitimate of resources. Thus the choice to consider a social problem as essentially or primarily economic, political, or scientific has

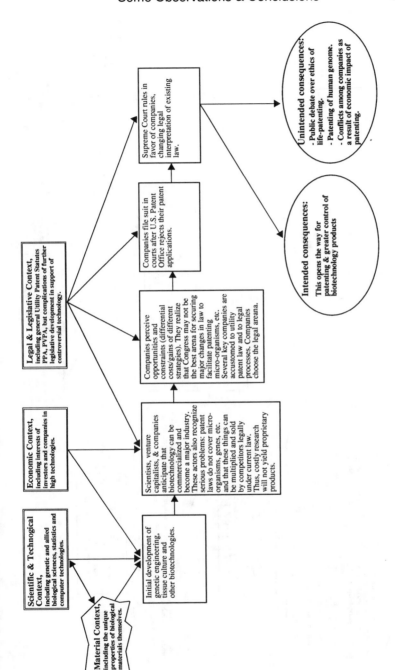

**Figure 4.** Background and Pursuit of Special Interpretations of Patent Laws in Courts

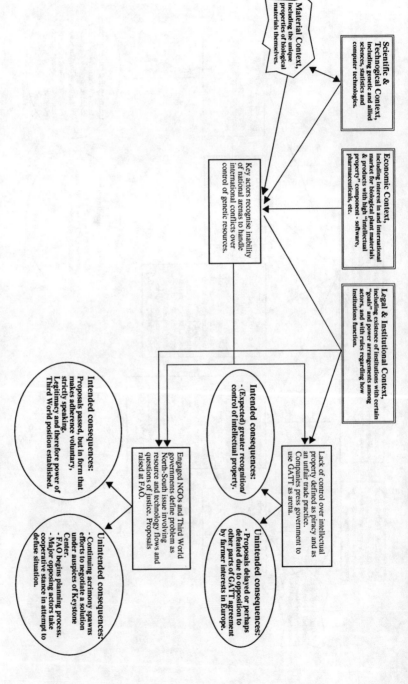

**Figure 5.** Background and Shifts to International Arenas

implications for the use of resources in the attendant conflicts . . . The social definition of an issue influences not only the relative value of resources . . . but also the kinds of argument that are considered appropriate and relevant.[5]

Struggles over policy therefore include not just the dynamics of action within a certain arena. They include how the problem is defined and how it comes to be dealt with in that arena as opposed to another. Actors tend to define problems in terms such that they can legitimately and more easily mobilize resources and exercise influence. They seek to have those problems dealt with in arenas which will be advantageous to their interests.[6]

In each case studied here, there are context-dependent patterns. These patterns have certain basic, abstract characteristics in common. But each case is unique and cannot be appropriately forced into a rigid mold. In each, the basic characteristics of the complex social processes must be examined, the connections and relationships between them uncovered. There is no equilbrium. We can see that law (or policy) proceeds as a history not of ideas, but of relationships.[7] What can we say about these relationships? The causal conditions are unstable[8] and it is difficult to know where the chain of causality begins. As Weber put it, the causal lines "run, at one time, from technical to economic and political matters, at another from political to religious and economic ones, etc. There is no resting point."[9] Still, within a general framework we can begin to make some sense of the empirical material. We can discern a number of patterns, but the number is not infinite.

Creative, effective actors occupy a central position in this study. But I have also spent much time identifying constraints to their actions. Has the context of action been adequately described? Has the emphasis been properly placed? Have the major processes been identified and the relationships between them elucidated? These are not matters that can be easily tested. In the end we are left with simple questions: Do we understand the subject more clearly now? Can this understanding be used to inform our research and our action further?

## PROPERTY RIGHTS AND BIOLOGICAL MATERIAL

There are many different rules relating people to resources. There can be collective ownership, situations in which no one owns, and other situations in which ownership is established with varying degrees of exactness and formality. Some rules can be applied better than others depending on the biological characteristics of the material owned or on other economic or political factors. The obvious subject matter of intellectual property rights laws is the inventive process and protection of the inventor.[10] In this study,

I have found that inventive processes can differ in important ways. In certain Third World areas, plant development appears to be a community effort. Frequently, seed selection is not made by individuals, but by groups after extensive discussion and observation. In such a context, it becomes difficult to identify an individual as the inventor. In contrast, inventors in industrialized countries often *appear* to be individuals, though their work certainly builds on that of others. Structures and hierarchies often exist which concentrate decision-making authority and responsibility in the hands of an individual plant breeder. And laws exist which officially recognize the individual or a legal person as the inventor.

Actors utilize and are affected by changes in technology and commercialization. The capabilities of plant breeders and commercial enterprises changed as the mysteries of inheritance were replaced by systematic knowledge. This affected how they viewed the biological material they dealt with and what they did with it. The wheat breeder could select characteristics and direct the course of evolution within the constraints of what was contained in the gene pool of wheat, at least until the 1980s. With genetic engineering techniques, inventors could begin to *design* new "made-to-order" plants, transferring genes from one species to another. This implied a different level of planning and expertise, with new possibilities of directing the course of evolution.

I have noted several times in this study that plants are not like light bulbs. The nature of the product reveals something about the inventive process as well as about the applicability and efficacy of property rights associated with that product. Most obviously, seeds reproduce themselves, light bulbs do not. In a sense, when breeders of new plant varieties sell seeds (the product), they also sell the "manufacturing" capability for producing more of the product. Furthermore, the raw materials used by the plant breeder are unlike those of the light bulb inventor. Tungsten is simply mined and processed before being used in the light bulb. The plant breeder, however, uses biological materials, often in the form of domesticated plants with valuable characteristics already discovered and developed by others. The light bulb inventor who incorporates a device invented by someone else into a new bulb in order to add a feature is, of course, beholden in some way to the other inventor. This is the normal conception of patent rights. In plant breeding this has not usually been the case, at least before 1980. Plant breeders were not obligated to recognize those who provided valuable genetic components which went into the new variety. These could be taken as "free resources." Finally we note that in plant breeding the distinction between discovery and invention can be blurry. Has the plant breeder who finds a mutation in the field (perhaps a flower with a new color), discovered a new plant or invented one? Is the new plant patentable or is it simply a product of nature? What, then, is the nature of the inventive process associated with living things?

There are different kinds of property, different kinds of property rights, and different kinds and degrees of control associated with those rights. When studying property rights, it is important to consider the nature of the property itself, as this affects those rights and their exercise. Some of the peculiarities of ownership and property rights over biological materials have already been alluded to above. Perhaps the first question to ask is: What, exactly, is it that is owned?

One can own both a light bulb and an apple tree. One form of ownership gives one the right to use each object and the right to exclude others from using the particular object. Typically these objects we own are also under our physical control. The plants are in our yard, the light bulb in our house. As noted above, these objects have different characteristics. The apple tree is making apples. The light bulb is only making light, not light bulbs. The usual right of ownership does not typically extend to controlling others' use of the fruits of the plants. Owning an apple tree does not mean we can presume to control how others use the fruit once possession is transferred. Our ownership of the tree certainly does not give us the right to determine how all apples of that variety will be used or whether they can be multiplied or sold as trees. We own an apple tree, not all apple trees of this particular variety. This simple example illustrates in a very basic way the notion of both personal ownership and common heritage. The norm of common heritage indicates that access to genetic resources should be unrestricted and that its use as a resource base of heritable characteristics is a right held by all.

The actor engaged in plant development and commercialization may well be interested in extending the simple property rights described earlier. The goal may be to extend control through an expansion of the scope of property rights to include use, for example. The type of control desired by the actor is context dependent, affected particularly by the capabilities of current technology and the commercial situation the actor faces.

In this study a number of commercial interests have wanted to obtain intellectual property rights for biological materials. To be effective these rights would have to prohibit the buyer of patented seed from multiplying the seed (which it does naturally) and then selling the seed *as seed*.[11] With wheat, for example, the product and the means of production are essentially the same. The control actually desired is far-reaching both in time and space, because the plant variety retains its ability to reproduce generation after generation and can be widely disseminated. In fact, it can be grown and its seed saved and replanted year after year. Minor genetic alterations will probably occur over the years. Is it still the same patented variety? Can it be legally sold as seed 15 years later? What is it that is owned?

In the 1930 and 1970 examples here, ownership is situated in the plant *variety*. One owns not the plant, not the genes, not the characteristics of the plant, but the unique *combination* of genes that constitutes the plant variety. (This is linked to but not quite the same as owning the unique combination of important characteristics.) Again the nature of biological material — particularly in the context of rapidly developing technologies — presents unique problems of control. Plants contain tens of thousands of genes. If a company owns a particular combination, can another actor make a minor alteration (one gene out of 100,000) and claim ownership of a "new" variety? If so, has the "original" owner not lost a measure of control even though we now technically have two distinct varieties? Is the company's real goal to control only that precise combination of genes or all varieties with those basic or unique (or market-valuable) characteristics? Assuming it is the latter, how is the "thing" that is owned now defined? In fact, is it *a* thing, *many* things, or a *concept*? How does this actor (a plant breeder or company, for example) define or justify the rights it desired as opposed to the rights that would be denied a Third World farming community for "their" varieties, genes, characteristics? This of course is a practical issue, but it brings us back to the question of how to define the object of protection and the nature of that protection when we deal with organisms which live, evolve and reproduce.[12]

This question becomes even more complicated in the 1980s with the rapid development of biotechnologies. The technology is being employed and literally thousands of patent applications are filed before a single product is on the market. Stock prices rise and fall dramatically on news of patent applications, or patent challenges. Venture capital flows into companies based on their patent position. Patent rights are bought and sold. Mergers are based on the strength of a firm's patent position in a certain market. At least one company is even formed which conducts no research but simply files patents and sues others for infringement. It would appear that in this legal and commercial context including powerful changes in technology, patents have themselves become a product, a commodity. This alters relationships, placing more importance on patents and the conditions for their production.

One further observation can be made pointing to difficulties some plant breeding enterprises may face in the future. In major crops, plant breeding goals among different corporations are generally similar in a given market. The various qualities desired by farmers and processors in the major commercial markets for wheat and corn, for example, are well known by breeders. Likewise, the genetic materials used by commercial breeders are impressively similar, almost identical.[13] To control their new varieties, company representatives talk of the need for protections against "derivative breeding," the use of protected varieties to produce new varieties that are almost the same. (I discussed above the dilemma regarding how similar two varieties must be before they are "too similar," and how similar they must be before they are considered the same.) Consider now an added twist to the problem: if both the breeding objectives and the genetic material are similar, plant breeders will almost inevitably produce varieties more and more similar as they fine-tune the same genetic material to the same goals. Thus, not even the seemingly easy question of what constitutes a different variety will have a clear answer. The degree of difference between two varieties (as a basis for intellectual property rights protection) may be a constantly moving *concept*, as opposed to a matter of precise genetic differences. As varieties become more and more similar in the future, smaller differences between them may have to become sufficient for legally distinguishing one variety from another. This would be due largely to the constraints imposed by the biological materials themselves[14] in this commercial and legal context. The problem with determining whether one variety is "essentially derived" from another becomes more and more acute as so many varieties become essentially "identical." Whether and how the law is changed will depend on how technology and commercial circumstances continue to change, on private sector actors' perceptions of their problems and alternatives, and on their ability to make legal changes within the context of the contemporary legal and political structures, as well as how scientific knowledge can be applied to clarify this concept. Revisions to the UPOV Convention reflect the problem of securing effective property rights to the moving targets of biological materials. But property rights problems can never be settled "once and for all." As we have seen throughout this study, they are not based on "timeless" norms which can be codified and left alone.

As indicated, there are different types of property and different types of control. An example was given in which someone might own a plant but not control the variety — or at least only exercise limited control. The perceived need to change rules regarding ownership is frequently tied to the more fundamental goal of the ability to control, which itself is related to changes in the economic, political and technological context. As an example, one can cite the distinction some seed industry representatives are now making between farmers' rights and farmers' privilege to harvest the seed of protected varieties and then replant it themselves. In this case, no changes or improvements in the inventive process are given as a rationale for an expansion of the property rights of plant breeders. There is however, a clear agenda of gaining more control and of forcing farmers to repurchase seed supplies in the marketplace. Such proposals to alter property rights are attempts to address problems and redefine social relationships.

With biological materials, control need not be connected solely to laws. In 1930, the segment of the seed industry that most used the technology and enjoyed the most control over its product was the one that had no legal protection whatsoever — the hybrid corn seed business. Hybrid seed is the product of the union of two inbred lines.[15] If farmers plant hybrid corn and harvest its seed, that seed is not the same. It is no longer the offspring of the inbred lines, but the offspring of a hybrid mother and a hybrid father. Farmers who plant this seed the following year risk an uncertain and potentially disastrous harvest, as the genetic qualities of their seed are no longer fixed. In the 1930s, hybrid corn companies had something that companies not dealing with hybrids still do not have — they had the ability to prevent other companies from copying and selling their varieties *and* they enjoyed a situation where farmers could not reuse their seeds. In other words, their control extended to the farm level, forcing farmers to return to the "inventor" yearly for more seed. Significantly, this control came through the biological properties of the seed and the technical properties of the hybridization process, not through legislation. This situation — the implications of which were well understood by early hybrid breeders[16] — eliminated a major incentive for seeking legal forms of protection.

What control actually means and the degree to which it is effective is also related to actors' ability to use (develop, exploit) the material in question. England's ability to develop and exploit rubber was radically different from that of the Indians of Brazil. The Brazilians may have owned their rubber trees, but they hardly controlled rubber. England controlled rubber because it had the ability to organize its collection, testing, propagation, dissemination, production, and sale in the international marketplace, while successfully discouraging serious competition for some time. With modern plant breeding, firms gain the ability to fashion new plant varieties of economic importance. Farmers or Third World governments may own the same plant materials or have all the genes necessary for creating a new, improved plant variety in their hands. But without the ability to fashion the new variety, their control over their biological material is limited; and without the ability to market new varieties, the usefulness of that control is circumscribed. The farmer's field with its unique genetic materials may simply become a "genetic Xerox machine" in the words of one biotech industry executive.[17] Those who do have control do not actually have to own the plant species they now use as raw material. They simply need access to the properties of the plants (through the genetic materials). Ownership specifies certain relationships. But it does not strictly determine how or whether those relationships can be used to increase power, make gains, or further goals. In other words, ownership can be a sterile and virually powerless attribute without the ability to exploit it. Such is the case of the Third World farmer and the risk of the Third World nation.

There are different forms of ownership (and ownership of different things or qualities) associated with biological materials. Depending on exactly what is owned, the question arises of how it is owned and *who* owns it. This question uncovers conflicts between different norms. Domesticated crops have such a long history as the results of manipulation by many generations of farmers that they are considered by some to be the "common heritage" of humanity. With the onset of agricultural commercialization and modern plant breeding, varieties which once may have had value only as food and/or seeds to the farmer-owners now can be seen as raw materials for research and development by the plant breeder or seed company. Yet, typically, raw materials are privately owned by specific actors. If, however, the materials are "common heritage," they are owned by everyone and no one. Very different *relationships* are implied between "owners" and "users" in these two cases, and these relationships are not neutral. They serve different interests. Collectors and developers of genetic resources utilize the concept of common heritage to justify free access to valuable resources physically possessed by others. On the other hand, farmers and governments in the Third World, rich in resources but often lacking the ability to exploit them, are disserved by this same norm, which makes it difficult for them to garner benefits from genetic resources.[18]

For much of this century, the great wealth of genetic diversity in the Third World was viewed as common heritage. In the farmer's field, it might be owned by an individual. Once collected, it technically became the property of the collector. The collector might deposit it in a gene bank, where it would become the property of the gene bank or the country which owned the gene bank. *If* the new owner so chose, it could be *treated* as "common heritage" and made freely available for others. But in the absence of any legal entity to hold it in trust for the world community, ownership over the physical biological material was never so general.[19] Controversies over such distinctions arose at FAO when, for example, the U.S. government endorsed the norm of common heritage while restricting access to its seed collections to particular countries. Was it common heritage in principal, but privately owned in reality?

The situation at FAO highlighted the fact that there can be conflicting property rights concepts. At FAO the question is broader than securing specific property rights. It involves the legitimacy of property rights over biological materials and the extent to which governments have rights (in addition to or over and above other actors) over this material.

During the FAO debates, the implications of common heritage were slowly uncovered. And this norm was seen to conflict with another— national sovereignty. The questions of what is owned and who owns it and who controls it are now joined. An individual may own a tomato plant or apple tree, but the properties of these plants and the right to have access to and use these properties is a matter of either national sovereignty or common heritage. Now the question of "who owns" is at least partially related to *where* the material is. And where the material is, influences *who* will make the determination of its status. Whether control (as opposed to ownership) is exercised is context-dependent in those states claiming national sovereignty. In the gene bank of Ethiopia, it is apparent that the material falls under national sovereignty, because that is the government's policy. Some coffee material which the government regards as important and potentially valuable is not exchanged. But the Ethiopian government can and does send other materials upon request. In the gene bank of a U.S. corporation, the material may be considered privately owned and not owned or controlled by the state. Each situation implies a different set of rules for prospective users of this material than if it were considered common heritage — that is, owned by all, or not owned by anyone. The United States considers its collections as common heritage except in certain circumstances when it reserves the right to exclude others from access. Thus, the United States exercises some form of unilateral control over what it acknowledges to be common heritage.[20] Can we continue to view the material as common heritage if certain interests have the right to set rules excluding others from access to this common property? Or does national sovereignty supersede common heritage? Does the U.S. position really differ from that of Ethiopia?

Biological materials, because of their peculiar characteristics, their history, their uses and various values, are quite distinct. Ownership and control of such materials are complicated by these factors. Struggles over ownership and control are therefore flavored by the unique nature of the material itself. Considered in its full social and biological context, the process of rule-making for biological materials is full of tensions and characteristically in flux.

Given the high degree of uncertainty (and the rapid *rate* of change)

**Table 11.** Mechanisms for Controlling Biological Materials[21]

| FORMS AND MECHANISMS OF CONTROL | ITEM TO BE CONTROLLED | | | | |
|---|---|---|---|---|---|
| | Species | Variety | Gene | Characteristic | "Farmer" Landrace |
| PHYSICAL AND BIOLOGICAL (control conditions) | 1. Isolated production | 1. Use of hybrids and non-access to inbred lines | 1. Non-access ("natural")<br>2. Non-use ("natural") | 1. Ignorance of charac-teristic | 1. Restricted access (either on site or in a collection) |
| LEGAL RULES | 1. Laws against removal of plants | 1. Plant Patent Act (1930)<br>2. Plant Variety Protection Act (1970), extended in 1980.<br>3. Utility patents (as interpreted after 1980).<br>4. Contracts<br>5. Federal Seed Act. | 1. Patents<br>2. Contracts (agreements with legal force) | 1. Patents<br>2. Contracts | 1. Contracts |
| CUSTOMS AND NON-LEGAL RULES | 1. Social division of labor | 1. Informal pacts within industry— social pressure<br>2. Marketing practices— being first to market, etc. | 1. To some extent, items listed under variety may apply. | 1. Limiting information about source | 1. FAO Undertaking (quasi-legal: not binding) |
| HUMANLY CONSTRUCTED BARRIERS | 1. Military or police control or action.<br>2. Isolation of production. | 1. Physical barriers such as fences. | 1. Corporate or scientific secrecy. | | |

surrounding new technologies and their introduction, seed and bio-technology companies as well as governments may be unsure of what their interests are. They may be ignorant of the newest technologies or ignorant of the effects these will have. This can lead to some confusion and to their pursuing goals for divergent reasons.

A number of questions have been raised in this conclusion about the nature of ownership and control over biological materials. Exactly what can be owned? Who owns and/or controls it? How? Some of these questions have been "answered" in recent years as actors have attempted to solve problems by developing new laws and fashioning new relationships, for instance. But such questions rarely get answered definitively or permanently, especially considering the complexity of problems of ownership and control of biological materials in inherently unstable and changing social contexts. Indeed there can be no predetermined or lasting solutions to such conflicts — no natural force to direct the course of events. People create new solutions for new conditions and cause new problems. People will continue to do this in defiance of our desires that history stop at least long enough for us to study it, write about it and enjoy momentary triumphs.

## NOTES

1. Giddens, Anthony, *The Constitution of Society*. Berkeley: University of California Press, 1984: p. 16ff.
2. Kloppenburg, Jack R., *First the Seed: The Political Economy of Plant Biotechnology, 1492–2000*. Cambridge: Cambridge University Press. 1988. For example, Kloppenburg speaks of hybridization furnishing "capital" with a means for circumventing the barrier which seed naturally presents to its commodification (p. 130). And he speaks of "capital's efforts to provide global conditions for its own expansion" (p. 170). Reflected in such terminology, inadvertently used by Kloppenburg perhaps, is a presumptive grant of agency to a disembodied concept. One might infer that it is capital itself (in contrast to actors) that has needs and capabilities. When employed, I suspect this linguistic and theoretical device insidiously distracts both writer and reader from more thoroughly examining and specifying real actors and their creative actions in particular situations within a conditioning and influential yet nondeterministic context. Such may account for the brief treatment afforded the actual battles and combatants in some of the struggles which lie at the heart of Kloppenburg's story. Without this, a long-standing social science debate concerning the connection between context and actor/action — a connection which, if made, would highlight questions of agency and determinism — is not joined.
3. These figures are tentative and are meant to assist the reader and encourage further discussion and elaboration. The figures allow one to see, at once, certain basic relationships, conditioning influences, major sequential events, etc. To serve our purpose, figures must be simplified. One should understand that not all relationships can or should be represented, nor can the complexity of relationships or events be completely captured. For example, intended and unintended consequences of human activity feed back into and affect contexts, as is obvious from the text of the book. And legal and legislative contexts are certainly connected with the economic context. The absence of

Some Observations & Conclusions     235

arrows indicating such links is not meant to imply that they do not exist. The figures should thus be used in conjunction with the text.

4. See Dietz, Thomas, Paul Stern, and Robert Rycroft, "Definitions of Conflict and the Legitimation of Resources: The Case of Environmental Risk," *Sociological Forum*, Vol. 4, no. 1, 1989. Though not the main theme of this paper, the authors' work nevertheless shows how problems can be conceptualized and defined in different ways by various actors and how these differences are socially embedded. More specifically, the orientations and goals of actors are related to (but nevertheless cannot be reduced to) their roles, positions, and occupations. Reliance on one universal notion of human behavior to the exclusion of others and as opposed to situating that behavior in a social context and studying it within that context is counterproductive to increasing theoretical specificity.

5. Ibid., p. 62–63.

6. See the Dietz, Stern and Rycroft article cited above, which studied the ways in which professionals from different fields and organizations defined certain environmental problems.

7. Milovanovic, op. cit.,p. 24

8. Giddens, op. cit., p. xxxii.

9. Weber, quoted in Milovanovic, op. cit., p. 16.

10. It is not, however, the only subject matter or "purpose" behind such laws. The American business magazine *Forbes* goes straight to the point and says that intellectual property "is the nearest thing on God's own earth to a perfect, unencumbered source of perpetual wealth." And they note that Elvis's brain is "alive and well, raking in over $15 million a year because of the value of 'intellectual property.'" Quote is from a letter to prospective subscribers to the magazine signed by the publisher, Malcolm S. Forbes, Jr. Undated (1991?): p. 3.

11. Here the matter of intent becomes important as there is essentially no difference between wheat and wheat seed. Does the seller intend that it be used as seed? Does the buyer intend that it be used as seed? What if a protected variety is purchased from a seed company, raised and harvested. The intention may be to sell the harvest as wheat. But what if the intention of the seller is to sell wheat, but the buyer's intention is to buy wheat seed? Does the corporate variety owner have recourse against the farmer buying the seed from someone else given that there was no direct transaction between the variety owner and that farmer? These are relationships which must be established somehow.

12. To a certain extent, genetic resources may be considered as pieces of information and genes as "instructions" for a plant to do something. As information, the resource is something more than just a renewable or nonrenewable resource, as I am indebted to Tom Dietz for pointing out (personal communication, November 23, 1992). As techniques of genetic manipulation become more and more sophisticated, a higher premium will be placed on what is done, on which pieces of information are moved into which species with what effect, than perhaps on the mechanisms of the transfer. Already, pharmaceutical companies have realized as well that missions to collect potential medicinal plants should attempt to ascertain what the local people know about the plant and its properties. The companies collect not just plants, but knowledge about the plants. In this situation, as pointed out earlier, it is the ability to use and develop the material, becomes important. This ability, of course, is affected by a number of factors, including property rights, technology.

13. National Academy of Sciences, *Genetic Vulnerability of Major Crops*, 1972. And personal discussion with Barry Greengrass, secretary general of UPOV, in Rome, 1991.

14. In particular, the degree of useful diversity available.

15. These inbred lines may themselves be the product of other inbred lines. See chapter 2.

16. See statements of Jones, chapter 2.

17. Carlson, Peter (vice president, Crop Genetics International), letter to Vic Althouse,

Member of Parliament (Canada), August 22, 1985, p. 3.
18. There is usually no market value, as the resource is considered a free good.
19. The FAO did, in fact, establish an "international network of gene banks" consisting of facilities already in existence, which agreed to store materials "under the auspices of the FAO," guided by the FAO undertaking. However, FAO has no ability to enforce any rules it might set regarding this material. Major collections exist outside the network. And it is clear that while FAO may technically constitute a mechanism through which materials could be placed in trust, it is not thought of or utilized in this way by many gene bank directors.
20. Legislation supporting the "common heritage" perspective was passed in 1990 (P.L. 101–624). In the past, embargoes and other restrictions have not targetted germplasm according to Henry Shands of the USDA. Germplasm has, however, been caught up in more general trade embargoes. In other words, in such times it is not automatically treated differently, i.e., as common heritage. The Department of Treasury has agreed *to consider* excluding germplasm in future embargoes, though the USDA will have to intervene at the writing of the embargo language. Thus, while the intention of many at USDA — most notably Shands himself — is to uphold the principle of common heritage, its status is not fully guaranteed, but is dependent on preventive action from USDA and a special exemption from the Department of Treasury. Efforts by Shands and others to obtain a more automatic exemption as a matter of standing policy have apparently not been fully successful.
21. This table is provided as a tentative formulation and as a basis for future research. It is not a process model and it does not imply or indicate a linear history. Some companies (Agrigenetics, for example) are considering a return to contracts with seed buyers to enforce varietal rights, a practice which predates the 1930 Plant Patent Act. At least one — Midwest Oilseeds — has instituted the practice.

# Loss of Genetic Diversity:
# The U.S. and the Third World

This appendix looks briefly at the loss of genetic diversity in the United States and then proceeds to touch on the commercialization of agriculture and subsequent "genetic erosion" which took place (and is still ongoing) in the Third World. Loss of genetic diversity has been a major side effect of the processes examined in chapter 2. Effects of this loss can be seen in certain political situations which arise and are discussed in chapter 6, for example.

Advances in plant breeding began to enable scientists after 1900 to direct the course of evolution in agricultural crops. In the *Yearbook of Agriculture* in 1936, Hambidge and Bressman noted:

> Now the breeder tends rather to formulate an ideal in his mind and actually create something that meets it as nearly as possible by combining the genes from two or more organisms . . . In this connection, he has a new confidence . . . he has a vision of creating organisms different from any now in existence, and perhaps with some remarkably valuable characters.[1]

The new techniques of plant breeding were factors in facilitating a change in the character of the breeding materials themselves. In a world where mass selection is the dominant technique and farmers are the breeders, nonproprietary varieties are where value is located. But if genes can be reliably and predictably transferred from one variety to another (through backcrossing, for example), then value shifts. It exists not only at the level of the variety, but also at the level of the gene, the characteristic.

Due to the Ice Age and other factors, genetic diversity in agricultural crops was mostly located in the fields of farmers in the Third World, though U.S. farmers used and developed an impressive amount of diversity brought in by immigrants and collecting efforts. This diversity contained the sum of all characteristics in the species. The possibility of using this diversity in a directed way transformed this diversity into a potential resource, a raw material. This occurred historically at the same time as the diversity itself became threatened. Ironically, but usually with justification, plant breeders (as well as many farmers) felt that their modern bred varieties were better than the old varieties they were replacing. Little concern, aside from Harlan and Martini's in the 1930s, was evident over the permanent loss of these old varieties and the diversity they contained.[2] At the beginning of the process of genetic erosion in this century, there was still so much diversity available for plant breeders that no constraints were felt, evidently.

Almost no solid data exists regarding the loss of genetic diversity over any substantial length of time. Little effort was made in the nineteenth century to catalog existing diversity within agricultural species. Without an inventory of what once existed, no accurate percentages can be provided of how much was lost. The lack of data is particularly acute for the Third World, where the greatest amount of diversity was located.

Virtually the only — and therefore the best — data comes from the United States, where the U.S. Department of Agriculture inventoried *varieties* being sold commercially in the nineteenth and early twentieth centuries.[3] Table 12 was constructed by comparing these USDA inventories with varieties now held in the National Seed Storage Laboratory (NSSL) in Fort Collins, Colorado. Varieties that appeared in the early USDA inventories but cannot be found today in U.S. collections are described as "lost" and "presumed extinct."[4] Table 12 thus indicates (quite conservatively) the extent of "farmer-bred" *varieties* which once existed in the United States as well as the extent of *their* disappearance through the processes of commercial agriculture and the introduction of new varieties as described in chapters 2, 3 and 4.

Different sources are used to estimate the loss of fruit varieties. Of 7098 varieties in use between 1804 and 1904, approximately 86 percent have been lost. Similarly, 87 percent of the 2683 pear varieties have been lost.[5] However, the sheer numbers of varieties in use is impressive. Even a cursory examination of the lists reveals the involvement of American families in the process of breeding and selecting these fruits. The overwhelming majority carry family names. In other words, the "breeders" gave the fruit the greatest honor they could — their names.

For various reasons, the above numbers are actually conservative. There were surely more varieties in use and countless types developed and selected by farmers for which no name was given and which the USDA had no way of counting in its surveys. Still, what the data shows is a dramatic separation of seed from farmer. Furthermore, it indicates how firmly the door was shut to any continued participation of farmers in breeding or selecting their own seed. The farm-level diversity of varieties which gave birth to American agriculture was essentially wiped out. It should be pointed out that for Native Americans this separation came much earlier. As they and their 200 native languages were killed, their

Table 12. U.S. Vegetable Varieties Lost (presumed extinct), 1903–83

| Vegetable | Total Number 1903 Varieties | 1903 Varieties in NSSL Collection | Varieties Lost (%) |
|---|---|---|---|
| Artichoke | 34 | 2 | 94.1 |
| Asparagus | 46 | 1 | 97.8 |
| Bean (Runner) | 14 | 1 | 92.9 |
| Bean (Lima) | 96 | 8 | 91.7 |
| Bean (Garden) | 578 | 32 | 94.5 |
| Beets | 288 | 17 | 94.1 |
| Mangel beet | 178 | 3 | 98.3 |
| Broccoli | 34 | 0 | 100.0 |
| Brussels sprouts | 35 | 4 | 88.6 |
| Burnet | 1 | 0 | 100.0 |
| Cabbage | 544 | 28 | 94.9 |
| Cardoon | 6 | 1 | 83.3 |
| Carrot | 287 | 21 | 92.7 |
| Cauliflower | 158 | 9 | 94.3 |
| Celeriac | 25 | 3 | 88.0 |
| Celery | 164 | 3 | 98.2 |
| Chervil | 8 | 0 | 100.0 |
| Chicory | 17 | 3 | 82.4 |
| Chives | 1 | 1 | 0.0 |
| Chufas | 2 | 0 | 100.0 |
| Collards | 25 | 5 | 82.1 |
| Corn (field) | 434 | 40 | 90.8 |
| Corn (popcorn) | 48 | 0 | 100.0 |
| Corn (sweet) | 307 | 12 | 96.1 |
| Corn salad | 21 | 1 | 95.2 |
| Cress | 39 | 2 | 94.9 |
| Cucumber | 285 | 16 | 94.4 |
| Cucumber (pickling) | 10 | 2 | 80.0 |
| Dandelion | 25 | 0 | 100.0 |
| Eggplant | 97 | 9 | 90.7 |
| Endive | 64 | 4 | 93.7 |
| Horseradish | 1 | 0 | 100.0 |

**Table 12.** (*continue*)

| | | | |
|---|---|---|---|
| Kale | 124 | 9 | 92.7 |
| Kohlrabi | 55 | 3 | 94.5 |
| Leek | 39 | 5 | 87.2 |
| Lettuce | 497 | 36 | 92.8 |
| Martynia | 4 | 0 | 100.0 |
| Muskmelon | 338 | 27 | 92.0 |
| Mustard | 44 | 5 | 88.6 |
| Okra | 38 | 4 | 89.5 |
| Onion | 357 | 21 | 94.1 |
| Orach | 5 | 1 | 80.0 |
| Parsley | 82 | 12 | 85.4 |
| Parsnip | 75 | 5 | 93.3 |
| Pea | 408 | 25 | 93.9 |
| Peanut | 31 | 2 | 93.5 |
| Peppers | 126 | 13 | 89.7 |
| Radish | 463 | 27 | 94.2 |
| Rampion | 1 | 0 | 100.0 |
| Rhubarb | 35 | 1 | 97.1 |
| Roquette | 1 | 0 | 100.0 |
| Rutabaga | 168 | 5 | 97.0 |
| Salsify | 29 | 2 | 93.1 |
| Scolymus | 1 | 0 | 100.0 |
| Skirret | 1 | 0 | 100.0 |
| Sorrel | 10 | 0 | 100.0 |
| Spinach | 109 | 7 | 93.6 |
| Spinach (New Zealand or Malabar) | 1 | 1 | 0.0 |
| Squash | 341 | 40 | 88.3 |
| Sunflower | 14 | 1 | 92.9 |
| Swiss chard | 23 | 1 | 95.7 |
| Tomato | 408 | 79 | 80.6 |
| Tomato (husk) | 17 | 2 | 88.2 |
| Turnip | 237 | 24 | 89.9 |
| Watercress | 2 | 2 | 0.0 |
| Watermelon & Citron | 223 | 20 | 91.0 |

seeds were also lost. A number of crops which Native Americans domesticated from indigenous plant material were driven into extinction and in other cases crops reverted back to their wild state.

The replacement of farmer-bred with professionally bred or commercially supplied varieties was already well advanced in the United States when some of the same actors involved in the upsurge in American agricultural research turned their attention to the Third World. Beginning with the establishment of the International Maize and Wheat Improvement Center in Mexico, the Rockefeller and Ford foundations together with assistance from the U.S. government and later the World Bank helped establish a network of crop breeding centers to bring the Green Revolution to the Third World.

The analysis of the Third World problem was strikingly similar to that which had been developed for the United States. William Myers, dean of the School of Agriculture at Cornell University and a Rockefeller Foundation trustee, returned from a trip to Mexico with John D. Rockefeller III in 1951, and observed that the Mexican economy was "handicapped by hundreds of thousands of uneconomic farm units . . ." In a letter to the president of the Rockefeller Foundation later that year, Myers reported that "these small farms cannot make use of improved agronomic practices because they have no surplus above family needs to sell to finance such improvements."[6]

From 1959 to 1971, research centers were established in Mexico, the Philippines, Colombia, Nigeria, Peru, India, Syria, and Liberia. Cornell received major grants from the Rockefeller Foundation to train Third World scientists and agricultural extension workers and a contract with the U.S. Mutual Security Agency to establish an agricultural university in the Philippines.[7]

For present purposes it is not necessary to go into detail, even though the establishment of the international agricultural research centers (IARCs) is crucial to any treatment of genetic resources. Suffice it to say that within a short period research institutions had been established, scientists hired, and local scientists and extension workers trained. In other words, the infrastructure was in place for a transformation of Third World agriculture.

The plant varieties produced by the IARCs are now famous, as much for their negative ecological and social effects as for their positive attributes. The new varieties, termed by some "high-yielding" and by others "high response" because of their use of fertilizers and water,[8] spread over Latin America and Asia with astonishing speed. In the process ancient centers of crop genetic diversity nearly disappeared. Through a variety of mechanisms, which even included force in some cases and often included withholding of credit, farmers were "encouraged" to adopt the new varieties.

In a twinkling of the evolutionary eye, the effects of thousands of years of crop evolution were wiped out.[9] As in the United States, loss of traditional farmer varieties meant that farmers were left without the very varieties best adapted to their ecology, culture, and economy. The economy, however, was being changed. As in the United States, uneconomical farming units were being eliminated, people were being brought into the market economy, and seed was becoming a commodity. The new varieties were often more appropriate in these commercial agriculture environments.

The genetic erosion caused by the green revolution was impossible to ignore. Over 100 million acres of new, uniform rices and wheats were soon being grown where tens of thousands of farmer varieties had once been found.[10] The modern varieties were replacing the resource upon which they were based and upon which their continued existence depended.

Sensing the danger, the U.S. Department of Agriculture established the National Seed Storage Laboratory (NSSL) in Fort Collins, Colorado, in 1958. Together with a system of plant introduction stations, NSSL sought to collect and store genetic diversity for future use in plant breeding. In fact, NSSL operated much the way botanical gardens had in previous centuries. Plant diversity was collected in the Third World, brought to the United States, stored in the gene bank, and then made available for commercial use to American corporations and public sector breeders. Sheer possession of and access to such diversity was of incalculable benefit to the seed industry as it built its own breeding programs. Here it is important to point out that access to diversity alone would not have been so important were it not for the industry's capacity to use that diversity. Thus the diversity was a key component (though nevertheless only one component) of a developed commercial system which could use this material profitably. That system included knowledge and techniques of scientific plant breeding as well as the organization infrastructure, including a marketing system and a clientele.

That the "Columbian Exchange" was at work again becomes even more evident when the IARCs are considered. The IARCs were not simply breeding and distributing new seed varieties. They were also amassing substantial collections of genetic diversity as their new varieties were replacing even more. More importantly, they were introducing commercialized agriculture. The new seeds, which "required" fertilizers, pesticides, and irrigation systems in order to reach their potential, created debt for the farmer which had to be repaid with money.[11] The increased production promised by the green revolution had to go to the marketplace where it could be sold. The farmer who accepted the new seeds was really being introduced to the market system.

The commercialization and subsequent mechanization of a sector of Third World agriculture created a huge new market for foreign agricultural input and machinery companies. The International Rice Research Institute estimated that the cash costs of farming using green revolution methods was eleven times higher than with traditional seeds. At one point, Massey-Ferguson farm equipment dealers had a twelve-year backlog of tractor orders in India. And in Asia alone, the Rockefeller Foundation estimated that 75–90 billion pounds of rice production had become dependent on imported petroleum supplies.[12]

During the green revolution, not only was an infrastructure of agricultural colleges and extension services built, but also a market for new seeds was created. This process destroyed much of the old system of seed-saving and farmer-breeding, and helped create a corporate infrastructure for the agricultural input and machinery business. Through this new infrastructure, proprietary, commercial seeds could begin to flow, at least theoretically. And finally, it made the old farmer-bred varieties rarer, and potentially more valuable.

## NOTES

1. Hambidge, Gove, and E. N. Bressman, "Forward and Summary," in *Yearbook of Agriculture, 1936.* Washington: U.S. Department of Agriculture. 1936: p. 130–131.
2. Harlan, H. V., and M. L. Martini, "Problems and Results in Barley Breeding," *Yearbook of Agriculture, 1936.* Washington: U.S. Department of Agriculture. 1936: p. 317.
3. Fowler, Cary, and Pat Mooney, *Shattering: Food, Politics and the Loss of Genetic Diversity.* Tucson: University of Arizona Press. 1990: p. 61ff. See this source for a full explanation of the limitations of this data and the methodology used in assembling table 12. See Fowler and Mooney, footnote 21, page 236, for complete references to the original sources used in constructing the table.
4. It should be understood that varieties are unique combinations of genes. It would theoretically be possible for many unique varieties to be lost without any unique genes being lost —all the genes in the lost varieties could be represented in different combinations in other, existing varieties. Table 12 shows tremendous losses of varieties. It cannot document the loss of genetic diversity. Furthermore, many of the varieties surveyed by the USDA disappeared before or shortly after the rediscovery of Mendel's laws, long before the development of accurate methods for mapping genes. Again, in terms of genetic diversity, we cannot say with precision how much was lost — or not lost — because no one knows for sure what there was to begin with. However, it is safe and reasonable to say that variety losses of over 90 percent — even in the United States — indicate a very real and perhaps substantial loss of genetic diversity. As future needs for diversity cannot be anticipated, the "costs" of these losses cannot be accurately estimat-

ed. See chapter 4 of *Shattering* by Fowler and Mooney for a much fuller treatment of the loss of genetic diversity, its causes and impacts.

5. Fowler and Mooney, op. cit., p. 63, 236.

6. Cleaver, Harry, "The Origins of the Green Revolution," Ph.D. dissertation, Stanford University. 1975: p. 327.

7. Fowler and Mooney, op. cit., p. 56ff.

8. Lester Brown, a prominent Green Revolution proponent, stated: "Most obviously, the new seeds demand an entirely different set of husbandry practices. If farmers are to realize the genetic potential of these seeds, they may need to increase the plant population or to change the time of planting or the depth of seeding; they must irrigate more frequently and with more precision; they must use fertilizer in large quantities and weed carefully lest the fertilizer be converted into weeds instead of grain." Quoted from *Seeds of Change: The Green Revolution and Development in the 1970's* by Lester Brown. New York: Praeger Publishers. 1973: p. 10.

9. There have been many causes of genetic erosion historically. (See chapter 4 of *Shattering* by Fowler and Mooney for a description and analysis of these.) Given the connection between traditional crop varieties and human cultures, one could argue that to some extent genetic erosion has advanced in tandem with the loss of languages and traditional forms of music and art. Indeed, were one to develop an "early warning system" for genetic erosion it might be useful to assume that genetic resources would be under threat in areas where traditional cultures and languages are experiencing pressure.

10. Fowler and Mooney, op. cit., p. 60.

11. Considerable debate still exists over whether the modern varieties were higher yielding in low-input Third World agricultural situations than the traditional varieties they replaced. Some research by Duvick (personal communication, June 26, 1992) indicates that for corn, the modern varieties were often better even under poor growing conditions. However, no one disputes that the new varieties were more responsive to inputs and, under the proper conditions and barring a mis-match of variety and environmental factors, could provide greater yields (albeit at higher costs) than traditional varieties. It is probable that in the beginning, IARC varieties were more "dependent" on these inputs and less inherently higher yielding (if higher yielding at all), because in later years IARCs were able to refine their breeding work and address pest, disease, and drought problems within the context of pursuing higher yields through high responsiveness. Thus, it may be fair to say that initially the modern varieties did, in fact, often "require" added inputs in order consistently or reliably to provide higher yields. (See Lester Brown's comment in footnote above.) For more on the question of the nature of high yielding varieties, see: Lappe', Frances Moore, and Joseph Collins, with Cary Fowler, *Food First: Beyond the Myth of Scarcity*. New York: Ballantine Books. 1977: p. 129ff.

12. Perelman, Michael, *Farming for Profit in a Hungry World*. Montclair, N.J.: Allanheld, Osmun & Co. 1977: p. 147ff.

# Sources of Information and Methodology

## GENERAL COMMENTS

Perhaps more than most topics, a study of mechanisms of control over and intellectual property rights to biological materials seems designed to challenge a scholar's versatility.

One must have a basic understanding of the biological material being controlled or protected — genes, varieties, gene complexes — and how it "works." Thus one must be familiar with the basic processes of evolution, selection, plant breeding and genetic engineering. Without this understanding one cannot hope to follow developments in the seed industry or intellectual property law. Furthermore, one could not possibly understand the changing significance of genetic resources. This "understanding," however, is a moving target and can never be complete in any case. Advances in genetic sciences and technologies are now so rapid that texts become dated at the printers, literally. Yet the influence of science and technology on the business of plant breeding and the formation of property rights is such that one must keep reasonably abreast of developments. While such materials do not figure prominently in the list of footnotes of this book, their influence should be apparent. Similarly, one must have a basic grasp of agriculture itself and of the farming endeavor. How do seeds fit into the practice of agriculture in different societies?

Economic considerations are clearly major motivations of many actors in this study. The impact of changes in science, technology, and law are often measured by the "bottom line." Marketing situations in the seed business change dramatically during the period covered by this study. New and different seeds also have an impact, both on farmers and the industry. Lack of understanding of such economic and structural changes would jeopardize any study.

One might make similar and equally valid claims about the importance of having a background in political science, law, and history, to name only the most obvious disciplines. As challenging as the task of gaining the necessary fluency in each of these fields is, the real difficulty lies in weaving the material and insights from these disciplines into something that enlightens the reader.[1] The subject of this book is admittedly complex, but this should not be used as an excuse either to eschew it altogether or to oversimplify it. Better understanding of the subject can only come from better attempts at integrating the various components of the story.

Due to the nature of task, it has been best to employ a number of different approaches to the research. No one methodology is appropriate for all situations.[2] Ideally, the methodology should fit the problem.

Chapters 1–3 deal with events which took place from roughly the 1600s to 1930. For the most part I have had to depend on secondary sources. As noted below, a considerable amount of data and information from the USDA and the U.S. Patent Office was also available. Where possible I have tried to go back to original sources used in the secondary material. (In such cases the original source is cited. If unavailable, I have normally cited the secondary source and made reference to the source it references.) A number of potential errors have been avoided in the process of searching out original sources, and more than one secondary source publication rendered suspect. When contradictory or confusing data/stories have arisen, it has almost always been a rewarding experience to search further to see if some sense cannot be made of the situation. It is easy to find a quote or a statistic to buttress what one wants to say, but the complexities and nuances of a story often lie entangled and obscured by surface contradictions in information. Data published by the USDA has served to clear up some mysteries and anchor many of the points made by authors of the period or modern-day historians.

Several different research methods were used in chapters 4–6, including interviews and participant-observation. Interviews were appropriate or necessary in cases where published materials were inadequate or nonexistent.

Participant-observation has a number of potential advantages. It can be open-ended, allowing for ongoing revision and updating of the study design.[3] It can enable the researcher to become aware of incongruous or unexplained facts and thus help the researcher avoid some errors.[4] As Schwartz and Jacobs argue, participant-observation can be a powerful method for examining the relationship between words and deeds, attitudes and behaviors.[5] It can be particularly suited to helping the researcher better understand the context of the phenomenon under study and to become aware of subtleties which may otherwise go unnoticed.[6]

Participant-observation also has a number of potential pitfalls as a method. Among them: (1) the researcher's focus on what is happening now may obscure important events which took place in the past; (2) informants may not be representative; (3) the behavior of those under observation may be altered as a result of the presence of the researcher; (4) the researcher may become overly involved and in the process "go native."[7] In addition, the participant-observer cannot be everywhere at once (in time or space) and thus cannot observe everything. And typically, there are parts of the social structure to which the researcher does not have access and cannot penetrate,[8] particularly if the researcher is "trapped" in a single role.

According to George McCall, plausibility is the first traditional test in evaluating data from participant-observation studies.[9] The second check is to see if it is consistent with other accounts and to evaluate constantly the material for internal and external consistency. The researcher's observations and interpretations can also be discussed with key informants from each of the various major factions.[10] Both the "problems" and "solutions" cited above bring into question the reliability of information collected through participant- observation. "The key to data quality control in participant observation," as McCall points out, "is, then, the thorough use of multiple indicants of any particular fact and an insistence on a very high degree of consonance among these indicants, tracking down and accounting for any contrary indicants."[11]

Participant-observers can vary in the degree to which they participate and observe. In my case, I was an active participant, indeed a partisan, in opposition to extension of the Plant Variety Protection Act in 1980. I continued this involvement through events at FAO and as a member of the Keystone Dialogue. Conceptualization of this book occurred after the legislative fight in 1980 was over, virtually all of the events at FAO discussed here had taken place, and the Keystone dialogue was well under way. These are the pieces of the history with which I was involved. Given the specifics of my situation (the fact that my participant-observation took place over a long period but largely prior to and outside the context of developing this book and that I had access to perhaps most key participants), some of the concerns generally voiced about this type of research may not be not applicable. The danger that the researcher might influence the subjects of research is, of course, unavoidable in this case.[12] Other concerns, however, are justifiable.

I have taken a number of precautions to mitigate the potential for bias, which so obviously exists. Although an active participant in events discussed in two chapters, I have not depended on these experiences as the sole source of information for important points. Frequent reference has been made to published materials which are available to other researchers. Since beginning focused research on this book in mid-1990, I have also conducted a number of formal and informal interviews. Participant-observation is thus only one of several methods used to obtain information. In this regard, it was most valuable as suggested above — as a way to understand the context of action more holistically, to uncover subtleties and to confirm or call into question information from other sources.

While most participant-observers play a particular role, I have, in fact, played a number of roles such as advocate, policy advisor, and mediator through several institutions. This has allowed me access to different actors and arenas and allowed me to observe and interact over a rather long period. It has given me the opportunity to talk with key individuals and to discuss my interpretations of events with them. I have discussed the general approach and findings of the book on numerous occasions with people currently involved with genetic resources and intellectual property rights issues.[13] (This has also been valuable in helping me deal with technical aspects of the science.) It has encouraged me to avoid oversimplifying the motivations and actions of certain actors, particularly those associated with the private sector. A substantial amount of contact with individuals from commercial seed companies and with government officials has given me a much clearer picture of how they perceive the context in which they act. I have had these contacts and experiences as a staff member of an "activist" nongovernment organization, as a member of the National Plant Genetic Resources Board (appointed by the U.S. secretary of agriculture), as a university faculty member, and as a long-term consultant to the UN Food and Agriculture Organization.[14] The last position was obtained with the endorsement of NGOs, several Third World governments, the U.S. government, and IBPGR — which I mention as it may indicate a certain evolving of my role and the degree to which I have been able to gain the trust of various actors.[15] In addition, the importance to this study of my participation in the Keystone dialogue (discussed below) should not be overlooked.

The risks of personal bias may have been further reduced by the fact that this study does not attempt to argue the various positions of the corporate or NGO actors, for instance.[16] It is less about the merits of their interests or particular proposals and more about the process of defining and pursuing those interests, and the course of events such as the passage of legislation or the outcome of court cases and particular negotiations.

Several other measures have been taken to protect against some of the shortcomings of the various methods used (though one of the main measures remains the use of multiple methods). Relevant portions of this book were reviewed prior to publication by people from different disciplines: sociology, political science, law, economics, genetics, and plant breeding (public and private sector), including several individuals intimately involved in events described here.

This study benefits from the numerous candid and often rather personal discussions I have had with key individuals "representing" various viewpoints in controversies discussed. Combined with the precautions mentioned above, I believe this type of interaction can produce important and perhaps even more reliable information than certain standard interview techniques, though it does not insure complete reliability. Data, no matter how obtained, are rarely free of all contaminants.[17] Reliability, however, is increased if the findings can be confirmed through additional sources. In this study the large number of interviews (formal and informal) conducted, together with the substantial volume and diverse types of published information used, made cross-checking of individual sources usually feasible and almost routine.

From its earliest stages, research for this book has been done under the guidance of Professor Tom Burns of the Institute of Sociology at Uppsala University in Sweden. Professor Burns has not been a participant in the issues discussed in the book and has therefore enjoyed a "distance" which was quite helpful in forcing me to examine, confront, and document certain assumptions I held. My interactions with Burns and with others noted above have certainly helped to mitigate some of the biases and shortcomings of the various research approaches in this book, particularly the participant-observer research.

I have chosen to footnote the text rather extensively. Frequently I have used the footnotes to elaborate on a point made in the text or to provide additional information concerning the source. The liberal use of footnotes should assist critics and/or future scholars in assessing my work and pursuing topics of their own interest.

Research for this book was carried out at a number of libraries, principally the University of North Carolina (Chapel Hill), North Carolina State University (Raleigh), the North Carolina Biotechnology Center (Research Triangle Park, N.C.), the University of California at Davis, and the National Agricultural Library (Beltsville, Maryland). Extensive use was made of interlibrary loan capabilities to locate materials not found in these libraries. The use of fine university libraries in different sections of the country was something of a fortuitous accident. The benefit of this emerged with the realization that they contained different and unique materials related to the agricultural history of their region. The North Carolina Biotechnology Center, among all state biotechnology centers, specializes as an information and documentation center. It holds materials (such as specialized consulting reports) virtually unavailable to the public elsewhere due to their high price. I was also able to draw upon the personal libraries of a number of individuals.

**COMMENTS BY CHAPTER**

Chapter 1 begins with an examination of the ownership and control of
biological materials primarily in the eighteenth and nineteenth centuries,
before the introduction of modern forms of intellectual property rights. I
have relied on Crosby for information concerning plant introductions.
This material was corroborated and supplemented by my research into the
origins and dispersal of crops, undertaken for the book, *Shattering: Food,
Politics and the Loss of Genetic Diversity*. Background material was also
obtained from my research associated with *Food First: Beyond the Myth
of Scarcity*. Brockway's study on the activities of Kew Gardens is a
masterpiece of historical research. The material is supplemented and
confirmed by accounts of people involved with Kew during the period
under discussion (such as William Bean, a Kew curator, and W. T.
Thiselton-Dyer, its third Director). Smith's piece on botanical gardens is
also useful as supportive information.

For the second section of chapter 1, early collection and dissemination
of seeds in the United States, yearly reports of the U.S. Patent Office and
later the U.S. Department of Agriculture (USDA) contained extensive and
detailed data on the procurement and introduction of exotic seeds. Inventories provide surprisingly detailed information on the characteristics of
individual introductions. Histories by people involved with seed introduction activities (e.g., Pieters, Ryerson) were also located. The use of these
biological materials by farmers for selection and breeding in the United
States has been largely ignored by most historians and agricultural scientists, though the phenomenon is well recognized with Third World farmers, for example. Some astute observers, such as Wallace, noted the skill
of ordinary farmers in selecting and developing varieties. And the descriptions of varieties found in USDA publications sometimes provide
pedigrees which substantiate the role of farmers in the apparently conscious development of genetic materials. Still this is an area which needs
more research, particularly by those with expertise in crop history and
evolution.

Chapter 2 dealt with the rationalization and commercialization of
American agriculture. Through this process we can trace the commodification of seeds. There is no scarcity of sources for use in setting the stage
for the focus of this chapter. The difficulty is in integrating the material
and keeping a focus. I tried to concentrate on the major changes being
experienced by farmers during this period as it might relate to seeds.
Kloppenburg and de Souza, both sociologists, were helpful in providing
an overview of this period. Agricultural histories and histories of west-

ward expansion are not difficult to locate. The journal *Agricultural History* proved a rich source of information, but a substantial number of other historical and agricultural journals were also used. The USDA itself is a prime source as it published a wide range of materials, including historical pieces. Data on crops, companies, and markets was used extensively, often to double-check other sources cited in the text. Further, more general corroborating information can be found in railroad histories and in statistics regarding the freight they hauled, as well as in unexpected sources such as individual city histories.

Focusing on the seed trade itself, the trade journal *Seed World* is particularly valuable. This publication provides an ongoing window on the commercialization of American agriculture and concomitant rise of the commercial seed industry and modern plant breeding.

Few histories of early seed or nursery companies exist. *The Stark Story* and the appropriately titled *Through the Patience of Job: The Story of a Family and a Family Business* (on the Wyatt-Quarles Seed Company) were published by the companies themselves and tend to focus on and laud the founding family. A refreshing exception is Fitzgerald's *The Business of Breeding* (about Funk Seeds), a rich account which makes use of early family and company documents. Unfortunately, no similar history of Pioneer Hi-Bred (ultimately the most influential company) exists. Pioneer's first corn breeder, Raymond Baker, though retired, still goes to work at Pioneer daily and should be interviewed in more detail than I was able to do about the company's history. Had time permitted, a more intensive study of early seed catalogs — which can be found in large quantity at the National Agricultural Library in Beltsville, Maryland — would have provided useful information. Due to the transitory nature of much of the "industry" in the early days, little information exists apart from what can be pieced together from accounts in agricultural journals. This situation is somewhat alleviated with the growth of the American Seed Trade Association and the publication of journals to serve the industry. Still it is the history of the corn-seed companies that is best known. Likewise, the scientific development of hybrid corn is well known, but the history of breeding efforts in other crops is much more obscure. Much more social science research could be done on the modern history of the development of vegetables and grain crops in the United States. The comments of Donald Duvick, retired vice president of research for Pioneer Hi-Bred, were particularly helpful as they brought in the perspective of a corporate plant breeder with a long history in the profession and a keen interest in the history. Though he is an expert in corn, Duvick's interests and knowledge are broader.

Horticultural histories, seed and nursery trade publications, and nursery company catalogs provided valuable background information for chapter 3 as well as chapter 2.

Regarding the immediate events surrounding passage of the 1930 Plant Patent Act in chapter 3, I have relied heavily on Robert Starr Allyn, a patent lawyer who took an interest in the act and wrote the only history of it to date. Allyn had access to some of the principals involved and his view is thus valuable. However, it also proved necessary to consult the actual record of the hearings, as some recent authors (Doyle and Terry) have erred on a few important points of the history. Allyn's account is extremely difficult to find — it was unavailable at the National Agricultural Library for example, but was finally secured with the help of the University of California at Davis, through the California university library system. (Attempts to locate relatives of Allyn in hopes that they might have other papers or articles of his were unsuccessful. However, a nephew of Harry Robb, perhaps the most prominent plant patent lawyer and a man who was probably quite involved in the actual drafting of the legislation, was found. He was able to provide some important information and seems interested in searching the records of his uncle's — and now his — law firm for more.) Similarly, some of the actual congressional committee reports and hearings appear not to exist due to curious referencing systems for some of the documents. Obviously, some of these documents are quite difficult to locate. Background materials on the politicians involved in sponsoring this act were found in several standard biographical references. Information on Paul Stark, a major industry figure in organizing support for the act, was located in a history of Stark Brothers Nursery and several articles and histories of the nursery industry. Private papers and "insider" accounts of the process of securing approval of this act are not known to exist and the prominent individuals involved are now dead. Family histories, privately owned or in state archives, may shed light on some of the personalities involved (e.g., Senator Townsend of Delaware), if they can be located. Additional materials may be uncovered at Stark Brothers Nursery, though the current president (a family member) was unaware of the existence there of any documents concerning the 1930 Plant Patent Act which were unknown to this researcher.

Analysis in chapter 4 of the 1970 Plant Variety Protection Act (PVPA) benefits from several pieces written over a period of some years by the chief architect and organizer for the act, the late Allenby White. But it suffers from the lack of any known account by others detailing his actions, motivations, etc. Biographical information on him is also scarce. Efforts (through colleagues at his company, Northrup-King) to locate his family were unsuccessful. A booklet published on PVP in 1964 by several professional organizations provides a fascinating and seemingly candid look at the obstacles within the plant breeding community which White and other proponents faced. It describes in some detail the problems as seen by the breeders and their analysis of various alternatives. It also gives the reader a glimpse into White's analysis and is particularly useful when employed for comparison with later statements.

In exploring the context for the PVPA, seed trade journals were very important once again. Studies by McMullen and by Butler were particularly important as background material on the seed industry. Several interviews with corporate executives from this period were also conducted. This was particularly helpful in gaining some understanding of the relationships between different types of seed companies and the commercial and political constraints and opportunities they perceived.

More detailed information on the hearings on the 1970 PVPA is available than from the 1930 act. A number of the principals involved in lobbying for the act were located. Harold Loden and John Sutherland, through telephone interviews, provided rich, detailed accounts of events leading up to passage of the bill. Both have kept personal papers and notes dealing with this history. At times, their stories conflicted and I was faced with seeking independent confirmation of particular points. Footnotes in chapter 4 discuss some of these problems and explain my interpretation of them. Furthermore, Sutherland acknowledged that he was withholding important information concerning the signing of the PVPA. In such circumstances, one must keep in mind that actors have certain ongoing interests that flavor how they tell their stories. The researcher is forced to assess the reliability of the informant using independent sources of information, the degree of candidness seemingly displayed by the informant (and past experiences with the individual), and other actors' impressions of the source. This difficulty is pointed out in footnotes, when and where I deemed that it might indicate a possible problem with the information itself.

Several individuals, such as Richard Lyng and possibly Richard Kleindienst, played seemingly important roles in the final passage of the PVPA. But unlike others (such as Loden), they were concerned with the PVPA for only a very brief time and it was probably not considered terribly important in their careers. It may have been only one of thousands of policy decisions or pieces of legislation with which they had contact. While these actors may have occupied crucial government positions and held great power, their memory of their own involvement in the PVPA is often fuzzy. This does not, I believe, necessarily indicate that their involvement was trivial. Instead it points to a methodological problem in studies such as this. To some extent, alternative sources (colleagues, others more actively involved in the issue, etc.) can be utilized. Still, important facts and insights may be lost.

Much of the background and analysis for the first part of chapter 5 dealing with the PVPA expansion of 1980 was based on participant-observation. In 1979 and 1980, as the initiator and organizer of opposition to the PVPA amendment, I was perhaps the most visible and vocal opposition spokesperson. This history subjects me to more than the usual influences of bias. I have tried to guard against this consciously. This effort was aided by the fact that chapter 5 is not primarily concerned with the merits of the case for or against PVPA, but with the process which led to its passage, with interactions and relationships. Questions such as the effect of PVPA on exchange of genetic resources are relevant and cannot be completely avoided. But questions of the act's effect on seed prices — a major issue at the time, for example — are not addressed in detail here. To the extent possible I have tried to avoid debating the merits of such legislation once again.

Others will have to judge whether I have correctly described my own role. In this regard, they may consult a number of sources, including published articles.[18] A substantial amount of published material can be found in industry trade sources as well. My conscious bias in writing has been to be conservative in interpreting the influence or importance of my actions. Arguably, more might have been said about my own background[19] and the "context" in which the opposition to the PVPA was mounted. During the last two years, tensions among adversaries have thawed and it has become possible to engage in friendly, detailed (and, I believe, rather candid) discussions of the history from 1980 onwards.

Involvement allowed me access to a great deal of literature — letters, pamphlets, internal papers — much of it unpublished. Some of this information — particularly that which I produced — has been used here without formal footnoting. Future researchers in search of this material may want to consult the archives of the National Sharecroppers Fund/Rural Advancement Fund (at the labor history library of the Wayne State University in Detroit, Michigan) or the working files of the Rural Advancement Foundation International (RAFI) in Pittsboro, North Carolina, or in Ottawa and Winnipeg, Canada. The account of Doyle (another participant) should be viewed as valuable backup material by future researchers.

For the second section of chapter 5, on biotechnology and the courts, I have drawn primarily from published accounts in legal and technical journals of the cases cited.

Chapter 6 begins with a section on GATT and other efforts to expand and reform patent law. Data and political and historical analysis from industry, legal, and business publications is rich and easily available. Furthermore, future researchers may be able to obtain interesting information on the U.S. government's position and on industry lobbying of the government through the Freedom of Information Act. GATT is a particularly complex arena involving many actors. Without more information, it seems appropriate to be modest and conservative in drawing conclusions.

The second section of this chapter on the UN Food and Agriculture Organization (FAO) concerns events with which I have personal knowledge. I was active in formulating and organizing support for the initiatives discussed here: the FAO commission, the undertaking, the FAO network of gene banks and the FAO fund. Many of the advantages and limitations of participant-observer research noted earlier also apply here. At the FAO however, many governments and other organizations were involved, somewhat complicating the extent to which one could learn about all their actions, and motivations, and the degree of influence any other actor or event had upon them.

I attended all FAO biennial conferences from 1981 through 1989 and was in attendance at all sessions of the FAO Commission on Plant Genetic Resources except one. FAO conferences are in session for about three weeks and give ample opportunity for observation of delegations and interactions with them, both formally and informally. Over the years personal and professional friendships were developed with a number of delegates, including I would guess most of the influential delegates from Third World countries. I participated in many of the planning, strategizing, and drafting sessions associated with efforts at the FAO. During the writing of this book I had access to hundreds of files assembled by myself and others, including much "gray" literature. As background material and to refresh my memory, I also made use of the rather extensive notes I took during each of the meetings at the FAO during the 1980s. Material in my possession may be made available on a case by case basis, subject to practical constraints.

In the early days of the decade, access to delegations from industrialized countries was limited. However, during this entire period I received information (written and oral) supplied by anonymous informants from several delegations and from the FAO and the International Board for Plant Genetic Resources (IBPGR). These sources sometimes provided their own particular "insiders" view of events. A significant and very valuable source of information on the U.S. government position as well as that of the seed industry and IBPGR comes from documents obtained

from the government as part of a law suit against the U.S. Department of
Agriculture by the Foundation on Economic Trends. These documents —
perhaps 150 pounds worth — were made available to me by the plaintiffs.
During the discovery phase of the suit, plaintiffs demanded all letters,
reports, memos, and other documents having to do with germplasm
related proposals at the FAO, with exchange and ownership of
germplasm, and with the care of that material under government auspices.
This proved to be extremely valuable material as it seemed to reveal the
thinking and planning of a number of actors and thus served as a useful
counterpart to my personal experience and documentation of "the other
side." (Copies of most of this material are held by the Rural Advancement
Foundation International in Pittsboro, N.C. The remainder is in my
possession.) The major difficulty in using this material proved to be one
of selection — maintaining a tight focus enabled many otherwise fascinating documents to be put aside. I note in the text that five documents
were withheld from attorneys, having been "classified" by the U.S.
Department of State.

Recently with a thawing of tensions I have been able to meet with and
talk to a number of the key American delegates to FAO about that history.
This has proven valuable in corroborating the above documentation,
particularly on the role of the ASTA in influencing American government
policy.

Furthermore, published information — particularly from the FAO — is
easily available to the researcher at FAO headquarters in Rome. There,
researchers will want first to contact the FAO Commission on Plant
Genetic Resources. Some of the more common documents may be available through FAO offices in individual countries. The so-called "verbatim" reports of debates/discussions during the meetings (available to
delegates and observers during the conferences) can be sources of a great
deal of information, though one must be careful when interpreting this
source as it can obscure positions and events. Interpretation benefits from
an understanding of the context, which virtually requires one's presence.

It should be noted that as this book entered its final editing stage, I
accepted a long term consulting job with FAO in Rome. I am overseeing
the planning process for the production of a report on the "State of the
World's Genetic Resources" and the development and negotiating of a
"Global Plan of Action" for the conservation and sustainable utilization of
plant genetic resources. I am also in charge of initial planning of the
diplomatic conference (tentatively scheduled for 1996) to consider adoption of the report and the global plan of action. The plan is intended to
elaborate on and operationalize relevant sections of the Convention on

Biological Diversity adopted at the UN Conference on Environment and Development (the "Earth Summit") in 1992. In addition to conservation measures, it is likely that the plan will address property rights issues, and questions of access and sharing of benefits. Virtually no substantive changes, however, have been made to the book since my assuming the position with FAO in the fall of 1992, and I do not believe it has had any significant impact on the book.

The third section of this chapter deals with the Keystone International Dialogue on Plant Genetic Resources. For personal reasons I was unable to attend the first plenary session of the dialogue though I was invited. I did however attend the next plenary session in Madras, India, as well as four working group sessions (two of which dealt exclusively with intellectual property rights issues) and the final plenary meeting in Norway (for which I participated in raising most of the funding through the Norwegian government). The Keystone dialogue allowed me unparalleled access to many of the major "players" in the intellectual property debate. During the two years of the dialogue I developed friendships with several "adversaries." As mentioned above, this facilitated discussion of issues and history and I believe encouraged the development of a more complex picture and richer analysis of events described here. This involvement also served to challenge quite strongly many of my own political positions on IPR issues and thus has helped to balance my own biases, I suspect.

Because Keystone meetings are held off the record and statements made therein are not for attribution, there are limits on how information I gained there can be used. Extensive notes taken during dialogue sessions proved invaluable as background material; in a few cases, interviews were conducted outside of Keystone sessions and I have felt freer to use this information.

Some of the risks and drawbacks of participant-observation research have already been noted. My experience is that analyses of events at FAO and Keystone by people who were not there or who were only marginally involved are often seriously flawed. Both FAO and Keystone operate on the basis of consensus. Documents arrived at by consensus cannot be relied on as accurate sources on the process or the real intentions or positions of actors. Furthermore, actors may have placed great stress in negotiating certain portions of the agreement and these sections may be "more agreed to" than other sections of the same consensus document. But such insights cannot be gleaned from reading the documents alone. Participation in events described has been helpful in eliminating the obvious errors and common misinterpretations which are associated with many analyses of FAO and Keystone.

Appendix IV lays the basic theoretical foundation for the study. I have relied on the work of Burns and Giddens extensively. Both recognize the importance of incorporating complexity into their analytical framework. Their theoretical work resists simple explanations and artificial certainty. Collins, Chambliss and Seidman, and others have proven valuable in interpreting the rationalization and legislative processes. Weber's work on rationalization was particularly helpful in setting the direction of research as well as the tone of chapter 2.

As this book is not primarily an exercise in social theory construction, the appendix on theory is brief. I have assumed and would assert that the value of theory is best revealed in its practice. It is in the formal chapters of this study that the theoretical underpinnings must be judged. Here, I think that Burns and Giddens have been particularly useful in helping me challenge unconscious "functionalism," which so easily creeps into modern thought, often in unnecessary and counterproductive ways. Burns's "actor-systems dynamics" model encourages one to examine the intricate relationships between actors and systems rather than to posit in one or the other the full power of causality.

## NOTES

1. The empirical difficulties of elucidating the interactions between society and law have often been noted. See, for example, Carl A. Auerbach, "The Relation of Legal Systems to Social Change," *Wisconsin Law Review*, 1980: p. 1229ff.
2. Trow, Martin, "Comment on 'Participation Observation and Interviewing: A Comparison,'" in McCall, George J., and J. L Simmons, *Issues in Participation Observation: A Text and Reader*. Reading Mass.: Addison-Wesley Publishing. 1969: p. 332.
3. Zelditch, Morris, Jr., "Some Methodological Problems of Field Studies, " in McCall and Simmons, op. cit., p. 19.
4. Becker, Howard and Blanche Geer, "Participant Observation and Interviewing: A Comparison," in McCall and Simmons, op. cit., p. 331.
5. Schwartz, Howard and Jerry Jacobs, *Qualitative Sociology: A Method to the Madness*. New York: Free Press, 1979: p. 46.
6. Becker and Geer, op. cit., p. 331.
7. Silverman, David, *Qualitative Methodology and Sociology*, Hants, England: Gower Publishing, 1985: p. 104–105.
8. Zelditch, op. cit., p. 13.
9. McCall, George, "Data Quality Control in Participant Observation," in McCall and Simmons, op. cit., p. 130.
10. Ibid., p. 132ff.
11. Ibid., p. 130. See also David Silverman, op. cit., p. 105.
12. Below, I provide a number of published sources which deal with my own involvement and I address this issue more directly in the text of this appendix and the chapters themselves, as appropriate.
13. Some of these people as well as those connected with specific disciplines are acknowledged in the preface.
14. My consulting job at the FAO is described later in the text.

15. John Lofland points out that "getting close to a setting requires that the observer be on reasonably good terms with the members of the setting." See *Analyzing Social Settings: A Guide to Qualitative Observation and Analysis*, Belmont, Calif.: Wadsworth Publishing, 1971: p. 99.

16. It is also apparent that there is currently less partisanship and conflict among many of the actors in this field than there once was. This has facilitated more questioning and self-criticism of past positions among a number of individuals, myself included. And it has also increased access to "opposing" actors. (Interviews with a number of corporate executives were set up by other corporate executives who "vouched" for me.) Like most actors engaged in activity, I have learned and changed. Thus, questions of personal bias should be less a concern today than they would have been in the early 1980s, for example. It might also be mentioned that being socialized in the family of a lawyer and judge has, I believe, made me sensitive to and appreciative of the value and appropriateness of playing different, distinct roles without overlapping them. While this is never completely accomplished, it is relevant to insert this personal note, because the personal characteristics of participant-observers are frequently cited ("belabored," according to Zelditch) as a problem in specific studies. See Zelditch, op, cit., p. 13.

17. McCall, op. cit., p. 131.

18. For example, see Anonymous, "Law Could Restrict Small Farm Crops," *Boston Globe*, September 7, 1979; Calais, Al, "Gardeners Beware . . . Seed Law is Growing," *Sacramento Bee*, November 5, 1979; Hornblower, Margot, "Controversy Sprouts Over Attempts to Patent Seeds," *Washington Post*, September 25, 1979; Walters, Charles, "Opposing that Corner on Seeds," *ACRES, USA*, February, 1980; Anonymous, "Seed Battle Hits Hill," *Family Farm Monitor*, April, 1980; Randal, Judith, "Plant Patenting Law Sowing Seeds of Controversy," *Grand Forks Herald*, May 4, 1980; Randolph, Eleanor, "Seed Patents: Fears Sprout at Grass Roots," *Los Angeles Times*, June 2, 1980; Crittenden, Ann, "Plan to Widen Plant Patents Stirs Conflict," *New York Times*, June 6, 1980; Oleck, Joan, "Seed Savers Seen as Saviors as Genetic Crop Diversity Falls," *Raleigh News & Observer* (North Carolina), February 12, 1984; Hackney, Rod, "Chatham Researcher Wins Swedish Award for Work," *Greensboro News and Record*, October 17, 1985; Henderson, Bruce, "Man Will Be Honored For Work To Preserve Varieties of Seeds," *The Charlotte Observer*, October 20, 1985; McIntire, Lynnette, "Work With Crops Will Be Cited," *Memphis Commercial Appeal*, October 27, 1985; Dunn, J.A.C., "The Seed Savor," *Carolina Gardner*, June, 1987; Quillin, Martha, "Doing Something, not just talking, about the tomatoes," *Raleigh News and Observer*, February 10, 1991. Various issues of seed trade publications such as *Seed World*, *Seedsmen's Digest* and *Seed Trade News* could also be consulted. Additionally, my own colleagues — particularly Hope Shand and Pat Mooney — now with RAFI could provide insights, as could certain of my seed company "adversaries" such as Harold Loden.

19. Some personal background is provided in the preface.

# Definitions of Technical Terms

## SOURCES FOR DEFINITIONS:

(a) Allard, R. W., *Principles of Plant Breeding*. New York: John Wiley & Sons. 1960.

(b) Committee on Managing Global Genetic Resources: Agricultural Imperatives, Board on Agriculture, National Research Council, *Managing Global Genetic Resources: The U.S. National Plant Germplasm System*. Washington: National Academy Press. 1991.

(c) Mayr, Ernst, *The Growth of Biological Thought: Diversity, Evolution and Inheritance,*.Cambridge, Mass.; Belknap Press of Harvard University Press. 1982.

(d) Mayr, Ernst, *One Long Argument: Charles Darwin and the Genesis of Modern Evolutionary Thought*. London: Penguin Books, 1991.

## clone

A group of genetically identical individuals that result from asexual, vegetative multiplication; any plant that is propagated vegetatively and that is therefore a genetic duplicate of its parent. (b)

## crossing

The act of fertilizing one plant with the pollen of the other. Such cross-pollination can be accomplished, for example, by humans, insects, or the wind, and can be intentional or not. When crossed by humans, however, some measure of intentionality is often assumed.

## cultivar

A cultivated variety.

## DNA

Deoxyribonucleic acid. The molecule which carries the genetic information (genes) in all organisms except the RNA viruses. (d)

**double cross**

A cross between two F$_1$ hybrids. See hybrid. (a)

**farmer variety**

See landrace.

**gene**

The basic functional unit of inheritance responsible for the heritability of particular traits. (b)

**gene bank**

For plants, normally a temperature- and humidity controlled facility used to store seed (or other reproductive materials) for future use in research and breeding programs. Also called seed banks.

**genetic diversity**

In a group such as a population or species, the possession of a variety of genetic traits and alleles that frequently result in differing expressions in different individuals. (b)

**genetic resources**

The term is essentially synonymous with germplasm as used in this book, except that it carries with it a stronger implication that the material has or is seen as having economic or utilitarian value. (b)

**germplasm**

Seeds, plants, or plant parts that are useful in crop breeding, research, or conservation. Plants, seed, or cultures that are maintained for the purposes of studying, managing, or using the genetic information they possess. (b)

**hybrid**

A cross between two species, races, cultivars, or breeding lines. (b) The first generation offspring of such a cross of inbred lines are called

$F_1$ hybrids, the second generation, $F_2$, and so on. In plants, hybrids typically display desirable characteristics, but the seed of hybrids cannot be replanted without loss of hybrid vigor or sometimes sterility.

### inbred line

A line produced by inbreeding. In plant breeding a nearly homozygous line usually originating by continued self-fertilization, accompanied by selection. See also "pure line." (a)

### inbreeding

The mating of individuals more closely related than individuals mating at random. (a)

### landrace

A population of plants, typically genetically heterogeneous, commonly developed in traditional agriculture from many years — even centuries — of farmer-directed selection, and which is specifically adapted to local conditions. (b)

### mutation

A sudden heritable variation in a gene or in chromosome structure. (a)

### pure line

A genetically uniform (i.e., homozygous) population. (c)

### species

A taxonomic subdivision; a group of organisms that actually or potentially interbreed and are reproductively isolated from other such groups. (b)

### variety

A plant type within a cultivated species that is distinguishable by one or more characters. When reproduced from seeds or by asexual means (e.g., cuttings) its distinguishing characters are retained. The term is generally considered to be synonymous with cultivar. (b)

# Theoretical Foundations: Human Agency, Technology, and Law

There can be (but is not always) a fundamental difference in the nature of "proof" offered in the social and natural, experimental sciences. The "laws" of social science vary in ways in which the laws governing the fall of Newton's legendary apple seem not to. Circumstances change. Actors' perceptions change. The material world changes. Over time and space these changes can be profound. One cannot expect that today's causes will be or can be tomorrow's. Tomorrow is a different day with different conditions which affect the given variables and change their qualities and relationships. Furthermore, experimentation in the social sciences is more limited. One may speak in general terms about "causes," but where do these causes end? If one examines the causal chain, it is tempting to stop at a certain stage and declare the last "cause" to be *the* cause. Mirages are discovered. Eventually more and more questions are raised.

Giddens observes: "The nature of the constraints to which individuals are subject, the uses to which they put the capacities they have and the forms of knowledgeability they display are all themselves manifestly historically variable."[1] He argues persuasively that "there are no universal laws in the social sciences, and there will not be any — not, first and foremost because methods of empirical testing and validation are somehow inadequate but because . . . the causal conditions involved in generalizations about human social conduct are inherently unstable . . ."[2]

We can attempt explanation, which can sometimes be accomplished simply with adequate characterization, according to Giddens.[3] This may involve the formulation of generalities, even of causal generalities. But we have to be content with the fact that no iron-clad laws can be generated. Instead, in this book I try to relate action to structure, intended to unintended consequences, and I explore the important influence of the context surrounding human action, in an attempt to provide a better understanding of my subject.

None of the classical sociological theories alone can adequately explain or characterize the topic under scrutiny in this book. (Nor can the narrow focus of any one discipline be sufficient.) A synthesis of theories however, is useful. The "actor-system dynamics" (ASD) theory, itself a synthesis, developed by Tom Burns and his colleagues has proven quite helpful as a starting point[4] and foundation, as has Giddens. Certain Weberian and Marxist approaches have also proven useful. These theoretical works provide a point of departure for my own theoretical formulations and applications.

Certain theoretical tendencies are criticized in the following pages, usually implicitly, sometimes explicitly. The inadequacies of functionalism and the rigidity of structuralism are noted, for example. But no attempt is made to construct theoretical straw men in order to engage in a war of theories. The purpose is not to critique functionalism. The theory underpinning this work will not be argued for theoretically, but will I hope find its proper place and its justification interwoven into the body of the book.

The concept of "actors" and "agency" is a prominent one in ASD theory and here. Actors can be individuals, groups, organizations, or networks. Actors are capable of purposeful activity. They cannot be reduced to the structure. Nor can they be fully explained by laws, be they economic, natural, or legislated.

This book proceeds on the assumption that actors are *social* actors, not simply a mass of individuals disconnected from social processes, relationships, and structures. They are capable of having different kinds of socially based motivations and values. Rational choice theories often posit the existence of one universal motivation, claiming that all actors pursue goals according to their own self-interest, typically economic or materialistic. Such theories assume a much different kind of actor and a much more constrained, determined, and static view of agency than is offered here. I cannot find or postulate "free" actors who are programmed with a uniform and universal system of values and motivations abstracted from the social world. Neither does my study support the view that understanding of a social event or process can always be furthered simply by uncovering the economic self-interests of those involved without reference to the surrounding social context.

Motivations and values are held by social actors. Like the actors themselves, their motivations and values do not exist outside of the social world. They exist in complex social contexts and, as a result, can exhibit different characteristics. We see clear instances of economic motivations among actors in this book. But we also see political motivations and examples of action based on values not so narrowly founded on self-interest, for example in the activities of some of the nongovernment organizations working at the Food and Agriculture Organization. Even when economic motivations appear strong — as in the appropriation and development of valuable plants by botanical gardens in the eighteenth and nineteenth centuries — one can find other motivations and values at work. Some actors see this activity in more political terms (building the empire), some in more career-oriented terms (rising in one's profession). Some may see the activity as promoting a social good, such as bettering the lives of people in the colonies. Actors may also be acting on the basis of a combination of motivations or even harbor unclear, poorly articulated, or conflicting motivations. And, of course, they may act on the basis of incomplete or incorrect information. In chapter 6 (part of which examines a negotiation process relating to the financing of genetic conservation and utilization programs in the Third World), we can see corporate executives pursuing social and political goals which are not strictly or completely in the economic interests of their employers even though these actors are highly influenced by and supportive of corporate interests. In this case it helps to understand the social history of these actors and the different influences on them — their farm backgrounds, religious and community influences, perhaps even how long they have before retirement. One may reduce such political, social, and interpersonal motivations and their combinations to the "economic," but only at the risk of obscuring the richness, diversity, nuances, and complexity of the actors and their purposes. We learn from rational choice theories that actors pursue their interests, but we are left without guidance as to how actors develop certain preferences which give substance to their interests.[5] Such reductionism does not help guide or direct the researcher in ways that uncover the complexity in human activity, elucidate relationships, explain peculiarities, or distinguish one situation and outcome from another. In the end, everything is explained by the same causal factor, which for the purposes of this book is too general to be sufficient.

Both actors and their motivations and goals are *socially embedded.* Actors' perceptions, modes of reasoning, judgments, and actions should be seen as, in part, social and cultural constructions.[6] Actors develop goals and purposes within a particular social context and through the process of acting upon that context and being affected by it. But this context is always in flux and in any case does not dictate or explicitly or precisely determine actors' goals and purposes. In the confluence of different contexts, ambiguities, uncertainty, confusion, dilemmas, and predicaments can arise. Actors interpret existing rules in new ways and engage in creative activity. When rules do not suit their purposes, they often attempt to change them, or change the arenas in which decisions are made in order to take advantage of the different rules and power relationships found there.[7]

As Sartre points out, actors make of themselves something more than they are made to be.[8] The notion of purposeful action implies a strong connection between actors, their intentions, and the future. It is not just the past or the present that influences human action, but the future as well.

While actors are capable of intentional action and of choice, they are not totally free. Their action takes place within a context. Indeed they are born into a context which is not of their own choosing. As actors construct the social reality around them, they are influenced by this reality. The obstacles which face them and the resources they possess are associated with the positions and the roles they have in society. The social and material world forms a context which constrains, enables, and shapes the actors which are a part of it. In the process of making, actors are themselves made.

The "choice" which is so crucial to a meaningful notion of agency is limited. The writings of Marx and Engels on the subject of freedom and determinism — on choice — have occupied the attention of theorists for many years. In the 1859 preface to "A Contribution to the Critique of Political Economy," Marx states: "The mode of production of material life conditions the social, political and intellectual life process in general. It is not the consciousness of men that determines their being, but, on the contrary, their social being that determines their consciousness."[9] Human beings make their own history, as Marx asserts, but not under conditions of their own choosing. Engels elaborates on Marx's statement from the 1859 preface by saying that "if somebody twists this into saying that the economic factor is the only determining one, he transforms that proposition into a meaningless, abstract, absurd phrase."[10] But in the end, Engels hardens the elaboration by saying that the economic "ultimately determines historical development."[11] More often than not, choice seems to be more theoretical than real, much more circumscribed than free. Agency remains unclear and theoretically undeveloped.[12]

Agency can now be further elaborated. Actors, as explained earlier, carry out intentional and purposeful action. This action can be effective —it can "make a difference." And it is not totally determined or totally predictable. Actors are capable of goal-oriented and problem-solving activity. They have different goals and they perceive their needs differently, in part as a "result" of their differing positions and roles in society. Actors "shape and alter material and social environments."[13] They in turn are shaped by these environments and this experience. The distribution of power and material resources is changed in the process. Learning takes place. Actors develop and try out new strategies to solve new problems. These processes of social transformation are largely governed by rule systems "that structure and regulate the behavior of the social agents involved" even as they try and often successfully manage to change such systems.[14] As Burns and Flam succinctly state: ". . . agents interact —struggle, form alliances, exercise power, negotiate, and cooperate — within the constraints and opportunities of existing structures, at the same time that they act upon and restructure these systems. The result is institutional change and development, but structurally conditioned."[15] This approach draws one to look at social actors within systems and action on systems and to the dynamics involved. It implies, correctly, that actor and system are in a reciprocal relationship with each affecting and changing the other.

The importance of purposive action has been noted. It must be assumed that purposive action often results in the achievement of the intended consequences. But invariably action results in unintended consequences. Actors can neither completely foresee nor completely control the results of their own actions.[16] As Shakespeare's Macbeth foresaw in an insightful soliloquy on his intended murder of King Duncan, the consequences of action escape us.[17] They enter into a larger, never fully understood social and material world. The successful introduction of modern, commercially bred varieties of agricultural crops, for example, displaced traditional varieties which were the basis, the raw material for the breeding of the new varieties. This unintended consequence of intentional activity changed the world and became an important part of the context which plant breeders came to experience. It created new problems and fed back into the conditions for future action.

All action occurs in context, some elements of which an actor may have created, and some not. The context enables and constrains. What one actor controls or creates may be experienced by another as something that "happens" to him, her, it, or us. "Many of the most delicately subtle, as well as the intellectually most challenging, features of social analysis derive from this," Giddens observes.[18]

If we think about it, some of the most gripping stories in western literature hinge on the power of context. The awakening of Frankenstein's monster provides a moment of intense action and drama. But it is sterile in effect without knowledge of the context. Indeed, in the end of Mary Shelley's story it is not so much the action that seems important, but the context — the tension and relationship between inventor and invention.[19] In the book it is Frankenstein not his "monster" who flees the laboratory, unable to take responsibility for his creation. It is not a "criminal brain" that prompts the monster to act aggressively, but the repeated failure of the doctor to help his creation fit into the social environment. What are the duties of the inventor to his invention? To what extent must the inventor be responsible for seeing that his new invention and the world into which it is brought are compatible? Frankenstein's creation, while offering to do his duty to the doctor if the doctor will only fulfill his obligations and care for him, is nevertheless ready to exact revenge if the doctor does not. The monster's murder of Frankenstein's bride on their wedding night must be set against Frankenstein's refusal to make a companion for the monster, a refusal to help fashion an appropriate environment for his invention. It is this context — one of tension over responsibilities — that drives the story as originally told. I use this example to demonstrate the importance of context in giving meaning and "understanding" to events and action. In the absence of firm laws governing social systems, we seek a fuller understanding of the "setting, circumstances, and springs" of action.[20] We look to the context to supply us with reasons for action, reasons which Giddens would argue are essentially causes in the social world.

Social rule systems form an important part of the context within which actors operate. And, of course, rules themselves are context-dependent. Rules and rule formation bridge actor and structure. They indicate who participates in a certain activity or process, as well as when, where and how they participate. "Social rule systems function as grammars" at the actor level in ASD theory.[21] They structure social transactions. They both apply to and are made in "concrete action settings." Various types of social rule systems are discussed here. At one level the book may seem to be about the making of laws. And it is. But the making of these laws involves processes of conflict and negotiation structured by other types of rule systems — norms, customs, traditions, and regulations, for example. Furthermore, these rules are themselves under stress. Actors with sufficient power, resources, and skill are in a better position to create rules to suit their needs and advance their interests. Other actors may initiate challenges using the skills and resources they can muster. In the process, the rules themselves are subject to challenge and can change. No permanent equilibrium exists in rule systems. Rules, which may be claimed by some actors to be essentially timeless and context-independent, are found to be human products and subject to the forces of politics, technological changes, and shifts in values.

Established rule systems cannot be easily and effectively applied to new problems or to old problems in new contexts.[22] The new biotechnologies which facilitate manipulation of individual genes give new value and importance to those genes. Old laws which do not provide for ownership of microorganisms are perceived to be an obstacle by those who wish to invest in the new technologies and control the fruits of that work. The attempt to establish new rules is met with opposition by actors who believe their interests threatened by the proposed changes.

In a commercial setting effective utilization of genetic diversity usually requires effective ownership or control.[23] As diversity is not spread equally around the globe and as it has not always been conserved, utilization also requires access to genetic diversity. Access, in turn, is often involved with questions of ownership and control. Certainly the distribution of benefits of genetic diversity is intimately related to who owns and controls that material.

Ambrose Bierce, the nineteenth century author of *The Devil's Dictionary*, defined the word "prehistoric" as "belonging to an early period and a museum." For some, his definition might also have applied to genetic resources. Commonly, these are seeds being stored in a botanical museum called a gene bank.[24] According to this view, genetic diversity is the "common heritage of mankind," something created in the past by everyone's ancestors. As such it is free for the collecting. Once collected and stored in a museum or gene bank it becomes the property of that facility, though it may be still be referred to as common property. American biologist Garrison Wilkes reflects this view arguing that "the payment to developing nations for the services of plant genetic resources would destroy the use of seed as part of our common heritage."[25] Wilkes asks rhetorically, "Why privitize a public good?"

For others, the question is more complicated. The return by Denmark of the *Flateyjarbok* and *Codex Regius* to Iceland in 1971 and the continuing controversy over the ownership of the Elgin (Parthenon) Marbles are but two well-known examples of disputes over ownership in the field of cultural property.[26] Should the cultural treasures of a society, be they books, works of art, or genes, really be "up for grabs?" Or do they constitute something over which nations should exercise sovereignty? In the view of the Indian scientist and activist, Vandana Shiva, "The 'value added' in one domain is built on the 'value robbed' in another domain . . . .The problem is that in manipulating life forms you do not start from nothing, but from other life forms which belong to others — maybe through customary law."[27]

In this situation we see virtually all of the basic elements outlined by Burns and Flam as conditions under which rule regimes and rule complexes are "likely to undergo reformulation and transformation," namely conditions where:

> power shifts and social control failures occur among established groups
> adhering to differing organizing principles and regimes;

new social agents or coalitions — movements, classes, professions, parties or political elites — emerge, advocating new organizing principles and regimes and possessing sufficient social power to introduce these;

the core technologies or resource base of established rule regimes are substantially altered.[28]

The question of ownership has long been determined by sheer physical control, whether it be over the spoils of war (as in the case of "Egypt's" Rosetta stone now on display in London) or the spoils of a peaceful plant collecting expedition (as in the case of high lysine sorghums collected in Ethiopia and now in the United States and the United Kingdom). The "laws of genes" are a recent outgrowth of a centuries-old conflict over the control of plants.

The Keystone negotiation forum is one in which the parties in conflict attempt to influence rule formation. The power of this negotiation comes from the legitimacy derived from the nature of the forum itself and its participants. It is too early to elaborate on this point. Suffice it to say that legitimation is important in securing wide acceptance of or inexpensive enforcement of rules.[29] In the case of genetic resources, where many actors wish to see a rule system which encompasses the entire world, the need for legitimation is clear.

The term technology is used in this book at various times to refer to objects or tools, knowledge about using them, or systems of knowledge. Technology is not simply the practical application of science. And it is "more than bits of disembodied hardware."[30] Technologies exist and are employed within society. Several implications follow from this, which Burns and Ueberhorst have outlined:

1. "Technology control and use are governed by social rule systems."[31] Of course there are also physical constraints and laws that apply as well, but agents develop social rules about technologies' use, ownership, access, and benefits.

2. "Technologies are instruments of social action with consequences. The introduction of new technologies and the development of technological systems entail more than setting up and using new machines and other physical artifacts. It entails social re-organizing and the making of new rules."[32] This point has been mentioned before in another context — changes in plant breeding technologies have opened up new possibilities of commercial exploitation of plant genetic resources, possibilities which could not be realized very profitably within current legal systems. New technologies, it can be observed, may not "fit" with existing social structures or rule systems.[33]

Major developments in plant breeding in this century (from the use of modern Mendelian techniques to the new biotechnologies) have been examples of this. The development of the technology thus implies the development by social change agents of the organizational and legal structures to facilitate its use. This leads to a third point.

3. "The social organization of technology suggests the concept of sociotechnical system. Social activities involving technology are organized and, to a greater or lesser extent, institutionalized in complex sociotechnical systems . . . Knowledge of technology-in-use presupposes knowledge of social organization and, in particular, knowledge of the organizing principles and rules of human institutions."[34]

Technologies structure human activity. Winner notes that they "settle important issues de facto without appearing to do so." The freedom or choice we may have in using the technology sometimes masks the "vast, centralized, complicated, remote and increasingly vulnerable artificial systems" which support them.[35] The choice about whether to use certain genetic engineering techniques and the various controversies over regulating the techniques and the introduction of genetically engineered organisms into the environment take on a different meaning when one notes the degree of corporate control over the commercial exploitation of these technologies and the sweeping legal reforms being suggested to facilitate their use. (This is not to ignore the fact that certain experiences with government control are hardly more encouraging.) How do we interpret "choice" when the choice to use a new technique in the laboratory seems to be part of a package which includes new rules and systems to privatize the most basic components of life — genes? Certain choices, it seems, involve a forfeiture of control, at least by certain actors. Such choices restructure the context and change power relationships.

Winner notes that "in a fundamental sense . . . determining things is what technology is all about. If it were not determining, it would be of no use and certainly of little interest."[36] But this is "determining" not in the sense that no choice or possibility of agency exists. Instead, it is "determining" in the sense of enabling and influencing. Milovanovic makes a useful distinction in pointing out that there can be two interpretations of determination. One can involve prediction, that is, that "some antecedent factor totally predicts, or totally controls — prefigures — subsequent activity."[37] The second type, which is implied in most cases in this book, is a determination which sets limits and exerts pressure. When Engels states that "we make our history ourselves, but, in the first place, under very definite assumptions and conditions," Milovanovic interprets this as employing the second type of determination. Without debating his interpretation, it is worth noting that Milovanovic's distinction would still allow for acts of will and purpose — that is, agency. This fits better with a dialectical method than a simple, one-way cause and effect relationship. Thus, while we can see in the technologies discussed in later chapters a powerful determining factor, we do not see the disappearance of agency. Agency, however, can vary in extent or effectiveness both over time and among actors. It can also vary from situation to situation with the same actor.

The individual inventor-genius model of technological development can only explain certain aspects of the developments discussed here. The scientific achievements, even the "breakthroughs," seem firmly tied to previous experience and work. As importantly, they are dependent on society's ability to use them. Mendel's breakthrough disappears in the 1860s, is "rediscovered" in 1900, but only becomes important through use some time later as other people refine and adapt it. The initial ideas are rarely the most important factor, though they often receive the greatest publicity. "It is," as Randall Collins points out, "the social conditions for their sustained development that is more central."[38]

This is strikingly evident in regard to the role that farmers have played in the creation and maintenance of genetic diversity. Do we have millions of isolated, independent, individual inventors (plant breeders)? Hardly. But we do have innovation and lots of it! We see the result of cooperation and joint labor and even of innovation at the community level as farmers build upon and develop the work of their neighbors. Interestingly, industry points to the hundreds of patents on apples as evidence of the encouragement patents give to innovation, but fails to explain the origin of the 7000 varieties being grown in the United States at the turn of the century long before patent protection was available. In this view inventors and inventions seem to disappear if they are denied legal recognition.

Technology exists within a context even as it constitutes part of the context experienced by social agents. Technologies can aid, constrain, and shape human activity. But technologies and the systems supporting them are human creations. Through technologies, people transform the natural world and in so doing are themselves transformed. The unintended consequences of the use of technologies is also an important factor to consider particularly in light of the control often exercised over technologies by small elites. Genetic erosion, for example, is a largely unintended consequence of modern plant breeding. This consequence, which has practical effects in the environment, takes on new meaning and importance when various actors struggle for control and ownership of genetic diversity. This is particularly highlighted when it is realized that the new biotechnologies which make possible valuable new uses of this diversity are largely controlled by elites.[39]

The role of technology within society means that the benefits and costs of technology are not always (or usually) equally shared. Furthermore, the unintended consequences — which are usually negative — can be experienced far after the "benefits" are derived. The costs, in fact, are often hidden in the beginning.[40] And many of those who will end up paying the costs are therefore unaware that costs are even involved. In such a setting, policy or technology alternatives are rarely formulated in a serious way.[41]

Though the alternatives may not be formulated in a serious way, they potentially exist. Choices are made of what policies to pursue based on the knowledge and interests of actors within context. In this book we spend a considerable amount of time looking at the formation of laws concerning property rights for biological materials. Having been raised in a society often described as one ruled "by laws, not men" (by a father who was a judge), I must resist the notion that laws are above "men." Chambliss correctly identifies three powerful myths about law: (1) that law simply codifies the values of the society; (2) that law describes how the system actually operates, how judges, lawyers, police, bureaucrats and public officials behave; and (3) that laws are applied in an unbiased way to new situations.[42]

Like technology, laws are enacted to solve problems. They are not neutral — they serve interests. The absence of laws — such as the absence of property rights laws which could be used by Third World people to protect their type of plant breeding — also represents a choice and furthers certain interests.

Laws, or the absence of laws, can have a deceptively neutral appearance. Laws which allow everyone to hire an attorney may seem to be utterly neutral. In fact, they serve the rich, who can afford lawyers or afford the best lawyers. A similar situation is found with patent and patent-like protection for biological materials. "Anyone" who "creates" a new variety can be protected. But in effect this protection, as well as the important power it gives in the marketplace, go not to the individual, "back-yard" breeder, but to giant corporations. In effect, the laws serve to protect and give rights not to individual innovators but to *systems* of innovation. They reward not so much creativity as large-scale systematic, problem-solving.

How is law invented? How does it change? The explanation that it changes because it is in the ruling class's interest for it to change is not satisfying.[43] Similarly one cannot say that it is forced into existence by economic determinism, though economics can be an important factor. As Weber argued, "economic situations do not automatically give birth to new legal forms; they merely provide the opportunity for the spread of a legal technique if it is invented."[44] One needs a theory that can recognize the strengths and weaknesses of the economic and the strength of certain actors — but one that does not give total or determining power to either. On the other hand, pluralist theories which give no power at all to these factors, must be rejected.

Law is not simply the embodiment of logic. What may seem like an orderly development in particular categories of law is not simply the unfolding of legal logic divorced from the interests, desires, and actions of actors. There is no inevitable "progress" to law and the notion that there is gives little explanatory assistance. A 1930 law in the United States giving patent protection to most (but not all) asexually reproducing plants does not automatically progress to laws which provide patents for microorganisms and individual genes. Law is more than ideas or the logical progression of ideas. Laws concern social relationships.[45] The assumption that laws both shape and are shaped by society underpins this study but is not new to it, having been expressed at least as early as Montesquieu.[46]

Property rights laws concern relations to objects as well as people. Chambliss notes the difference between saying that "the book is brown," and "the book is mine." The first describes. The second also prescribes; it gives me the authority to exclude others from touching or using my book. It indicates how others should act toward me and the object I own. It indicates a number of potentially enforceable relationships.[47]

Legal control through patent and patent-like laws becomes important as the practicality of immediate physical control over resources recedes. In the strictest sense, patent laws serve to exclude others from imitating, manufacturing, using, or selling a product or utilizing a patented matter or process (without permission). So defined, they are a means of allocating ownership, assigning control, regulating access, and apportioning benefits. They reflect power relationships in a very concrete manner.

These laws are shown to be time-bound, corresponding to a certain state of societal development (including its technological development).[48] Their passage indicates a perceived need and a desire on the part of some actors to change old social relations and create new ones. Conversely, opposition to these patent regimes implies criticism of current social relations. The legal ideology of patent law is not separate from social relations which include business and political interests of competing groups. Biological patent law has not yet achieved the kind of legitimacy that other types enjoy. The instability in this area of law is a reflection of rapid changes in technology, changing business needs, and political debates among conflicting interests. Such law is still very much in the process of being created by actors. The lack of legitimacy tied to the participation of new and different actors raises new issues not previously thought to be connected to the question of patents. For example, it is important whether or not patents are connected to exploitation of Third World peoples. But whether or not the patent system and its allies are affected by this question has to do with social forces and the power of other actors to make it an issue.

Patent laws are an attempt to gain legal control when other methods of control are inefficient or unavailable. In recent times the superseding of old patent laws with new ones has been influenced heavily by advances in technology and new commercial and marketing situations. Old arenas of decision-making lose their applicability. Can we see why that happens? New arenas are sought. Can we see how and why they are chosen? New actors with different interests can then emerge, and do. How can we understand this development by looking at the issues and the actors and their interplay within a broader social, historical, and technological context?

Intellectual property rights (patent and patent-like), such as those passed in the United States in 1930 and 1970, were designed and created for a purpose by actors acting with certain constraints — the level of technological development, the needs of the business community, legal precedent, the support and opposition of friends and foes, and the economy. They were not passed because an all-powerful social system dictated that they be passed. But the context within which they emerged is crucial to understanding not only why plant patent laws came into being, but what peculiar forms they took, and how these served as the backdrop for further struggle.

In analyzing particular events as regards intellectual property rights for plants, we cannot fail to be impressed by the importance of changes in arenas. The growth of technology and the expanding scope of the seed industry mean that property rights secured in the United States are not secure at all to a company operating internationally. The fight for patents becomes global, pushing the proponents of patents across the American border to international institutions. This arena change allows for and is also the product of new actors on the scene — actors with opposing views who realize that a change of venue is to their advantage. Commercial interests in pursuit of their goals favor different arenas. The debate and struggle becomes established in multiple arenas, calling for different skills and resources from the various actors, and producing risk and uncertainty. New actors change the rules, shake things up, introduce new issues, and involve the public. The patent system becomes more vulnerable as actors attempt to engineer its growth and internationalization. The perceived need for new legal structures precedes the ability of the actors to create them, thus adding to the intensity of the fight.

Decisions once made by the experts in safe arenas have now become public decisions debated in more hostile arenas. The rules have suddenly changed with the arrival of new actors, new resources, new interests. These changes in turn call for a response and an alteration in the game plan of those who previously acted in a more confined and controllable setting. One avenue is to incorporate the dissidents into the system and reprivatize the debate. This approach alters relationships and again changes the rules and creates uncertainty. How does it affect the outcome?

Interestingly, in colonial days power stemmed from having direct control over the plants themselves. With the advent of modern plant breeding and more so with biotechnology, power has come from control over information and plant parts (genes). That control is offered and secured by patents. Companies no longer need to defend physical territory or particular physical seeds. If reciprocal patent rights are granted, control can be worldwide. Yet, biotechnology now makes plant diversity potentially more valuable, though how that value is determined, assigned, safeguarded, and realized is extremely problematic and contentious. (It is even questionable whether all actors appreciate its value and act with this understanding.)

Individual characteristics and genes have become very important. The new technology indirectly has the effect of giving (potentially) great value to genes. In trying to maintain legal control through the patent system, industry encounters a serious problem. The genes it needs to control are often located in the Third World. If they are not located in the Third World, they could easily be taken there to establish production systems in legal competition to those "protected" by patents in industrialized countries.

Physical control could again become crucial as it provides a possible bargaining chip for "Third World interests" in debates over the restructuring and expanding of the international patent system as well as for bilaterial agreements and contracts. Such developments have spurred certain interests to put pressure on old rule systems. Previously, crop genetic resources have been termed "the common heritage of mankind." This term "explained" and "justified" the fact that in other words, they were economically free. But, if they are so valuable, should they be so free? The notion that somehow genetic resources are different from most other resources and should be freely and openly available to all comers is one that serves some interests while it disserves others. The resistance to this notion now threatens an overhaul in the way genetic resources are viewed . . . and made available, or not.

Historically, "common heritage" has been promoted as a political principle even by those who would stand to gain little from its implementation. They did so as a way of attacking the patent system which already applies to the biological materials of companies, for instance, but does not apply to the categories of genetic resources in which the Third World is so rich. The argument was: "If our resources are common heritage, then so should yours be." The argument was effective momentarily and in certain fora as a political or educational tool. But the patent system for plants survived. Soon, however, the argument was reversed: "If your resources are private, why should ours not be?" How deep is the new understanding of the resource, its qualities, uses, values, and vulnerabilities, however? And how "correct?"

Can we be surprised that current challenges arise at a time when technology is adding tremendous (but uncompensated) value to Third World genetic resources, and when changes in arena might allow for Third World participation in the debate over ownership and control of plant genetic resources? The history and developments outlined in this book were not the inevitable results of omnipotent social or economic laws or the byproducts of technological pressures. Neither will the future be so determined. Challenges and the form they take may be understandable without being considered inevitable. We have explored ways of furthering our understanding of these events and relationships. The importance of agency, and the capabilities and limits of agency within context, are some of the more important theoretical considerations examined. Burns observes that "the relative importance in human action and development of freedom of choice as opposed to determinism is more a matter of emphasis or orientation rather than a testable hypothesis or proposition."[49] The test of this book then is how this emphasis is placed and how well the dynamic is characterized and explained.

## NOTES

1. Giddens, Anthony, *The Constitution of Society: Outline of the Theory of Structuration.* Berkeley: University of California Press. 1984: p. 219.
2. Ibid., p. xxxii.
3. Ibid., p. 216.
4. Burns, Tom, Thomas Baumgartner, and Philippe Deville. *Man, Decisions, Society: The Theory of Actor-System Dynamics for Social Scientists.* New York: Gordon and Breach. 1985. Subsequent developments concerning evolutionary theory by Tom Burns and

Thomas Dietz are also interesting but do not depart radically from previous work. Their evolutionary theories draw attention to and highlight slightly different matters than ASD. Following evolutionary theories in biology, they note that success is not guaranteed and that the direction of change toward optimality is not automatic. To simplify the presentation to the reader, I have chosen not to introduce the additional terms employed in Burns and Dietz's writings on evolutionary theory, though many of the points made in their writings are covered here. See Burns, Tom R., and Thomas Dietz, "Cultural Evolution: Social Rule Systems, Selection and Human Agency, *International Sociology*. Vol. 7, no. 3. September, 1992.

5. Burns, Tom, "Two Conceptions of Human Agency: Rational Choice Theory and the Social Theory of Action," in Piotr Sztompka (ed.) *Human Agency and the Reorientation of Social Theory*. New York: Gordon and Breach (in press). As Burns notes: "game and rational choice theories, in spite of their many valuable contributions to social science, are simply unable to take into account or analyze, at least in any systematic way, the social basis of preference structures, action alternatives, decision principles, and human interaction patterns at the same time that human agents shape and reshape their social basis [as] part of the historical development of social institutions and societies."

6. Granovetter, M., "Economic Action and Social Structure," *American Journal of Sociology*, Vol. 50. 1985.

7. Burns, Tom, E. Griffor, and L. D. Meeker, *The Theory of Social Interaction and Games*, manuscript, 1993.

8. Sartre, Jean-Paul, *Search for a Method*. New York: Vintage Books. 1968: p. 91.

9. Quoted in Milovanovic, Dragan. *Weberian and Marxian Analysis of Law: Development and Functions of Law in a Capitalist Mode of Production*. Aldershot, U.K.: Avenbury. 1989: p. 42.

10. Ibid., p. 42.

11. Ibid., p. 43.

12. Rational choice theorists also stress agency in theoretical debates on freedom and determinism. It is not necessary to delve into a critique of this position. In its "pure" form, it finds limited support among sociologists today. Suffice it to say that this tendency ignores the very real constraints to action which Marxists, for example, would correctly identify. It fails to recognize the dynamic between actors and system. In the final analysis, it fails to explain why certain choices exist and not others, and how actors may structure their choice situations. In general, the role of elites and the existence and use of power seem strangely missing. See, for example, the discussion of "power" and structural constraints in Dietz, Thomas, and Tom Burns, "Human Agency and the Evolutionary Dynamics of Culture," *Acta Sociologica*. Vol. 35, 1992: p. 190.

13. Burns, Baumgartner, and Deville, op. cit., p. 11.

14. Ibid., p. xiii.

15. Burns, Tom, and Helena Flam, *The Shaping of Social Organization: Social Rule System Theory with Applications*. London: Sage Publications. 1987: p. 2.

16. Giddens, op. cit., p. 218.

17. Shakespeare, William, "Macbeth," in *The Complete Works of William Shakespeare*. New York: Avenel Books. 1975: p. 1050. Macbeth states:

> If it were done when 'tis done, then 'twere well
> It were done quickly. If the assassination
> Could trammel up the consequence, and catch,
> With his surcease, success; that this blow
> Might be the be-all and the end-all here...
> But in these cases
> We still have judgment here; that we but teach
> Bloodly instructions, which being taught, return
> To plague the inventor: this even-handed justice
> Commends the ingredients of our poison'd chalice
> To our own lips.

18. Giddens, op. cit., p. 346.
19. There are a number of published editions of the story, entitled *Frankenstein, or the Modern Prometheus.*
20. Elton quoted in Giddens, op. cit., p. 360.
21. Burns and Flam, op. cit., p. 13.
22. Burns and Flam, op. cit., p. 385.
23. Utilization, here, refers to the use that plant breeders make of different genetic characteristics to breed new varieties and to market those varieties.
24. When the seeds from a collecting expedition enter the bank they typically do so as the property of the bank itself. Unlike a commercial bank, the seeds are not being stored for those who donated them. The seeds are the sole property of the facility — not of the farmer or farm community that produced them. Most large gene banks are government facilities. However, private companies hold important "working" collections of diversity of the crops they actively breed. Government facilities often regard their collections as "common property," the practical effect being that scientists and plant breeders are given access to the materials.
25. Wilkes, H. G. "Plant Genetic Resources: Why Privitize a Public Good?" *BioScience.* March, 1987: p. 217.
26. Greenfield, Jeanette, *The Return of Cultural Treasures.* Cambridge: Cambridge University Press. 1989: p. 10ff.
27. Shiva, Vandana, "The Seed and the Spinning Wheel: Biotechnology, Development and Biodiversity Conservation." Draft of paper presented to the International Conference on Conservation of Genetic Resources for Sustainable Development. Røros, Norway. 1990: p. 25.
28. Burns and Flam, op. cit., p. 386.
29. Burns and Flam, op. cit., p. 371.
30. Rosenberg, quoted in Burns, Tom, and Reinhard Ueberhorst, *Creative Democracy: Systematic Conflict Resolution and Policymaking in a World of High Science and Technology.* New York: Praeger. 1988: p. 22.
31. Burns, Tom R., and Reinhard Ueberhorst, *Creative Democracy: Systematic Conflict Resolution and Policymaking in a World of High Science and Technology.* New York: Praeger. 1988: p. 19.
32. Burns and Ueberhorst, op. cit., p. 20.
33. Burns and Flam, op. cit., p. 299. (Note also the example of Frankenstein above!)
34. Burns and Ueberhorst, op. cit., p. 21.
35. Winner, quoted in Burns and Flam, op. cit., p. 294.
36. Winner, Langdon, *Autonomous Technology: Technics-out-of-Control as a Theme in Political Thought.* Cambridge: MIT Press. 1987: p. 75.
37. Milovanovic, op. cit., p. 43.
38. Collins, Randall, *Weberian Sociological Theory.* Cambridge: Cambridge University Press. 1986: p. 115.
39. This is not just a problem of technology, narrowly defined. It also concerns "specialization," as Tom Dietz points out (personal communication, November 23, 1992). The degree of specialization involved in a task or a technology affects the ability of, the incentive for, and the likelihood of other actors to make improvements or alterations to it.
40. Dorner, Peter, "Technology and U.S. Agriculture," in Gene F. Summers (ed.), *Technology and Social Change in Rural Areas.* Boulder, Colo.: Westview Press. 1983: p. 84.
41. Burns and Ueberhorst, op. cit., p. 50.
42. Chambliss, William, and Robert Seidman, *Law, Order, and Power.* Second Edition. Reading, Mass.: Addison-Wesley. 1982: p. 7.
43. Auerbach, Carl A., "The Relation of Legal Systems to Social Change," *Wisconsin Law Review.* 1980: p. 1245. Auerbach notes the difficulty of Marxist theory in explaining the mechanism by which the economy is the causal factor in creating law.
44. Weber quoted in Milovanovic, op. cit., p. 36.
45. Milovanovic, op. cit., p. 24.

46. Auerbach, op. cit., p. 1237.
47. Auerbach, op. cit., p. 1237.
48. Tigar, Michael E., and Madeleine R. Levy, *Law and the Rise of Capitalism*. New York: Monthly Review Press. 1977: p. 277, 288.
49. Burns, Baumgartner, and Deville, op. cit., p. 8.

# Bibliography

Allard, R. W., *Principles of Plant Breeding*, New York: John Wiley & Sons, 1960.

Allyn, Robert Starr, "Plant Patent Queries: A Patent Attorney's Views on the Law," *The Journal of Heredity*, **Vol. 24**, no. 2, February, 1933.

Allyn, Robert Starr, *The First Plant Patents: A Discussion of the New Law and Patent Office Practice*. Brooklyn: Educational Foundations, Inc. 1934.

Alsberg, Carl, "The Objectives of Wheat Breeding." *Wheat Studies*. **Vol. 4**, no. 7. 1928.

American Seed Trade Association, "ASTA Position Statement on Intellectual Property Rights for the Seed Industry." Approved by the ASTA Board of Directors, June 29, 1990. Washington: ASTA. 1990.

American Seed Trade Association, "Position Paper of the American Seed Trade Association on FAO International Undertaking on Plant Genetic Resources." Washington: ASTA. May 5, 1984.

American Seed Trade Association, *Proceedings of the American Seed Trade Association*, 1909. Hartford, Conn.: Hartford Press. 1909.

Anderson, Jack, "Stewart Is Yet To Answer Questions About Ethics," Syndicated newspaper column. October, 1980.

Anonymous, "Beating the Farmer at His Own Game," *Seed World*. **Vol. 5**, no. 6. April 18, 1919.

Anonymous, "Better Seed Grains and the Seedsman," *Seed World*. **Vol. 3**, no. 6. June 5, 1917.

Anonymous, *Business Week*. November 21, 1970.

Anonymous, *Changes in Farm Production and Efficiency, 1978*. Washington: U.S. Department of Agriculture. January, 1980.

Anonymous, "Discourage Home Seed Saving," *Seed World*. **Vol. 5**, no. 5. April 4, 1919.

Anonymous, "Editorial." *Seed World*, **Vol. 3**, no. 4. April 5, 1917.

Anonymous, "Editorial." *Seed World*. **Vol. 61**, no. 18. September 19, 1947.

Anonymous, "Farm Bill Could Make Growing of Some Vegetable Varieties Illegal," *The Farmers Forum*, Fargo-Moorhead, September 7, 1979.

Anonymous, "Good Seed Cannot be Grown by Amateurs," *Seed World*. **Vol. 5**, no. 3. March 7, 1919.

Anonymous, "Home Seed Saving Again a Factor," *Seed World*. **Vol. 6**, no. 4. August 16, 1919.

Anonymous, *Journal of the Plant Variety Protection Office*, U.S. Department of Agriculture. Various issues.

Anonymous, "Law Could Restrict Small Farm Crops," *Boston Globe*, September 7, 1979.

Anonymous, "Patenting of Plants Promises Big Profits — and Big Problems," *Business Week*, August 26, 1931.

Anonymous, "Pay Attention to Patents, Says Management Expert." *Research & Development*. December, 1988.

Anonymous, Plant Patents with Common Names. Washington: American Association of Nurserymen. 1963.

Anonymous, "Pleasing the Mail Order Customer," *Seed World.* **Vol 5**, no. 2. February 5, 1919.

Anonymous, "Quandary over Plant Patenting Brings Diverse Group of Experts Together." *Diversity.* **Vol. 5**, no. 2 & 3. 1989.

Anonymous, "Seed Battle Hits Hill," *Family Farm Monitor.* April, 1980.

Anonymous, "What the War Has Done for the Seed Trade," *Seed World.* **Vol 5**, no. 9. June 6, 1919.

Associated Seed Growers, "Old Favorites Can Be Well Bred Too!" *Seed World.* **Vol. 51**, no. 5, March 6, 1942.

Auerbach, Carl A., "The Relation of Legal Systems to Social Change," *Wisconsin Law Review.* 1980.

Bailey, Liberty H., *Annals of Horticulture in North America for the Year 1889.* New York: Rural Publishing Co. 1890.

Bailey, Liberty H., *Annals of Horticulture in North America for the Year 1893.* New York: Orange Judd Co. 1894.

Barbee, David Rankin, "Bill Before Hoover Grants Plant Patents," *Washington Post*, May 25, 1930.

Bean, William J., *The Royal Botanic Gardens, Kew: Historical and Descriptive.* London: Cassell & Co. 1908.

Beck, Frank Victor, *The Field Seed Industry in the United States: An Analysis of the Production Consumption and Prices of Leguminous and Grass Seeds.* Madison: University of Wisconsin Press. 1944.

Becker, Howard, and Blanche Geer, "Participant Observation and Interviewing: A Comparison," in G. J. McCall and J. L. Simmons, *Issues in Participant Observation; A Text and Reader*, Reading Mass.: Addison-Wesley Publishing, 1969.

Beetham, David, *Max Weber and the Theory of Modern Politics.* Cambridge: Polity Press. 1985.

Beier, F. K., and J. Straus, "Patents in a Time of Rapid Scientific and Technological Change: Inventions in Biotechnology," in Beier, F. K., R. S. Crespi, and J. Straus (eds.), *Biotechnology and Patent Protection.* Paris: Organization for Economic Cooperation and Development, 1985.

Berenbeim, Ronald, "Safeguarding Intellectual Property." Research Report 925. New York: The Conference Board. 1989.

Berg, Trygve, Åsmund Bjørnstad, Cary Fowler, and Tore Skrøppa, *Technology Options and the Gene Struggle.* NORAGRIC Occasional Papers Series C. Ås: Norwegian Centre for International Agricultural Development. Agricultural University of Norway. March 1991.

Berman, Larry, *The Office of Management and Budget and the Presidency, 1921–1979.* Princeton: Princeton University Press. 1979.

Bhagwati, Jagdish, "It's the Process, Stupid," *The Economist.* **Vol. 326**, no. 7804, March 27, 1993: p. 83.

Bishop, W. D., Report of the Commissioner of Patents for the Year 1859. 36th Congress, 1st Session, Senate, Ex. Doc. no. 11. Washington: U.S. Government Printing Office. 1860.

Bradley, A. Jane, "Intellectual Property Rights, Investment, and Trade in Services in the Uruguay Round: Laying the Foundations," in *Stanford Journal of International Law.* no. 23. 1987.

Brockway, Lucile, *Science and Colonial Expansion: The Role of the British Royal Botanic Gardens.* New York: Academic Press. 1979.

Brown, E., "How Seed Testing Helps the Farmer," *Yearbook of Agriculture,* 1915. Washington: Government Printing Office. 1916.

Brown, George, Jr., Letter to Representative Kika de la Garza dated November 8, 1979.

Brown, Lester, *Seeds of Change: The Green Revolution and Development in the 1970's.* New York: Praeger Publishers. 1973.

Brown, Louis Joseph, "The United States Patent Office and the Promotion of Southern Agriculture, 1850-1860." M.A. thesis, Florida State University. June, 1957.

Brush, Steve, "Genetic Diversity and Conservation in Traditional Farming Systems," *Journal of Ethnobiology,* Vol. **6,** no. 1. Summer 1986.

Bryant, Keith L., Jr., *History of the Atchison, Topeka and Santa Fe Railway.* New York: Macmillan Publishing. 1974.

Burns, Tom, "Two Conceptions of Human Agency: Rational Choice Theory and the Social Theory of Action," in Piotr Sztompka (ed.) *Human Agency and the Reorientation of Social Theory.* New York: Gordon and Breach (forthcoming).

Burns, Tom, Thomas Baumgartner, and Philippe Deville, *Man, Decisions, Society: The Theory of Actor-System Dynamics for Social Scientists.* New York: Gordon and Breach. 1985.

Burns, Tom R., and Thomas Dietz, "Cultural Evolution: Social Rule Systems, Selection and Human Agency," *International Sociology.* Vol. **7,** no. 3. September, 1992.

Burns, Tom, and Helena Flam, *The Shaping of Social Organization: Social Rule System Theory with Applications.* London: Sage Publications. 1987.

Burns, Tom, E. Griffor, and L. D. Meeker, *The Theory of Social Interaction and Games,* manuscript, 1993.

Burns, Tom R., and Reinhard Ueberhorst, *Creative Democracy: Systematic Conflict Resolution and Policymaking in a World of High Science and Technology.* New York: Praeger. 1988.

Burrill, G. Steven, with the Ernst & Young High Technology Group, *Biotech 90: Into the Next Decade; Fourth Annual Survey of Business and Financial Issues in America's Most Promising Industry.* New York: Mary Ann Liebert, Inc. 1989.

Burrill, G. Steven, with the Ernst & Young High Technology Group, "From the Double Helix to the Human Genome," in *Biotech 90: Into the Next Decade; Fourth Annual Survey of Business and Financial Issues in America's Most Promising Industry.* New York: Mary Ann Liebert, Inc. 1989.

Butler, L. J., and B. W. Marion, *The Impacts of Patent Protection on the U.S. Seed Industry and Public Plant Breeding.* Research Division, College of Agricultural and Life Sciences, University of Wisconsin-Madison. September, 1985.

Buttel, Frederick, and Randolph Barker, "Emerging Agricultural Technologies, Public Policy, and the Implications for Third World Agriculture: The Case of Biotechnology," *American Journal of Agricultural Economics.* Vol. **66,** no. 2. December, 1985.

Calais, Al, "Gardeners Beware . . . Seed Law is Growing," *Sacramento Bee,* November 5, 1979.

Carew, John, "Germ Plasm Control as it Would Affect Variety Improvement and Release of Vegetables and Flowers," in H. L. Hamilton (ed.), *Plant Breeder's Rights*. ASA Special Publication Number 3. Denver: Crop Science Society of America in cooperation with the American Society for Horticultural Science, the American Seed Trade Association, the International Crop Improvement Association and the National Council of Commercial Plant Breeders. March, 1964.

Carlson, Peter (vice president, Crop Genetics International), letter to Vic Althouse, Member of Parliament (Canada), August 22, 1985.

Carter, William B., "Speaking Out on Vegetable Seed Prices," *Seed World*. Vol. **90**, no. 7. April 13, 1962.

Cavanagh, H. M., *Seed, Soil and Science: The Story of Eugene D. Funk*. Chicago: Lakeside Press. 1959.

Chambliss, William, and Robert Seidman, *Law, Order, and Power*. Second Edition. Reading, Mass.: Addison-Wesley. 1982.

Chaney, James W., "A National Plant Variety Protection System," *Seed World*. Vol. **106**, no. 1. January 9, 1970.

Cipolla, Carlo, M., *Before the Industrial Revolution: European Society and Economy, 1000–1700*. New York: Norton. 1976.

Cipolla, Carlo, M., *Guns and Sails in the Early Phase of European Expansion*. London: Collins. 1965.

Clark, A. Bryan, "Breeders' Rights and Breeders' Freedom," *Seed World*. Vol. **93**, no. 12. December 27, 1963.

Clark, A. Bryan, "Shall The ASTA Take A New Tack?" *Seed World*. Vol. **94**, no. 11. June 12, 1964.

Cleaver, Harry, Jr., *The Origins of the Green Revolution*. Ph.D. dissertation, Stanford University. 1975.

Cleaver, Harry, "Contradiction of the Green Revolution." *Monthly Review*. June, 1972.

Cochrane, Willard W., *The Development of American Agriculture: A Historical Analysis*. Minneapolis: University of Minnesota Press. 1979.

Collins, J. H., "The Food Problem and the Seed Catalogue," *Seed World*. Vol. 3, no. 11. November 5, 1917.

Collins, Randall, *Max Weber: A Skeleton Key*. Beverly Hills: Sage Publications. 1986.

Collins, Randall, *Weberian Sociological Theory*. Cambridge: Cambridge University Press. 1986.

Committee on Managing Global Genetic Resources: Agricultural Imperatives, Board on Agriculture, National Research Council, *Managing Global Genetic Resources: The U.S. National Plant Germplasm System*. Washington: National Academy Press. 1991.

Committee on Registration of the Peninsula Horticultural Society, "Registration of New Fruits," *The American Garden*. Vol. **XII**, no. 6. June, 1891.

Consultative Group on International Agricultural Research, *Annual Report — CGIAR*, 1988/89. Washington: CGIAR. 1989.

Cook, Arthur G., "Patents as Non-Tariff Trade Barriers," *TIBTECH*. October, 1989.

Cook, O. F., Inventory no. 1, Foreign Seeds and Plants Imported by the Section of Seed and Plant Introduction, Numbers 1–1000. Washington: U.S. Department of Agriculture, Division of Botany. undated (1898).

Cook, Robert, "Other Plant Patents," *Journal of Heredity*. **Vol. XXIV**, no. 2. February, 1933.

Correa, Carlos M., "TRIPs: An Asymmetric Negotiation," Unpublished draft, June, 1993.

Cox, Thomas S., J. Paul Murphy, and Major M. Goodman, "The Contribution of Exotic Germplasm to American Agriculture," in Jack Kloppenburg (ed.), *Seeds and Sovereignty: The Use and Control of Plant Genetic Resources.* Durham: Duke University Press. 1988.

Crabb, A. Richard, *The Hybrid-Corn Makers: Prophets of Plenty.* New Brunswick: Rutgers University Press. 1947.

Crawford, Wm. H., "Treasury Circular," reprinted in Rasmussen, Wayne D., *Agriculture in the United States: A Documentary History.* Vol. 1. New York: Random House. 1975.

Crittenden, Ann, "Plan to Widen Plant Patents Stirs Conflict," *New York Times.* June 6, 1980.

Crosby, Alfred W., Jr., *The Columbian Exchange: Biological and Cultural Consequences of 1492.* Westport, Conn.: Greenwood Press. 1972.

Cullinan, G., *The Post Office Department.* New York: Praeger. 1968.

Dahlberg, Kenneth, "Testimony before House Subcommittee on Department Investigations, Oversight, and Research on H.R. 999." Washington. April 22, 1980.

Danhof, Clarence H., *Change in Agriculture: The Northern United States, 1820–1870.* Cambridge, Mass.: Harvard University Press. 1969.

Demuth, Richard, Letter to Quentin Jones, March 8, 1985.

de Souza Silva, Jose, *Science and the Changing Nature of the Struggle Over Plant Genetic Resources: From Plant Hunters to Plant Crafters.* Ph.D. dissertation, University of Kentucky. 1989.

Dietz, Thomas, and Tom Burns, "Human Agency and the Evolutionary Dynamics of Culture," *Acta Sociologica*, **Vol. 35**, 1992.

Dietz, Thomas, Paul Stern, and Robert Rycroft, "Definitions of Conflict and the Legitimation of Resources: The Case of Environmental Risk," *Sociological Forum*. **Vol. 4**, no. 1. 1989.

Dietz, Thomas, Robert W. Rycroft, and Paul C. Stern, "Framing and Power in Policy Systems: The Case of Environmental Risk," unpublished draft. October 23, 1992.

Dorner, Peter, "Technology and U.S. Agriculture," in Gene F. Summers (ed.), *Technology and Social Change in Rural Areas*, Boulder, Colo.: Westview Press. 1983.

Dorsey, John G., "U.S. Laws and Regulations on Protection of Varieties and Juridical Requirements for Breeders' Rights" in H. L. Hamilton (ed.) *Plant Breeders' Rights*, ASA Special Publication Number 3, Denver: Crop Science Society of America in cooperation with the American Society for Horticultural Science, the American Seed Trade Association, the International Crop Improvement Association and the National Council of Commercial Plant Breeders. March, 1964.

Doyle, Jack, *Altered Harvest: Agriculture, Genetics and the Fate of the World's Food Supply.* New York: Viking. 1985.

Dreyer, Peter, *A Gardener Touched with Genius.* New York: Coward, McCarn & Geoghegan. 1975.

Dunn, J. A. C., "The Seed Savor," *Carolina Gardner*, June, 1987; Quillin, Martha, "Doing Something, not just talking, about the tomatoes," *Raleigh News and Observer*, February 10, 1991.

Dwyer, Paula, "The Battle Raging Over Intellectual Property." *Business Week*. May 22, 1989.

East, Edward M., and Donald Jones, *Inbreeding and Outbreeding: Their Genetic and Sociological Significance*. Philadelphia: J. B. Lippincott Co. 1919.

Edler, George C., "Seed Marketing Hints for the Farmer," Farmers' Bulletin no. 1232, USDA, Washington: Government Printing Office. October, 1921.

Edminster, T. W., (Administrator USDA), Letter to Richard Demuth, Chairman, IBPGR, January 19, 1977.

Edwards C. R. (Acting chief, Seed Branch, USDA Consumer and Marketing Service), letter to Paul Kulp, Planning and Evaluation Staff, USDA, December 18, 1970.

Elder, Walter, *The Cottage Garden of America*, Philadelphia: Moss & Brother, 1854.

Elgin, J. H., "Briefing Paper — Impact of the 1991 Revised UPOV Convention." Unpublished USDA internal document. April 5, 1991.

Emergency Committee for American Trade, "The Role of the Multinational Corporation in the United States World Economies," Sections A-1 and A-2 in Subcommittee on International Trade of the Senate Finance Committee, Multinational Corporations, 93.

Esquinas-Alcazar, Jose T., "Plant Genetic Resources: A Base for Food Security," *Ceres*, no. 118. 1987.

Fairchild, David, "The Fascination of Making a Plant Hybrid." *Journal of Heredity*. **Vol. XVIII**, no. 2. February, 1927.

Farney, Dennis, "Meet the Men Who Risked Their Lives to Find New Plants," *Smithsonian*. June, 1980.

Fitzgerald, Deborah, *The Business of Breeding: Hybrid Corn in Illinois, 1890–1940*. Ithaca: Cornell University Press. 1990.

Fogel, R. W., *Railroads and American Economic Growth: Essays in Econometric History*. Baltimore: Johns Hopkins Press. 1964.

Folger, J. C., and S. M. Thomson, *The Commercial Apple Industry of North America*. New York: Macmillan Co. 1921.

Food and Agriculture Organization of the United Nations, "International Undertaking on Plant Genetic Resources." Document C 83/II REP/4, 5. 1983.

Forbes, Malcolm, Jr., Open letter, undated (1991?)

Fortmann, H. R., "Plant Variety Protection Legislation: The State-Federal Viewpoint," *Seed World*. **Vol. 105**, no. 8. November 28, 1969.

Fowler, Cary, "A Brief Guide to the Issues Involved in Plant Patenting and Amendments to the Plant Variety Protection Act (H.R. 999, and S. 23) Which Would Expand Coverage of Our Plant Patenting Law." (Unpublished) National Sharecroppers Fund: 1980.

Fowler, Cary, *The Graham Center Seed Directory*. Wadesboro, N.C.: National Sharecroppers Fund/Rural Advancement Fund. 1979.

Fowler, Cary, Open letter dated July 4, 1979.

Fowler, Cary, "The Progressive Farmer," *Southern Changes*. July, 1979.

Fowler, Cary, "Seeds of Life or Destruction?" Nashville, Tenn.: Agricultural Marketing Project, Vanderbilt University Medical School. 1977.

Fowler, Cary, "Testimony" before the Senate Agriculture Subcommittee on Agricultural Research and General Legislation on S. 23, An Amendment to the Plant Variety Protection Act. Washington. June 17, 1980.

Fowler, Cary, Eva Lachkovics, Pat Mooney, and Hope Shand, "The Laws of Life: Another Development and the New Biotechnologies." *Development Dialogue.* Uppsala: Dag Hammarskjöld Foundation. Nos. 1–2. 1988.

Fowler, Cary, and Pat Mooney, *Shattering: Food, Politics and the Loss of Genetic Diversity.* Tucson: University of Arizona Press. 1990.

Frundt, Henry, *American Agribusiness and U.S. Foreign Agricultural Policy.* Ph.D. dissertation, Rutgers University. 1975.

Gadbaw, R. Michael, and Rosemary E. Gwynn, "Intellectual Property Rights in the New GATT Round," in Gadbaw, R. M. and T. J. Richards (eds.), *Intellectual Property Rights; Global Consensus, Global Conflict?* Boulder, Colo.: Westview Press. 1988.

Gadbaw, R. Michael, and Timothy J. Richards, "Introduction," in Gadbaw, R. M. and T. J. Richards (eds.), *Intellectual Property Rights; Global Consensus, Global Conflict?* Boulder, Colo.: Westview Press. 1988.

Galloway, B. T., Distribution of Seeds and Plants by the Department of Agriculture. USDA Bureau of Plant Industry Circular no. 100. Washington: Government Printing Office. 1912.

Gates, Paul Wallace, "The Promotion of Agriculture by the Illinois Central Railroad, 1855–1870," *Agricultural History.* Vol. V, no. 1. January, 1931.

General Accounting Office, "The Department of Agriculture Can Minimize the Risk of Potential Crop Failures," Report to the Congress by the Comptroller General, GAO, April 10, 1981.

Giddens, Anthony, *The Constitution of Society: Outline of the Theory of Structuration.* Berkeley: University of California Press. 1984.

Goodman, Louis, with Arthur Domike, and Charles Sands, *The Improved Seed Industry: Issues and Options for Mexico.* Washington: Center for International Technical Cooperation. 1982.

Goodwyn, Lawrence, *The Populist Moment: A Short History of the Agrarian Revolt in America.* Oxford: Oxford University Press, 1978.

Granovetter, M., "Economic Action and Social Structure," *American Journal of Sociology,* Vol. 50. 1985.

Greenfield, Jeanette, *The Return of Cultural Treasures.* Cambridge: Cambridge University Press. 1989.

Hackney, Rod, "Chatham Researcher Wins Swedish Award for Work," *Greensboro News and Record,* October 17, 1985.

Hambidge, Gove, and E. N. Bressman, "Forward and Summary," in *Yearbook of Agriculture, 1936.* Washington: U.S. Department of Agriculture. 1936.

Hamilton, H. L. (ed.), Plant *Breeders Rights's Rights,* ASA Special Publication Number 3. Denver: Crop Science Society of America in cooperation with the American Society for Horticultural Science, the American Seed Trade Association, the International Crop Improvement Association and the National Council of Commercial Plant Breeders. March, 1964.

Harlan, H. V., and M. L. Martini, "Problems and Results in Barley Breeding," in *Yearbook of Agriculture, 1936.* Washington: U.S. Department of Agriculture. 1936.

Harlan, Jack, "Genetics of Disaster." *Journal of Environmental Quality.* Vol. 1, no. 3. 1972.

Harlan, Jack, "Our Vanishing Genetic Resources," *Science*, May 1975.

Hastings, Donald M., "Vegetable Seed Novelties and New Important Seed Strains," *Seed World*, Vol. 32, no. 2. July 22, 1932.

Haughton, Claire Shaver, *Green Immigrants*. New York: Harcourt Brace Jovanovich. 1979.

Hays, Willet M., "Address by Chairman of Organization Committee," *Proceedings of First Meeting of American Breeders' Association* held at St. Louis, Mo. Washington, D.C.: American Breeders' Association. 1905.

Hays, Willet M., "Distributing Valuable New Varieties and Breeds," *Proceedings of First Meeting of the American Breeders' Association* held at St. Louis, Mo. Washington, D.C.: American Breeders' Association. 1905.

Hayter, Earl W., "Horticultural Humbuggery Among the Western Farmers, 1850–1890." *Indiana Magazine of History*. Vol. XLIII, no. 3. September, 1947.

Hayter, Earl W., "Seed Humbuggery Among the Western Farmers." *Ohio Archaeological and Historical Quarterly*, Vol. LVIII, 1949.

Hedrick, U. P., *A History of Horticulture in America to 1860*. Portland, Oregon: Timber Press. 1988 (original copyright, 1950, Oxford University Press).

Hedrick, U. P., *The Small Fruits of New York.*, Report of the New York Agricultural Experiment Station. Albany: J.B. Lyon Co. 1925.

Heitz, Andre, "History of the UPOV Convention and the Rationale for Plant Breeders' Rights" in *Proceedings, UPOV Seminar on the Nature of and Rationale for the Protection of Plant Varieties under the UPOV Convention*. Geneva: Union for the Protection of New Varieties of Plants. 1990.

Henderson, Bruce, "Man Will Be Hornored For Work To Preserve Varieties of Seeds," *The Charlotte Observer*, October 20, 1985.

Henderson & Co., Peter, "Manual of Everything for the Garden," (catalog) New York: 1899.

Henretta, James A., "Families and Farms: Mentalité in Pre-Industrial America." *William and Mary Quarterly*. Vol. XXXV, no. 1. January, 1978.

Hepper, F. N., *Royal Botanic Gardens, Kew: Gardens for Science and Pleasure*. London: Her Majesty's Stationery Office. 1982.

Hicks, John D., *The Populist Revolt: A History of the Farmers' Alliance and the People's Party*. Minneapolis: University of Minnesota Press. 1931.

Hightower, Jim, *Eat Your Heart Out: Food Profiteering in America*. New York: Crown. 1975.

Hightower, Jim, *Hard Tomatoes, Hard Times*. Cambridge, Mass.: Schenkman Publishing. 1973.

Hjort, Howard, "Final Impact Statement" (on amendment to PVPA). USDA. January 9, 1979.

Ho, Ping-ti, "The Introduction of American Food Plants into China," *American Anthropologist*, 57. 1959.

Hofstadter, Richard, "The Myth of the Happy Yeoman," *American Heritage*. Vol. 7. April, 1956.

Hopkins, John A., *Changing Technology and Employment in Agriculture*. Washington: U.S. Government Printing Office/USDA Bureau of Agricultural Economics. May, 1941.

Hornblower, Margot, "Controversy Sprouts Over Attempts to Patent Seeds," *Washington Post*. September 25, 1979.

International Biotechnology Association, "Backlog in Biotechnology Patent Applications," IBA Reports. July–August, 1988.

Jabs, Carolyn, The Heirloom Gardener. San Francisco: Sierra Club Books. 1984.

Jefferson, Thomas, Thomas Jefferson: Garden Book, edited by Edwin Morris Betts. Philadelphia: American Philosophical Society. 1944.

Jones, C. Clyde, "The Burlington Railroad and Agricultural Policy in the 1920's." Agricultural History. Vol. 31. no. 4. October, 1957.

Jones, Donald F., "Selection in Self-Fertilized Lines as the Basis for Corn Improvement," Journal of the American Society of Agronomy. Vol. 12, no. 3. March, 1920.

Jones, E. L., "Creative Disruptions in American Agriculture 1620–1820," Agricultural History. Vol. XLVIII, no. 4. October, 1974.

Jones, Quentin, Draft for the IBPGR Executive Committee Meeting in Leuven, Belgium on IBPGR and the FAO Undertaking. August 6, 1984.

Jones, Quentin, Draft Report on FAO Undertaking. Internal USDA document. May 3, 1984.

Kalton, Robert R., "The Impact of Commercial Research Programs on Field Seeds," Seed World. Vol. 92, no. 7. April 12, 1963.

Kasler, Kirk, Max Weber: An Introduction to His Life and Work. Cambridge: Polity Press. 1988.

Katzenbach, Nicholas deB., "The International Protection of Technology: A Challenge for International Law Making," Technology in Society. Vol. 9. 1987.

Kenney, Martin, Biotechnology: The University-Industrial Complex. New Haven: Yale University Press. 1986.

Kenney, T. B., Administrator, USDA, in telegram to George Dietz, First Secretary at the U.S. Mission to UN-FAO. April 19, 1984.

Keystone Center, "Final Report of the Keystone International Dialogue on Plant Genetic Resources: Session I; Ex Situ Conservation of Plant Genetic Resources." Keystone, Colo.; Keystone Center. August 15–18, 1988.

Keystone Center, "Final Consensus Report of the Keystone Internatinal Dialogue Series on Plant Genetic Resources: Madras Plenary Session." Keystone, Colo.: Keystone Center. January 29–February 2, 1990.

Keystone Center, Keystone International Dialogue Series on Plant Genetic Resources, "Final Consensus Report: Global Initiative for the Security and Sustainable Use of Plant Genetic Resources." Oslo Plenary Session. Prepublication draft. Keystone, Colo.: Keystone Center. June 21, 1991.

Kimmelman, Barbara A., "The American Breeders' Association: Genetics and Eugenics in an Agricultural Context, 1903–13," Social Studies of Science. Vol. 12. 1983.

King, Ronald, Royal Kew. London: Constable & Co. 1985.

Klein, Andrew, "Statement" (Synnestvedt and Lechner, Patent Lawyers/ABA) to the Subcommittee on Departmental Operations, Committee on Agriculture, U.S. House of Representatives. Hearings on proposed Plant Variety Protection Act. June 10, 1970.

Kloppenburg, Jack Ralph, Jr., First the Seed: The Political Economy of Plant Biotechnology, 1492-2000. Cambridge: Cambridge University Press. 1988.

Kloppenburg, Jack R. Jr., Seeds and Sovereignty: The Use and Control of Plant Genetic Resources. Durham: Duke University Press. 1988.

Klose, Norman, America's Crop Heritage: The History of Foreign Plant Intro-

*duction by the Federal Government*. Ames, Iowa: Iowa State College Press. 1950.

Kneen, Orville H., "Patent Plants Enrich Our World," *National Geographic*. March, 1948.

Lacy, William, and Lawrence Busch, "The Changing Division of Labor Between the University and Industry: The Case of Agricultural Biotechnology," in Molnar, Joseph, and Henry Kinnucan (eds.), *Biotechnology and the New Agricultural Revolution*. Boulder, Colo.: Westview Press for the American Association for the Advancement of Science. AAAS Selected Symposium 108. 1989.

Lambert, Wade, and Arthur S. Hayes, "Investing in Patents to File Suits Is Curbed," *Wall Street Journal*. May 30, 1990.

Lappe´, Frances Moore, and Joseph Collins, with Cary Fowler, *Food First: Beyond the Myth of Scarcity*. New York: Houghton Mifflin. 1977.

Lappe´, Marc, *Broken Code: The Exploitation of DNA*. San Francisco: Sierra Club Books. 1984.

Learmond, Douglas, *Journal of Commerce*. November 24, 1971.

Lemmon, Kenneth, *Golden Age of Plant Hunters*. Cranbury: A. S. Barnes and Co. 1968.

Lemon, James T., *The Best Poor Man's Country: A Geographical Study of Early Southeastern Pennsylvania*,. Baltimore: Johns Hopkins Press. 1972.

Loden, Harold, "Breeders' Rights, Plant Patents and Variety Protection," *Seedsmen's Digest*. January, 1969.

Loden, Harold D., "Speaking Out On Research In The Seed Industry," *Seed World*. Vol. **93**, no. 10. November 22, 1963.

Loden, Harold, "Report on Developments of Breeder's Rights for Commercially Developed Cotton Varieties Through Certification and Patent System." Annual Meeting, Texas Certified Seed Producers, Inc. in Dallas, Tex. January 9, 1967.

Loden, Harold, "Statement" (as director of research ACCO Seed, Anderson, Clayton) to the Subcommittee on Departmental Operations, Committee on Agriculture, U.S. House of Representatives. Hearings on the proposed Plant Variety Protection Act. June 10, 1970.

Loden, Harold, "Statement" on House Bill 294 Before the Senate Agriculture Committee at Austin, Tex., March 18, 1969.

Loden, Harold, "Statement" to the House Interim Agriculture Committee Hearing, Lubbock, Tex., July 26, 1966.

Lofland, John, *Analyzing Social Settings; A Guide to Qualitative Observation and Analysis*. Belmont, Calif.: Wadsworth Publishing. 1971.

Long, B. A. W., *Mail by Rail: The Story of the Postal Transportation System*. New York: Simmons-Boardman Publishing. 1951.

Manks, Dorothy S., "How the American Nursery Trade Began," *Plants & Gardens: Origins of American Horticulture*. Brooklyn: Brooklyn Botanic Garden. Vol. **23**, no. 3. Autumn, 1967.

Mann, Susan A., and James A. Dickinson, "State and Agriculture in Two Eras of American Capitalism." in Frederick H. Buttel and Howard Newby (eds.), *The Rural Sociology of the Advanced Societies: Critical Perspectives*. Montclair, N.J.: Allenheld, Osum. 1980.

Mansfield, Edwin, "Intellectual Property, Technology and Economic Growth" in Francis W. Rushing and Carole Ganz Brown (eds.), *Intellectual Property*

*Rights in Science, Technology, and Economic Performance: International Comparisons*, Boulder, Colo.: Westview Press, 1990.

Marti, Donald B., *Historical Directory of American Agricultural Fairs*. New York: Greenwood Press. 1986.

Mason, Charles, Report of the Commissioner of Patents for the Year 1854. 33d Congress, 2d Session, House of Representatives, Ex. Doc. no. 59. Washington: U.S. Government. 1855.

Mayr, Ernst, *The Growth of Biological Thought: Diversity, Evolution, and Inheritance*. Cambridge: Harvard University Press. 1982.

Mayr, Ernst, *One Long Argument: Charles Darwin and the Genesis of Modern Evolutionary Thought*, London: Penguin Books, 1991.

McAuliffe, Sharon, and Kathleen McAuliffe, *Life for Sale*. New York: Coward, McCann & Geoghegan. 1981.

McCall, George, "Data Quality Control in Participant Observation," in G. J. McCall and J. L. Simmons, *Issues in Participant Observation; A Text and Reader*, Reading, Mass.: Addison-Wesley Publishing, 1969.

McIntire, Lynnette, "Work With Crops Will Be Cited," *Memphis Commercial Appeal*, October 27, 1985.

McMullen, Neil, *Seeds and World Agricultural Progress*. Washington: National Planning Association. 1987.

Merrill, M., "Cash is Good to Eat: Self-Sufficiency and Exchange in the Rural Economy of the United States," *Radical History Review*. no. 3. 1977.

Midyette, J. W., Jr., "Compulsory Registration of Varieties," *Seed World*. Vol. **90**, no. 8. April 27, 1962.

Miller, Cloy, "Germ Plasm Control As It Would Affect Variety Improvement and Researse of Asexually Produced Crops" in H. L. Hamilton (ed.), *Plant Breeder's Rights*, ASA Special Publication Number 3, Denver: Crop Science Society of America in cooperation with the American Society for Horticultural Science, the American Seed Trade Association, the International Crop Improvement Association and the National Council of Commercial Plant Breeders. March, 1964.

Milovanovic, Dragan, *Weberian and Marxian Analysis of Law: Development and Functions of Law in a Capitalist Mode of Production*. Aldershot, U.K.: Avenbury. 1989.

Mody, Ashoka, "New International Environment for Intellectual Property Rights" in Francis Rushing and Carole Ganz Brown (eds.), *Intellectual Property Rights in Science, Technology, and Economic Performance: International Comparisons*. Boulder, Colo.: Westview Press, 1990.

Mooney, Pat Roy, "The Law of the Seed." *Development Dialogue*. no. 1–2. Uppsala: Dag Hammarskjöld Foundation. 1983.

Mooney, Pat, Letter to Michael Lesnick and John Ehrmann (executive vice presidents of the Keystone Center), May 7, 1991.

Mooney, Pat, *Seeds of the Earth: Private or Public Resource?* Ottawa: Canadian Council for International Co-operation and the International Coalition for Development Action. 1979.

Moore, J. N., "Small Fruit Breeding — A Rich Heritage, A Challenging Future," *HortScience*. Vol. **14**, no. 3. June, 1979.

Morton, J. Sterling, Report of the Secretary of Agriculture, 1894. Washington: U.S. Department of Agriculture/ U.S. Government Printing Office. 1894.

Murphy, Charles and Quentin Jones, "Briefing Paper." Internal USDA document. October 26, 1983.

Nabhan, Gary, *Enduring Seeds: Native American Agriculture and Wild Plant Conservation.* San Francisco: North Point Press. 1989.

National Academy of Sciences, *Genetic Vulnerability of Major Crops.* Washington: National Academy of Science. 1972.

Neely, Wayne Caldwell, *The Agricultural Fair.* New York: Columbia University Press. 1935.

Newman, Peter, "A Modest Proposal for European Patents," *Bio/Technology*, Vol. 7. January, 1989.

Nichols, Harry E., "Iowa," in W. H. Upshall (ed.), *History of Fruit Growing and Handling in United States of America.* University Park, Penn.: American Pomological Society. 1976.

Nixon, W. H., "Vegetable Breeding Is Important," *Seed World.* Vol. 32, no. 1. July 8, 1932.

North, Douglas C., "International Capital Flows and the Development of the American West," *Journal of Economic History.* Vol. XVI, no. 4. 1956.

Oleck, Joan, "Seed Savers Seen as Saviors as Genetic Crop Diversity Falls," *Raleigh News & Observer* (North Carolina). February 12, 1984.

Olmo, H. P., "California," in W. H. Upshall (ed.), *History of Fruit Growing and Handling in United States of America and Canada.* University Park, Penn: American Pomological Society. 1976.

Page, Earl M., "Compulsory Registration of Varieties," *Seed World.* Vol. 90, no. 3, February 9, 1962.

Page, Earl M., "Garden Seed Breeding And Production in the United States," *Seed World.* Vol. 92, no. 10, May 24, 1963.

Parker, William N., and Stephen J. Decanio, "Two Hidden Sources of Productivity Growth in American Agriculture, 1860–1930." *Agricultural History.* Vol. 56, no. 4. October, 1982.

Peng, Martin Khor Kok, "Transnational Corporations: The Interests Behind GATT." *The Ecologist.* Vol. 20, no. 6. November-December, 1990.

Peoples' Business Commission, Parker v. Chakrabarty, Brief in the Supreme Court of the United States, October Term, 1979, no. 79–136.

Perelman, Michael, *Farming for Profit in a Hungry World.* Montclair, N.J.: Allanheld, Osmun & Co. 1977.

Pfister Seed Co., "Pfister Hybrids Are Different," *Wallace's Farmer.* August 13, 1938.

Pieters, A. J., *Yearbook of Agriculture for 1899.* U.S. Department of Agriculture. Washington: Government Printing Office. 1900.

Pinkett, Harold T., "Records of the First Century of Interest of the United States Government in Plant Industries," *Agricultural History.* Vol. 29, no. 1. January, 1955.

Quillin, Martha, "Doing Something, not just talking, about the tomatoes," *Raleigh News and Observer*, February 10, 1991.

Ragan, W. H., *Nomenclature of the Apple: A Catalogue of the Known Varieties Referred to in American Publications from 1804 to 1904.* Bureau of Plant Industry, Bulletin no. 56. Washington: U.S. Government Printing Office. 1926.

Randal, Judith, "Plant Patenting Law Sowing Seeds of Controversy," *Grand Forks Herald.* May 4, 1980.

Randolph, Eleanor, "Seed Patents: Fears Sprout at Grass Roots," *Los Angeles Times*. June 2, 1980.

Rasmussen, Wayne D. (ed.), *Agriculture in the United States: A Documentary History*. Vol. 1 & 2. New York: Random House. 1975.

Reeve, Eldrow, "Statement" (Campbell Soup Co.) to the Subcommittee on Departmental Operations, Committee on Agriculture, U.S. House of Representatives. Hearings on the proposed Plant Variety Protection Act. June 10, 1970.

Richards, Paul, *Coping With Hunger: Hazard and Experiment in an African Rice-Farming System*. London: Allen & Unwin. 1986.

Ripley, Randall B., and Grace A Franklin, *Congress, the Bureaucracy, and Public Policy*. Homewood, Illinois: Dorsey Press. 1976.

Robb, Harry C., "Plant Patents," *Journal of the Patent Office Society*. Vol. XV, no. 10. October, 1933.

Robertson, Thomas E., "Memorandum for Secretary of Commerce R. P. Lamont," March 8, 1930.

Rochester, Anna, *Why Farmers Are Poor: The Agricultural Crisis in the United States*. New York: International Publishers. 1940.

Rome, Adam Ward, "American Farmers as Entrepreneurs, 1870–1900." *Agricultural History*. Vol. **56**, no. 1. January, 1982.

Rosenburg, Charles, *No Other Gods: On Science and American Social Thought*. Baltimore: Johns Hopkins University Press. 1976.

Rosenberg, S. H. (ed.), *Rural America A Century Ago*. St. Joseph, Mich.: American Society of Agricultural Engineers. 1976.

Rossiter, Margaret, "Graduate Work in the Agricultural Sciences, 1900–1970." *Agricultural History*. Vol. **60**, no. 2. Spring, 1986.

Rossman, Joseph, "Plant Patents," *Journal of the Patent Office*, Vol. **XIII**, no. 1. January, 1931.

Rourke, Francis E., *Bureaucracy, Politics, and Public Policy*. Second Edition. Boston: Little, Brown & Co. 1976.

Royal Botanic Gardens, "Centenary of the Royal Botanic Gardens," *Kew Bulletin of Miscellaneous Information*. 1941.

Royal Botanic Gardens, "List of the Staffs of the Royal Gardens," *Kew Bulletin of Miscellaneous Information*. no. 29. 1889.

Runge, C. Ford, "The Developing Countries and the Uruguay Round." *Staff Paper*. St. Paul, Minn.: University of Minnesota Institute of Agriculture, Forestry and Home Economics. February, 1991.

Ryerson, Knowles A., "History and Significance of the Foreign Plant Introduction Work of the United States Department of Agriculture," *Agricultural History*. Vol. **7**, no. 2. April, 1933.

Ryerson, Knowles A., "The History of Plant Exploration and Introduction in the United States Department of Agriculture," in *Proceedings of the International Symposium on Plant Introduction*, Escuela Agricola Panamerican, Tegucigalpa, Honduras. Nov. 30–Dec, 2, 1966.

Sartre, Jean-Paul, *Search for a Method*. New York: Vintage Books. 1968.

Schaub, James, W. C. McArthur, et. al., *The U.S. Soybean Industry*. U.S. Department of Agriculture, Economic Research Service, Agricultural Economic Report No. 588. Washington: U.S. Government Printing Office. May, 1988.

Schmidt, Louis Bernard, "Some Significant Aspects of the Agrarian Revolution in the United States," *Iowa Journal of History and Politics*. Vol. **XVIII**. July,

1920.
Schmidt, Louis Bernard, "The Westward Movement of the Wheat Growing Industry in the United States," *Iowa Journal of History and Politics*. **Vol. XVIII.** July, 1920.
Schwartz, Howard, and Jerry Jacobs, *Qualitative Sociology: A Method to the Madness*, New York: Free Press, 1979.
Scott, Roy V., "Railroads and Farmers: Educational Trains in Missouri, 1902–1914." *Agricultural History*. **Vol. 36**, no. 1. January, 1962.
Sears, E. R., "Genetics and Farming," in *Science and Farming: Yearbook of Agriculture, 1943–1947*. Washington, D.C.: U.S. Government Printing Office/USDA. 1947.
Shafritz, Jay M., *The Dorsey Dictionary of American Government and Politics*. Chicago: Dorsey Press. 1988.
Shakespeare, William, "Macbeth," in *The Complete Works of William Shakespeare*. New York: Avenel Books. 1975.
Shands, Henry (USDA), Letter to Foundation on Economic Trends attorneys, May 25, 1988.
Shannon, Fred A., *The Farmer's Last Frontier: Agriculture, 1860-1897*. **Vol. V**, *The Economic History of the United States*. New York: Farrar & Rinehart. 1945.
Sherwood, Morgan, "The Origins and Development of the American Patent System," *American Scientist*. **Vol. 71.** September–October, 1983.
Shiva, Vandana, "The Seed and the Spinning Wheel: Biotechnology, Development and Biodiversity Conservation." Draft of paper presented to the International Conference on Conservation of Genetic Resources for Sustainable Development. Røros, Norway. 1990.
Silverman, David, *Qualitative Methodology and Sociology*, Hants, England: Gower Publishing, 1985.
Smith, Curtis Nye, "Seed Legislation," *Seed World*. **Vol. 5**, no. 9. June 6, 1919.
Smith, Henry Justin, *Chicago's Great Century: 1833-1933*. Chicago: Consolidated Publishers. 1933.
Smith, J. Ritchie, Testimony on PVPA to U.S. House of Representatives, Subcommittee on Departmental Operations, Ninety-First Congress, Second Session, June 10, 1970.
Smith, Marvanna (ed.), *Chronological Landmarks in American Agriculture*. Washington: U.S. Department of Agriculture. 1979.
Smith, Nigel J. H., "Botanic Gardens and Germplasm Conservation," Harold L. Lyon Arboretum Lecture Number Fourteen. Honolulu: University of Hawaii Press. February 6, 1985.
Somer, Margaret Frisbee, *The Shaker Garden Seed Industry*. Old Chatham, New York: The Shaker Museum. (M.A. thesis University of Maine — Orono, 1966) 1972.
Stark Brothers Nursery, *Stark Yearbook*, 1930. Louisiana, Mo.: Stark Brothers Nursery. 1930.
Stark, Paul, "Statement" (as senior vice president, Stark Brothers Nurseries) to the Subcommittee on Departmental Operations, Committee on Agriculture, U.S. House of Representatives. Hearings on the proposed Plant Variety Protection Act. June 10, 1970.
Stewart, Senator Donald, "Statement." Hearings before the Subcommittee on Agricultural Research and General Legislation of the Committee on Agricul-

ture, Nutrition, and Forestry, United States Senate, on S. 23, S. 1580 and S. 2820. June 17, 1980.

Stone, A. L., "20 Years of State Seed Laws," *Seed World*. **Vol. 27**, no. 6. March 21, 1930.

Stover, J. F., *History of the Illinois Central Railroad*. New York: Macmillan Publishing. 1975.

Straus, Joseph, "Biotechnology and its International Legal and Economic Implications." Undated draft.

Studebaker, John, "PVP: Where Are We Going From Here?" *Seed World*. July, 1991.

Taylor, William A., "The Influence of Refrigeration on the Fruit Industry," *Yearbook of Agriculture, 1900*. Washington: U.S. Government Printing Office/USDA. 1901.

Terry, Dickson, *The Stark Story: Stark Nurseries 150th Anniversary*. St. Louis: Missouri Historical Society. 1966.

Taylor, William A., "The Influence of Refrigeration on the Fruit Industry," in *Yearbook of Agriculture*, 1900. Washington: U.S. Government Printing Office/USDA. 1901.

Thiselton-Dyer, W. T., "Introduction," in William J. Bean, *The Royal Botanic Gardens, Kew: Historical and Descriptive*. London: Cassell & Co. 1908.

Tigar, Michael E., and Madeleine R. Levy, *Law and the Rise of Capitalism*. New York: Monthly Review Press. 1977.

Tindall, George, *The Emergence of the New South, 1913-1945*. Baton Rouge: Louisiana University Press, 1948.

Tracy, W. W., Jr., *American Varieties of Vegetables for the Years 1901 and 1902*. Bureau of Plant Industry, Bulletin no. 21, U.S. Department of Agriculture. Washington, D.C.: Government Printing Office. 1907.

Trow, Martin, "Comment on 'Participation Observation and Interviewing: A Comparison,'" in McCall, George J., and J. L. Simmons, *Issues in Participation Observation; A Text and Reader*, Reading Mass.: Addison-Wesley Publishing, 1969.

True, Alfred Charles, *A History of Agricultural Experimentation and Research in the United States, 1607-1925*. Miscellaneous Publication no. 251, USDA. Washington: U.S. Government Printing Office. 1937.

Turrill, W. B., *The Royal Botanic Gardens Kew: Past and Present*. London: Herbert Jenkins. 1959.

United Nations, Convention on Biological Diversity, adopted May 22, 1992.

United States Patent Office, "Patent 4,237,224: Process of Producing Biologically Functional Molecular Chimeras." Washington: U.S. Patent Office. 1980.

U.S. Department of Agriculture, "Farmers in a Changing World," *The Yearbook of Agriculture*, 1940. Washington: Government Printing Office. 1940.

U.S. Department of Agriculture, "Foreign Seeds and Plants: Inventory no. 1." Washington, D.C.: U.S. Government Printing Office. 1899.

U.S. Department of Agriculture, *Seed Reporter*. U.S. Department of Agriculture, Bureau of Markets. **Vol. 2**, no. 2. August 10, 1918.

U.S. Department of Commerce, Bureau of the Census, *Historical Statistics of the United States: Colonial Times to 1970, Part 2*. Washington: U.S. Government Printing Office. 1975.

U.S. Department of State, "U.S. Position on FAO Undertaking and Commission on Plant Genetic Resources." March, 1985.

U.S. Embassy — Rome. Telegram to Secretary of State, U.S. Department of State. October 1, 1984.

U.S. House of Representatives Committee on Agriculture, "Report to Accompany S. 3070." Report no. 91-1605, 91st Congress, 2nd Session. Oct. 13, 1970.

U.S. House of Representatives Committee on Patents, 59th Congress, Hearings on HR 13570 "Authorizing the Registration of the Names of Horticultural Products and to Protect the Same." Washington: Government Printing Office. March 28, 1906.

U.S. House of Representatives Committee on Patents, Report to Accompany H.R. 11372. Report no. 1129. April 30, 1930.

U.S. House of Representatives Congressional Record, May 5, 1930.

U.S. Senate Committee on Patents, "Report from the Committee on Patents on S. 4015." Report 315, 71st Congress, 2nd Session. April 2, 1930.

U.S. Senate Committee on the Judiciary, Plant Variety Protection Act, Report to Accompany S. 3070. Washington: U.S. Government Printing Office. September 29, 1970.

U.S. Senate, Hearings before the Subcommittee on Agricultural Research and General Legislation of the Committee on Agriculture, Nutrition, and Forestry, on S. 23, S. 1580, and S. 2820. June 17, 1980.

U.S. Senate Congressional Record, April 17, 1930.

UPOV, Diplomatic Conference for the Revision of the International Convention for the Protection of New Varieties of Plants. "Final Draft, International Convention for the Protection of New Varieties of Plants." Geneva: Union for the Protection of New Varieties of Plants. March 19, 1991.

Van den Belt, Henk, and Arie Rip, "The Nelson-Winter-Dosi Model and Synthetic Dye Chemistry," in Bijker, Wiebe, Thomas Hughes, and Trevor Pinch, (eds.), *The Social Construction of Technological Systems; New Direction in the Sociology and History of Technology.* Cambridge, Mass.: MIT Press. 1987.

Van den Broeck, Julien, *Public Choice.* Dordrecht, The Netherlands: Kluwer Academic Publishers. 1988.

Vaupel, James W. and Joan P. Curhan, *The World's Multinational Enterprizes: A Sourcebook of Tables.* Boston: Harvard Business School. 1973.

Wallace, Henry (ed.), "Corn Breeding Plot," *Wallace's Farmer.* March 29, 1918.

Wallace, Henry (ed.), "Corn Breeding," *Wallace's Farmer.* February 26, 1915.

Wallace, Henry (ed.), "The Story of Hybrid Corn," *Wallace's Farmer,* August 13, 1938.

Wallace, Henry A. and William L. Brown, *Corn and Its Early Fathers.* East Lansing: Michigan State University Press. 1956.

Wasserman, Harvey, *Harvey Wasserman's History of the United States.* New York: Harper. 1972.

Watson, J. D. and F. H. C. Crick, "Molecular Structure of Nucleic Acids: A Structure for Deoxyribose Nucleic Acid," *Nature.* Vol. 171. 1953.

Weber, Max, "Science as a Vocation," In H. H. Gerth and C. Wright Mills (eds.), *From Max Weber: Essays in Sociology.* New York: Oxford University Press. 1969.

Weber, Max, *The Theory of Social and Economic Organization,* edited by Talcott Parsons. New York: Oxford University Press. 1947.

Webster Co., Mel L., "Specialists," Advertisement in *Seed World.* Vol. 5, no. 3. March 7, 1919.

Weiss, Martin G, "Public-Industry Position on Plant Variety Protection." *HortScience.* **Vol. 4**, no. 2. Summer, 1969.
Weissman, Robert, "Prelude to a New Colonialism: The Real Purpose of GATT." *The Nation.* March 18, 1991.
White, Allenby L., "The Effect of Breeders' Rights on the Seed Trade," in H. L. Hamilton (ed.), *Plant Breeder's Rights,* ASA Special Publication Number 3, Denver: Crop Science Society of America in cooperation with the American Society for Horticultural Science, the American Seed Trade Association, the International Crop Improvement Association and the National Council of Commercial Plant Breeders. March, 1964.
White, Allenby, "Statement" (as chairman of the Breeders' Rights Study Committee, American Seed Trade Association), to the Subcommittee on Departmental Operations, Committee on Agriculture, U.S. House of Representatives. Hearings on the proposed Plant Variety Protection Act. June 10, 1970.
White & Co., James, *The National Cyclopedia of American Biography.* Clifton, N.J.: James T. White & Co. 1982.
White, Richard P., *A Century of Service: A History of the Nursery Industry Associations of the United States.* Washington: American Association of Nurserymen. 1975.
Wickson, Edward J., *California Nurserymen and the Plant Industry: 1850–1910.* Los Angeles: California Association of Nurserymen. 1921.
Wilkes, H. G., "Hybridization of Maize and Teosinte in Mexico and Guatemala and the Improvement of Maize," *Economic Botany.* **Vol. 31.** July-September, 1977.
Wilkes, H. G., "Plant Genetic Resources: Why Privitize a Public Good?" *BioScience.* March, 1987.
Williams, J. T., (IBPGR), Letter to George White (USDA). November 30, 1982.
Williams, J. T., (IBPGR), Letter to Quentin Jones (USDA). June 19, 1984.
Winner, Langdon, *Autonomous Technology: Technics-out-of-Control as a Theme in Political Thought.* Cambridge, Mass.: MIT Press. 1987.
Wolf, Howard, and Ralph Wolf, *Rubber, A Story of Glory and Greed.* New York: Covici Friede. 1936.
Wood, David, Letter addressed to "Genetic Resources Units: IARC's," Annex. September 15, 1987.
Woolley, C. L., *The Sumerians.* Oxford: Clarendon Press. 1930.
Wyatt, Joann Carlson, *Through the Patience of Job: The Story of a Family and a Family Business. 1881-1981.* Raleigh, N.C.: Edwards & Broughton Company. 1981.
Yoo, John, "Biotech Patents Become Snarled in Bureaucracy," *Wall Street Journal.* July 6, 1989.
Zelditch, Morris, Jr., "Some Methodological Problems of Field Studies," in G. J. McCall and J. L. Simmons (eds.), *Issues in Participant Observation; A Text and Reader.* Reading Mass.: Addison-Wesley Publishing, 1969.

# Index